ETHICAL DILEMMAS IN EMERGENCY MEDICINE

The emergency department is a place of challenging ethical dilemmas and little time and resources to solve them. *Ethical Dilemmas in Emergency Medicine* provides invaluable information, perspectives, and solutions to common ethical dilemmas in emergency medicine. It addresses important topics seen in the emergency department, including triage, medicolegal issues, privacy and confidentiality, social media, difficult patients, minors, research, patient safety, disasters, suicide, and end-of-life issues.

The accompanying educational modules provide a unique educational opportunity for resident and staff education on ethical issues in emergency medicine. Featuring twenty-three layers of ethical dilemmas in emergency medicine, along with corresponding multimedia resources, including media presentations, case-based discussions, and multiple-choice questions, this book is an invaluable resource for residents in training as well as practicing physicians.

Catherine Marco, MD, FACEP, is a professor at Wright State University in the Department of Emergency Medicine. She has been active in the education, research, and writing arenas. She has written numerous research manuscripts and book chapters on medical ethics, resuscitation, and pain management.

Raquel M. Schears, MD, MPH, FACEP, is a full-time clinician and scholar at the Mayo Clinic. Currently, she is an associate professor in the Department of Emergency Medicine. Dr. Schears has written peer-reviewed articles, taught in several residency programs, and has conducted clinical research. Her publications reveal career interests in the ethical dilemmas of life-sustaining interventions, including advance directives, organ donation and informed consent.

D0905558

Ethical Dilemmas in Emergency Medicine

Catherine Marco

Wright State University Department of Emergency Medicine

Raquel Schears

Mayo Clinic Department of Emergency Medicine

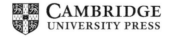

CAMBRIDGE
UNIVERSITY PRESS

32 Avenue of the Americas, New York, NY 10013-2473, USA

Cambridge University Press is part of the University of Cambridge.

It furthers the University's mission by disseminating knowledge in the pursuit of education, learning, and research at the highest international levels of excellence.

www.cambridge.org
Information on this title: www.cambridge.org/9781107438590

© Cambridge University Press 2015

First published 2015

Printed in the United States of America

A catalog record for this publication is available from the British Library.

Library of Congress Cataloging in Publication Data
Ethical dilemmas in emergency medicine / [edited by] Catherine Marco,
Raquel Schears.
    p.   ;   cm.
Includes bibliographical references and index.
ISBN 978-1-107-43859-0 (alk. paper)
I. Marco, Catherine A., editor.   II. Schears, Raquel, editor.
[DNLM: 1. Emergency Medicine – ethics.   2. Patient Rights – ethics. WB 105]
RC86.95
174.2'96025–dc23   2015020960

CONTENTS

CONTRIBUTORS

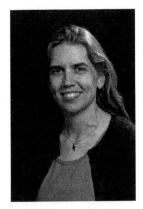

SHELLIE ASHER, MD
Albany Medical College
Albany, New York
AsherSh@mail.amc.edu

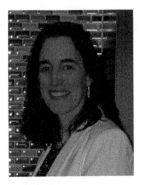

EILEEN F. BAKER, MD, FACEP
Assistant Professor
University of Toledo College of Medicine and Life Sciences
Riverwood Emergency Services, Inc.
Perrysburg, Ohio
uhemsdoc@earthlink.net

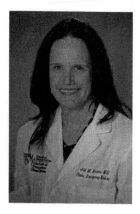

JILL M. BAREN, MD, MBE, FACEP, FAAP
Professor and Chairman
Department of Emergency Medicine
Perelman School of Medicine
Chief, Emergency Services University of Pennsylvania Health System
Philadelphia, Pennsylvania
barenj@uphs.upenn.edu

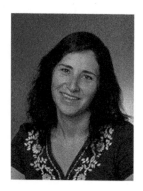

KELLY BOOKMAN, MD, FACEP
Associate Professor
School of Medicine
University of Colorado
Aurora, Colorado
Kelly.Bookman@ucdenver.edu

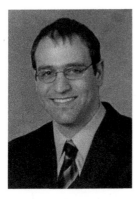

JAY M. BRENNER, MD, FACEP
Associate Professor
Department of Emergency Medicine
Center for Bioethics and Humanities
SUNY-Upstate Medical University
Syracuse, New York
brennerj@upstate.edu

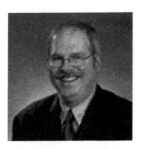

JAMES E. BROWN, MD, MMM
Professor and Chair
Department of Emergency Medicine
Wright State University Boonshoft School of Medicine
Dayton, Ohio
james.e.brown@wright.edu

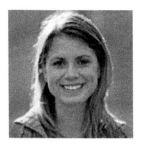

SARAH C. CAVALLARO, MD
Perelman School of Medicine
University of Pennsylvania
Philadelphia, Pennsylvania
Sarah.Cavallaro@uphs.upenn.edu

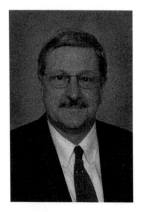

ARTHUR R. DERSE, MD, JD, FACEP
Director, Center for Bioethics and Medical Humanities
Professor of Bioethics and Medical Humanities, and
Professor of Emergency Medicine
Medical College of Wisconsin
Milwaukee, Wisconsin
aderse@mcw.edu

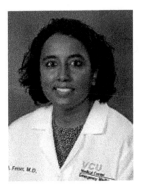

V. RAMANA FEESER, MD
Virginia Commonwealth University
Richmond, Virginia
vrfeeser@aol.com

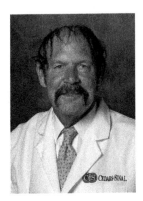

JOEL MARTIN GEIDERMAN, MD
Co-Chairman and Professor of Emergency Medicine
Ruth and Harry Roman Emergency Department, Department of Emergency Medicine
Center for Healthcare Ethics, Burns and Allen Research Institute
Cedars-Sinai Medical Center
Los Angeles, California
geiderman@cshs.org

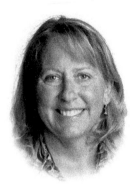

DIANE L. GORGAS, MD
Associate Professor
Department of Emergency Medicine
Executive Director
Office of Global Health
The Ohio State University's Wexner Medical Center
Columbus, Ohio
diane.gorgas@osumc.edu

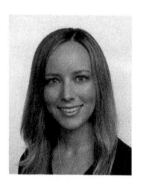

JOY HARDISON, MD, MPH
Vivace Health Solutions
Cardiff by the Sea, California
joy.hardison@vivacehealthsolutions.com

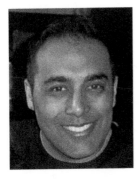

JAVAD T. HASHMI, MD
Center for Bioethics
Harvard Medical School
Boston, Massachusetts
javad.hashmi@gmail.com

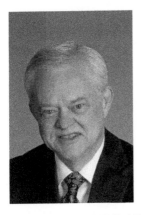

GREGORY L. HENRY, MD, FACEP
Clinical Professor
Department of Emergency Medicine
The University of Michigan
Ann Arbor, Michigan
Past President
The American College of Emergency Physicians
Risk Advisor, The Emergency Physicians Medical Group
Ann Arbor, Michigan
ghenry@epmg.com

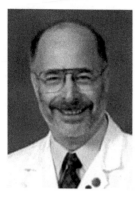

KENNETH V. ISERSON, MD, MBA
Professor Emeritus, Emergency Medicine
The University of Arizona
Tucson, Arizona
kvi@u.arizona.edu

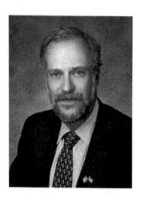

GABOR KELEN, MD
Johns Hopkins University
School of Medicine
Department of Emergency Medicine
Baltimore, Maryland
gkelen@jhmi.edu

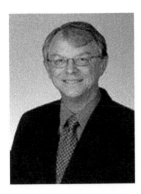

WALTER E. LIMEHOUSE, JR, MD, MA, FACEP
Medical University of South Carolina
Charleston, South Carolina
wlimehouse@comcast.net

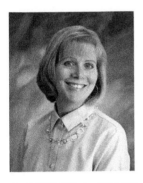

CATHERINE A. MARCO
Professor
Department of Emergency Medicine
Wright State University
Dayton, Ohio
Catherine.Marco@wright.edu

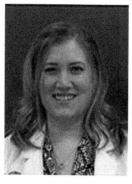

JILLIAN MCGRATH, MD
Department of Emergency Medicine
The Ohio State University's Wexner Medical Center
Columbus, Ohio
Jillian.mcgrath@osumc.edu

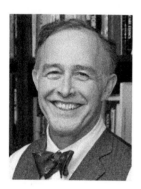

JOHN C. MOSKOP, PHD
Wake Forest School of Medicine
Winston-Salem, North Carolina
jmoskop@wakehealth.edu

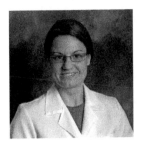

JENNIFER NELSON, MD
Department of Emergency Medicine
Allegheny Health Network
Pittsburgh, Pennsylvania
jnelson7@wpahs.org

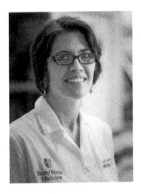

ERIKA NEWTON, MD, MPH
Department of Emergency Medicine
Stony Brook University
Stony Brook, New York
Erika.Newton@stonybrookmedicine.edu

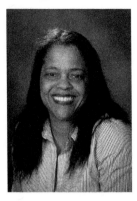

TAMMIE E. QUEST, MD
Director, Emory Palliative Care Center
Roxann Arnold Professor in Palliative Care
Associate Professor
Department of Emergency Medicine
Emory University School of Medicine
Atlanta, Georgia
tquest@emory.edu

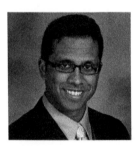

KARTIK RAO, DO
Department of Emergency Medicine
Wright State University
Dayton, Ohio
kraodo@gmail.com

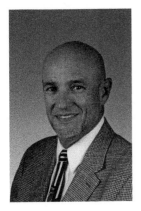

PAUL P. REGA, MD, FACEP
Assistant Professor
Department of Public Health and Preventive Medicine
Department of Emergency Medicine
University of Toledo
College of Medicine
Toledo, Ohio
ndmsmd@aol.com

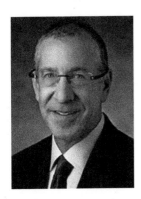

RICHARD ROTHMAN, MD, PHD
Johns Hopkins University
School of Medicine
Department of Emergency Medicine
Baltimore, Maryland
rrothma1@jhmi.edu

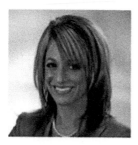

LYDIA MARIE SAHLANI, MD
Assistant Professor
Department of Emergency Medicine
The Ohio State University's Wexner Medical Center
Columbus, Ohio
lydia.sahlani@osumc.edu

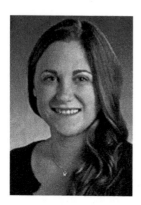

LAUREN SAUER, MSC
Johns Hopkins University
School of Medicine
Department of Emergency Medicine
Baltimore, Maryland
lsauer2@jhmi.edu

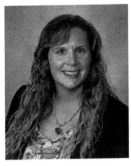

RAQUEL M. SCHEARS, MD, MPH, FACEP
Associate Professor
Department of Emergency Medicine
Mayo Clinic Health System
Rochester, Minnesota

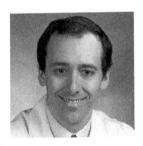

JEREMY R. SIMON, MD, PHD, FACEP
Columbia University
New York City, New York
jrs3@nyu.edu

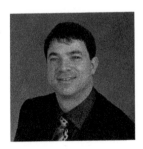

ADAM J. SINGER, MD
Professor and Vice Chairman for Research
Department of Emergency Medicine
Stony Brook University
Stony Brook, New York
Adam.singer@stonybrook.edu

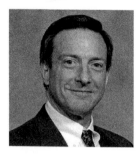

ROBERT C. SOLOMON, MD
Allegheny General Hospital
Pittsburgh, Pennsylvania
rcsmd82@comcast.net

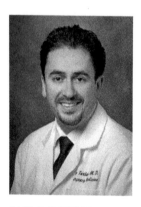

SAM S. TORBATI, MD, FAAEM, FACEP
Co-Chairman and Associate Professor of Emergency Medicine
Department of Emergency Medicine
Cedars-Sinai Medical Center
Los Angeles, California
Sam.Torbati@cshs.org

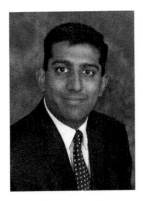

ARVIND VENKAT, MD, FACEP
Department of Emergency Medicine
Allegheny Health Network
Pittsburgh, Pennsylvania
arvindvenkat@hotmail.com

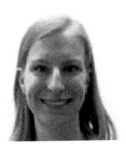

LESLIE R. VOJTA, MD
Assistant Professor
Department of Emergency Medicine
Wright State University Boonshoft School of Medicine
Dayton, Ohio
leslievojta@gmail.com

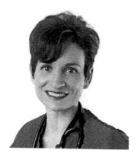

MONICA WILLIAMS-MURPHY, MD
Huntsville Hospital Emergency Physician
Medical Director for Advanced Care Planning and End of Life Education
Programs
Clinical Assistant Professor
Internal Medicine
UAB School of Medicine
Huntsville Campus
Birmingham, Alabama
mwmur007@aol.com

PREFACE

The practice of emergency medicine is a complex mission. Successful practice includes emergency stabilization, patient assessment, diagnostic tests, and medical interventions. The Accreditation Council for Graduate Medical Education and the American Board of Emergency Medicine have established the Emergency Medicine Milestone Project, a framework for assessment of residents in training in twenty-three milestones, from Emergency Stabilization to Teamwork.

In this complicated environment, ethical dilemmas frequently arise. The complex, time-pressured environment makes the assessment and management of ethical dilemmas challenging. Thus, a study of ethical issues and principles guiding their application in the clinical environment is essential.

This book includes twenty-three chapters, analogous to the twenty-three Emergency Milestones, and in respect to the specialty of Emergency Medicine, the twenty-third recognized medical specialty by the American Board of Medical Specialties. Each chapter addresses an important ethical topic in emergency medicine, including issues, controversies, and a summary of Ethics Takeout Tips. Available online are educational modules for use in teaching ethical principles at any level. It is our hope that this book will serve as a valuable resource to emergency providers and educators.

ACKNOWLEDGMENTS

The editors wish to thank the authors, who have dedicated their time and expertise to the education and application of principles of medical ethics to the practice of emergency medicine.

Principles of Medical Ethics

KENNETH V. ISERSON, MD, MBA

WHAT IS BIOETHICS?

Bioethics, a subset of ethics, applies ethical principles and decision-making methods to actual or anticipated moral dilemmas facing clinicians in order to find reasoned and defensible solutions. Given the nature of our pluralistic society, we derive these moral precepts from a variety of sources including general cultural values, philosophical and religious moral traditions, social norms embodied in the law, and professional oaths and ethical codes. All of these sources claim moral superiority. The goal of bioethics is to help us understand, interpret, and weigh these competing moral values (American College of Emergency Physicians Ethics Committee, 1997). The clinical application relies on case-based (casuistic) reasoning, usually giving most weight to patients' autonomy and values.

In contrast to professional etiquette, which relates to standards governing the relationships and interactions between practitioners, bioethics involves basic moral values and patient-centered issues (Arras, 2001). Specifically, bioethics deals with relationships between providers and patients, providers and society, and society and patients.

As Arras wrote, the purpose of medicine's professed morality is "to give physicians an identity as professionals, rather than as self-interested tradespeople, and a basic education in some key medical virtues" (Arras, 2011). Arras goes on to say that ethics as it is applied to medical practice should

- emphasize those duties (like confidentiality) that help to make the practice of medicine possible;
- incorporate traditional maxims that are useful as general rules of thumb (e.g. "Do no harm"); and

- adopt a set of fiduciary responsibilities with a strict duty to place patients' welfare ahead of one's own financial (or other) interests (Beauchamp & Childress, 1989).

BIOETHICS AND EMERGENCY MEDICINE

Although ethical issues abound in emergency medicine, they often go unrecognized. These issues stem from pre-hospital and emergency department (ED) clinicians' four imperatives: to save lives when possible, to relieve pain and suffering, to comfort patients and families, and to protect staff and patients from injury. This is complicated by emergency physicians' typical lack of prior relationships with their patients, whose trust is based on institutional and professional assurances rather than on an established personal relationship (American College of Emergency Physicians Ethics Committee, 1997). In addition, patients often arrive with acute illnesses or injuries requiring immediate interventions, and emergency physicians have little time to gather additional data, consult with others, or deliberate about alternative treatments. Patients with acute mental status changes may be unable to participate in decisions regarding their health care.

This chapter addresses the relationship of law, religion, and bioethics; foundational ethical theories and the derived principles; values and virtues; ethical oaths and codes; applying bioethics to clinical situations; and bioethics committees and consultants.

RELATIONSHIP BETWEEN LAW, RELIGION, AND BIOETHICS

How does bioethics differ from law? Both give us rules of conduct to follow based on societal values. But although good ethics often makes good law, good law does not necessarily make good ethics (Beauchamp & Childress, 1989). Emergency physicians often look to the law for answers to thorny dilemmas. Yet, except in the rare cases of "black-letter law," wherein very specific actions are mandated, these issues are best served by turning to bioethical reasoning, using bioethics consultations, or applying previously developed institutional bioethics policy (see Chapter 2).

Whereas, in homogenous societies, organized religions see themselves as keepers of society's values, most Western societies are multicultural, with no single religion holding sway over the entire populace (Arras, 2001). Since ED patient populations practice a number of religions, a patient-value-based approach to ethical issues is necessary. The question physicians must ask is, "What is the patient's desired outcome for medical care?" (Arras, 2001). It is important to note that religion influences modern secular bioethics, which uses many religion-originated decision-making methods, arguments, and ideals. In addition, clinicians' personal spirituality may allow them to relate better to patients and families in crisis (Beauchamp & Childress, 1989).

Most religions have a form of the Golden Rule – "Do unto others as you would have them do unto you" – as a basic tenet. Problems surface, however, when trying to apply religion-based rules to specific bioethical situations. For example, nearly all religions accept the dictum, "Do not kill." However, the interpretation of the activities that constitute killing, active or passive euthanasia, or merely reasonable medical care vary with the world's religions, as they do among various philosophers.

FOUNDATIONAL ETHICAL THEORIES

Foundational ethical theories represent grand philosophical ideas that attempt to coherently and systematically answer the fundamental questions "what ought I do?" and "how ought I live?" Philosophers continue to elaborate or reconstruct fundamental ethical theories, many with elements from ancient ethical systems developed in India and China, and within the Jewish, Christian, Islamic, and Buddhist religions.

The "mid-level" ethical principles that guide clinical practice and bioethical thought stem from these foundational theories. While ethicists generally appeal to these principles when defending a particular action or proposing public policy, it is worthwhile having a passing familiarity with the nature of the foundational theories – some of which are quite contradictory. There are two main "foundational" theories of ethics: utilitarianism and deontology.

Utilitarianism, based on John Stuart Mill's and Jeremy Bentham's writings, is one of the more functional and commonly used ethical theories. Sometimes called *consequentialism* or *teleology*, it promotes good or valued results rather than using the right means to achieve those results. This theory promotes outcomes that most advantage the majority in the most impartial way possible. (Simplistically, it may be said to propose achieving the greatest good for the greatest number of people.) It is often advocated as the basis for broad social policies. Nevertheless, trying to define what is "good" or who comprises the affected community exposes major problems with this theory (Iserson, 1993).

Deontology holds that the most important aspects of our lives are governed by certain unbreakable moral rules. Deontologists (*deon* is the Greek word for duty) believe in rules that prescribe right actions (duties). One example of a list of "unbreakable" rules is the Ten Commandments. Adherents hold that these rules may not be broken, even if following the rule leads to results that may not be "good." The philosopher Immanuel Kant is often identified with this theory.

Other commonly cited ethical theories include:

Natural Law. This system, often attributed to Aristotle, suggests that man should live life according to an inherent human nature, in contrast to man-made or judicial law. Yet the two are similar since both may change over time despite the frequent claim that natural law is immutable. Natural law is often associated with particular religious beliefs, especially Catholicism. The claim that the medical profession has an inherent morality mirrors natural law.

Virtue Theory. This theory asks what a "good person" would do in specific real-life situations. It stems from the writings of Aristotle, Plato, and Thomas Aquinas in which they discussed such timeless and cross-cultural character traits as courage, temperance, wisdom, justice, faith, and charity. The Society for Academic Emergency Medicine adopted a virtue-based Code of Conduct.

Some modern philosophers have proposed "anti-theories," including various combinations of casuistry, narrative ethics, feminism, and pragmatism. Unlike the foundational "top-down" theories, they favor the "bottom-up," case-based approach, emphasizing each case's messy uniqueness and challenging *principilism*, a system of ethics based on the moral principles of autonomy, beneficence, nonmaleficence, and justice (Iserson, 2000). This approach addresses, to some extent, the main problems with foundational theories, which are so general and abstract that they are difficult to apply to actual cases. Still, as with all unifying ethical theories, it is unclear which theory or combination of theories clinicians should use (Iserson, 1993). Fortunately for non-philosophers, "the boundaries between these rival methodologies have blurred significantly in the intervening years, so much so that all of these methods might now be said to be mutually complementary, non-exclusive modes of moral inquiry for doing ethics in the public domain" (Iserson, 2000). The situation becomes even clearer using mid-level bioethical principles.

MID-LEVEL PRINCIPLES

"Mid-level principles" derived from ethical theories are less general and abstract than theories. These ethical principles are "action guides," role-specific duties that physicians owe to patients and consist of various "moral rules" that comprise a society's values (Iserson, 2011). For example, when examined closely, the principle of autonomy (respect for persons) includes the values of dealing honestly with patients; fully informing patients before procedures, therapy, or becoming involved in research; and respecting patients' personal values.

How Have We Derived Modern Bioethical Principles?

Rather than drawing from one foundational theory, the bioethical principles we use stem from multiple sources. The most widely accepted principles were developed from extensive experience followed by the public and legal debate generated by controversial cases. Bioethicists select elements from well-known philosophers' writings to bolster or refute arguments; they reject or ignore the rest. As Jonsen wrote, "Bioethics has no dominant methodology, no master theory. It has borrowed pieces from philosophy and theology . . . (and) fragments of law and the social sciences have been clumsily built onto the bioethical edifice" (Iserson, Biros, & Holliman, 2012). The resulting ideas are then adapted to the needs of the modern medical environment.

For example, bioethicists often quote Emanuel Kant when discussing patient autonomy and respect for persons. Kant's philosophical theory, which he molded from elements of his predecessors' theories, was again remolded by the National Commission for the Protection of Human Subjects. To fit Kant's ideas into a modern setting, they took "a sliver from the timber of Kant's mind and reconceptualized it in the context of the problem posed by research with human subjects" (Iserson et al., 2012). This is not Kant, but a derivation: Kant would have rejected individualistic self-rule, the basis for modern ethics' idea of "autonomy."

Likewise, other core bioethical principles stem from various bits and pieces of classic philosophy and historical precedent. Beneficence generally comes from the consequentialist theory of utilitarianism, nonmaleficence strongly relates to medicine's historical professionalism, and the idea of distributive justice stretches from Plato to Rawls.

Melding medicine's goals with societal morality, law, religious values, and societal expectations for the profession, Beauchamp and Childress popularized the most commonly cited mid-level principles: autonomy, beneficence, nonmaleficence, and distributive justice. These four principles provide a handy medical ethics template and a practical, although often difficult-to-apply checklist when considering the moral implications of specific cases (Iserson, 1993, 2011).

Physicians and some philosophers claim that medicine has its own internal set of moral rules, sometimes referred to as "internalism." These have been defined as:

- "'Essentialism,' according to which a morality for medicine is derived from reflection on its 'proper' nature, goals or ends.
- 'The practical precondition account,' according to which certain moral precepts are derived as preconditions of the practice of medicine.
- 'Historical professionalism,' according to which the norms governing medicine are decided upon solely by the practitioners of medicine; an ethic about physicians, by physicians, and for physicians. And, an
- 'Evolutionary perspective,' according to which professional norms in medicine evolve over time in creative tension with external standards of morality" (Arras, 2011).

A question that naturally arises is whether ethical principles are universal or local constructs for medical purposes. For individual clinicians, the bioethical principles they follow and the values that stem from them do not change because of geography. Clinicians practicing or teaching within cultures other than their own have a responsibility to continue applying their core ethical principles while being sensitive to the local population's values (Iserson & Heine, 2013).

COMMON ETHICAL PRINCIPLES

Beneficence. Beneficence is doing good. Most health care professionals enter their career to apply this principle; it has been one of the medical profession's long-held and universal tenets. Physicians demonstrate beneficence when they treat or prevent disease or injury.

Nonmaleficence. The basic tenet that all medical students are taught is nonmaleficence: *primum non nocere* (First, do no harm). It stems from recognizing that physicians can harm, as well as help, their patients. This principle also includes preventing harm and removing harmful conditions.

Justice. The concept of comparative or distributive justice (in contrast to the judicial system's retributive and compensatory justice) encourages clinicians to act with impartiality or fairness, suggesting that comparable individuals and groups should share similarly in the society's benefits and burdens. Although it forms the basis for many society-wide policy decisions about the allocation of limited health care resources, it is not the basis for ad hoc physician–patient decisions at the bedside. Triage decisions conform to this principle when they are applied uniformly and impartially to all patients (Iserson et al., 2008).

Autonomy. For several decades, patient autonomy has been the overriding professional and societal bioethical value in most Western countries. It is the counterweight to the medical profession's long-practiced paternalism (or parentalism), wherein a practitioner acts on what he believes is "good" for the patient, whether or not the patient agrees. Grounded in the moral principle of respect for persons, autonomy recognizes the right of adults with decision-making capacity to accept or reject recommended health care interventions, even to the extent of refusing potentially lifesaving care. Physicians have a concomitant duty to respect their choices (Arras, 2001).

One important and often misunderstood aspect of autonomy is that individuals with decision-making capacity can voluntarily and verbally assign decision-making authority to other people (e.g. family) for a specific decision or time period, such as when they are in the ED. Since patients may exercise their autonomy only if they have decision-making capacity, emergency clinicians must be able to determine this at the bedside so that surrogate decision-makers may, if necessary, become involved (see Chapters 7–10 for specifics). Basic bioethical research principles (Chapter 12) stem primarily from the basis for autonomy, the respect for persons as individuals.

OTHER PRINCIPLES

Communitarianism. A counterbalance to autonomy, communitarianism considers the larger picture of the patient's life, including his or her family and his or her community, when puzzling through a bioethics case or developing public policy. The principle generally holds that the community's good and welfare outweighs an individual's rights or good and that deliberations should involve communal (e.g. family, elders) discussions (Iserson, 1993). Many cultures rely on communitarian deliberations when making medical choices and use this pattern for public policy decisions. When making bedside ethical decisions, physicians should determine, whenever possible, not only their patient's individual values, but also whether their patient subscribes to an individualistic or communitarian ethic (Beauchamp & Childress, 1989).

Confidentiality. Based on a respect for persons (as is autonomy), patient confidentiality has been a cornerstone principle of the medical profession since antiquity. It presumes that what patients tell physicians during the medical encounter will not be revealed to any other person or institution without the patient's permission (Beauchamp & Childress, 1989). Various U.S. federal and state laws have both emphasized and carved out exceptions (mandatory reporting; see Chapter 4). With the advent of minimally secure electronic medical records, the ability to maintain patient confidentiality has become even more difficult.

Privacy. Often confused with confidentiality, privacy is a patient's right to sufficient physical and auditory isolation so that he or she cannot be seen or heard by others during interactions with medical personnel (Beauchamp & Childress, 1989). ED crowding, patient and staff safety issues, and ED design limit patient privacy in many cases. The increasing use of telemedicine to render advice and guide procedures and the common practice of filming ED patients places a strain on both patient privacy and confidentiality (Iserson, 2006).

VALUES AND VIRTUES IN EMERGENCY MEDICINE

Values describe the standards that individuals, institutions, professions, and societies use to judge human behavior. They are the moral rules derived from ethical principles. Virtues describe admirable personal behavior that Aristotle and other philosophers claim is derived from natural internal tendencies (Jonsen, 2007).

Values

Values, the standards by which human behavior is judged, are learned, usually at an early age, through indoctrination into the birth culture, from observing behavior, and through secular (including professional) and religious education. They are moral rules, promoting those things we think of as good and minimizing or avoiding those things we think of as bad. Societal institutions incorporate and promulgate values, often attempting to solidify old values even in a changing society. In pluralistic societies, clinicians must be sensitive to alternative beliefs and traditions because they treat people with multiple and differing value systems. Not only religious, but also family, cultural, and other values contribute to patients' decisions about their medical care; without asking the patient, there is no way to know what decision they will make.

Although many people cannot answer the question "What are your values?" physicians can get concrete expressions of patients' uncoerced values by asking what they see as their goal of medical therapy and why they want specific interventions. In patients who are too young or are deemed incompetent to express their values, physicians may need either to make general assumptions about what a normal person would want done or to rely on surrogate decision-makers.

Institutional, Organizational, and Clinician Values. Institutions, including health care facilities and professional organizations, have their own value systems. Health care facilities often have specific value-related missions. Religiously oriented or affiliated institutions may be the most obvious of these, but charitable, for-profit, and academic institutions also have specific role-related values. Professional organizations' values often appear in their ethical codes (Arras, 2001).

Clinicians also have their own ethical values, based on religious, philosophical, or professional convictions. Although conscience clauses permit clinicians to "opt out" when they feel that they have a moral conflict with professionally, institutionally, or legally required actions, they are generally required to provide timely and adequate medical care for the patient – which may be particularly difficult to achieve in emergency medicine.

Virtues

Virtues, as Aristotle described them, stem from natural internal tendencies. The *virtuous person concept* can be summed up with the ancient saying: "In a place where there are no men, strive to be a man" (Kuczewski, 1998). Virtuous behavior stems from a sense of duty and the perception that it is the right thing to do, rather than from a desire to garner personal benefits. These ideal, morally praiseworthy character traits (e.g. showing kindness) are evident across many situations throughout the person's lifetime. Virtues that may be inherent in emergency medicine clinicians include courage, safety, impartiality, personal integrity, trustworthiness, and justice (American College of Emergency Physicians Ethics Committee, 1997).

Courage allows one to carry out an obligation despite reasonable personal risk. The courageous clinician also advocates for patients against incompetent practitioners and those who attempt to deny them care, autonomy, or confidentiality. Emergency clinicians also exhibit courage when they assume reasonable personal risk to care for violent or contagious patients and during disaster responses.

Safety balances unreasoned courage. In both in the pre-hospital and ED settings, clinicians must face not only environmental hazards, but also potentially dangerous patients, visitors, and bystanders. In these situations, emergency clinicians' first priorities must be their own safety and that of their coworkers. This does not imply that clinicians should ignore patient safety, but only that they should first ensure their own safety if they or their colleagues are at risk (Arras, 2001). Whether emergency physicians should respond to major disasters relies on considering this virtue and carefully analyzing the risks involved (Larkin et al., 2009).

Impartiality prompts the emergency physician to provide unbiased, unprejudiced, and equitable treatment to all patients, no matter their race, creeds, customs, habits, or lifestyle preferences – most of which will differ from those of the clinician. This virtue extends to the many ED patients who are poor, intoxicated, and have poor hygiene, little education, mental disturbances and value systems at odds with those of the physician. A difficult aspect of this virtue is treating perpetrators of violent crime with the same regard as victims.

Personal integrity spurs clinicians to adhere to their own reasoned and defensible set of values and moral standards, which is basic to thinking and acting ethically. This virtue incorporates *trustworthiness*, which prompts the clinician to protect his or her sick and often vulnerable emergency patients' interests through exercising ethical principles.

Truth-telling remains a somewhat controversial virtue within the medical community (Arras, 2001). Although many champion absolute honesty to the patient, honesty must be tempered with sensitivity and compassion; honesty does not equate to brutality. In recent years, poor role models, a lack of training in interpersonal interactions, and bad experiences may have diminished the perception of truth-telling as a physician virtue. However, if clinicians withhold information strictly for their emotional, legal, or financial benefit, this behavior suggests serious ethical deficits.

ETHICAL OATHS AND CODES

Since ancient times, medical practitioners have formulated and established professional rules of behavior. Although its precepts clash with modern bioethical thinking, the existing part of the Hippocratic Oath served as the medical profession's standard for countless generations (Arras, 2001).

Many medical professional societies' ethical codes (and the associated oaths) promote moral standards that their members presumably agree with and should follow. The interpretation of those principles often evolves as the larger society changes. The American Medical Association's Code of Ethics is one example; it has mutated over time in response to societal changes and legal challenges. For example, although the Code was first published in 1847, it was only in 2001 that it stated that the physician's primary responsibility should be to the patient for whom he or she is caring. While existing medical professional codes differ markedly (Table 1.2), all try to give a "bottom line" – that is, a minimally acceptable course of action.

Yet, how does professional agreement about behavior morally justify it? This is especially concerning because these codes or the behaviors they engender also affects outside parties, such as patients and third-party payers (Arras, 2011). In addition, many current medical ethical codes have been criticized for primarily addressing professional etiquette (interactions among practitioners) rather than bioethics (relationships between practitioners and patients, practitioners and society, and society and patients).

TABLE 1.1. *Relationship between the law and bioethics*

Bioethics	Function	Law
✓	Case-based (casuistic)	✓
✓	Has existed since ancient times	✓
✓	Changes over time	✓
✓	Strives for consistency	✓
✓	Incorporates societal values	✓
✓	Basis for health care policies	✓
	Some unchangeable directives	✓
	Formal rules for process	✓
	Adversarial	✓
✓	Relies heavily on individual values	✓
✓	Interpretable by medical personnel	
✓	Ability to respond relatively rapidly to changing environment	✓

From Iserson, K. V. (1999). Principles of biomedical ethics. In Marco, C. A. & Schears, R. M. (Eds.). Ethical issues in emergency medicine. *The Emergency Clinics of North America* 17(2), 283–306.

TABLE 1.2. *Comparing ethics codes for emergency medicine organizations*

	AAEM/AMA	ENA	SAEM	AOA/AOCEP	ACEP
Protect patient confidentiality	X	X		X	X
Professional excellence through CME	X		X	X	X
Be a good citizen	X		X		
Change laws to be in patients' best interests	X			X	X
Obtain consultation when necessary	X	X		X	
Choose whom to serve except in emergencies	X			X	
Avoid discriminatory practices	X		X	X	X
Promote highest quality of health care	X	X	X		X
Protect patient welfare	X	X	X		X
Honesty	X		X		X
Respect the law	X			X	X
Respect patient autonomy	X			X	X
Report clinical research honestly	X		X	X	
Prevent patient exploitation		X	X		X
Encourage public health through education	X	X	X		
Protect patient dignity	X	X	X		
Full disclosure to patients	X			X	X
Expose incompetent/dishonest physician	X				X
Patient free choice of physician	X			X	
Do not abandon patients	X			X	
Perform duties objectively/ accurately	X	X			
Promote harmony with other health professionals	X				X
Assure death with dignity	X				
Transplant/donation conduct	X				
No participation in torture/ inhumane practices	X				

This table is a comparison of five ethical codes used by emergency medicine professional organizations: the American Medical Association (AMA) used by the American Academy of Emergency Medicine, the Emergency Nurses Association (ENA), the Society for Academic Emergency Medicine (SAEM), the American Osteopathic Association (AOA) used by the American Osteopathic College of Emergency Physicians, and the American College of Emergency Physicians (ACEP).

APPLYING BIOETHICAL METHODS

To apply bioethical principles to a clinical situation, one first must recognize that a bioethical problem exists, which is not always an easy task. Once it has been identified, addressing the problem brings its own challenges. Clinicians adhere not only to basic bioethical principles, but also, at least tacitly, to a number of professional, religious, and social organizations' ethical oaths, codes, and statements. This complexity can produce a confusing array of potentially conflicting bioethical imperatives.

When dealing with bioethics cases, clinicians need to use ethical reasoning, which includes the application of foundational theories, mid-level principles, and case-based reasoning (casuistry). These methods for approaching ethical dilemmas, which balance perceptions of particular cases with more general levels of reflection, help us systematically identify elements within moral problems that we otherwise might overlook.

In practice, it can be difficult to identify and extract the most appropriate and useful principle to apply to a particular case. Principles may be too vague, or several may seem to apply to a given case even while conflicting with one another. The key is to prepare for bioethical problems as one would for critical medical events – by reading about, reflecting on, and discussing how to face these issues. This leads not only to increased personal preparation, but also to more general policies that help guide clinicians when faced with difficult bioethical issues.

Prioritizing Conflicting Principles: The Bioethical Dilemma
Applying bioethical principles may be confusing. When two or more seemingly equivalent principles or values seem to compel different actions, a bioethical dilemma exists. This situation is often described as being "damned if you do and damned if you don't," where any potential action appears, on first reflection, to be an option between two seemingly equivalent "goods" or "evils." While we theoretically have a duty to uphold each bioethical principle, none routinely "trumps" another, so the clinician must find a solution.

Working through bioethical dilemmas generally requires a case-based approach. The key is to use *paradigm* and *analogy* (the first step in the *rapid decision-making model*, described later). When faced with a troubling case, one should identify relevant mid-level principles and alternative courses of action. Then, compare its features with similar but much clearer paradigms; that is, cases with resolutions with which virtually any "reasonable person" will agree. Identifying such cases may be difficult and relies on experience and a significant knowledge base – which can be increased by using a bioethics committee approach or case-based bioethics and legal databases (Iserson, 1993).

Application to Emergency Medicine: The Rapid Decision-Making Model
When faced with bioethical dilemmas, emergency clinicians often must make ethical decisions with little time for reflection or consultation. Ethical problems, like clinical problems, require *action* for resolution. For that reason, a rapid decision-making model (Arras, 2001) was developed, based on accepted bioethical theories and techniques (Figure 1.1). It provides guidance for emergency medicine practitioners who are under severe time pressures and wish to make ethically appropriate decisions (Moskop & Iserson, 2007).

When using this approach, the clinician must first ask: "Is this an instance of a type of ethical problem for which I have already worked out a rule?" Or, at least, is it similar enough to such cases that the rule could be reasonably extended to cover it? In other words, if there had been time in

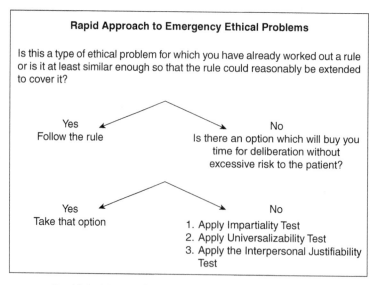

FIGURE 1.1. Rapid decision-making model.
Modified from Iserson, K. V. (1995). An approach to ethical problems in emergency medicine. In K. V. Iserson, A. B. Sanders, & D. Mathieu (Eds.), *Ethics in emergency medicine*, 2nd ed. Tucson, AZ: Galen Press.

the past to think coolly about the issues, discuss them with colleagues, and develop some rough guidelines, could they be used in this case? If the case in question does fit under one of those guidelines arrived at through critical reflection, and there is not time to further analyze the situation, then the most reasonable step would be to follow that rule, if it is still appropriate. In ethics, this step follows from *casuistry*, or case-based reasoning.

If the case does not fit under any previously generated ethical rule, the practitioner should consider if there is an option that will buy time for deliberation. If there is such an option, and it does not involve unacceptable patient risks, then it would be the reasonable course to take. Using a delaying tactic may afford time to consult with other professionals, the bioethics committee, and the family.

If there is no acceptable delaying tactic, the clinician should weigh what she considers the best option using a set of three tests, drawn from three different philosophical theories, to help make a decision. These are the:

Impartiality Test. "Would you be willing to have this action performed if you were in the other person's (the patient's) place?" A version of the Golden Rule, it helps correct one obvious source of moral error – partiality, or self-interested bias.

Universalizability Test. "Would you be comfortable if all clinicians with your background and in the same circumstances act as you are proposing to do?" This generalizes the action and asks whether developing a universal rule for the contemplated behavior is reasonable – an application of Kant's categorical imperative. This helps eliminate not only bias and partiality, but also short-sightedness.

Interpersonal Justifiability Test. "Can you give reasons that you would be willing to state publicly? Will peers, superiors, or the public be satisfied with the answers?" This uses a theory of consensus values as a final screen.

When ethical situations arise in which no time exists for further deliberation, it is probably best to go ahead and act on the rule or perform the action that allows all three tests to be answered in the affirmative with some degree of confidence. Once the crisis has subsided, clinicians can hone their ethical decision-making abilities by reviewing the decision with colleagues and bioethicists.

BIOETHICS COMMITTEES AND CONSULTANTS

Multidisciplinary bioethics committees have been developed in most large hospitals to help resolve bioethical dilemmas. Many smaller hospitals now have bioethics consultants. The four roles that bioethics committees should perform are concurrent case reviews (consultations) often mediating between dissenting parties, retrospective case reviews, policy development, and education.

In every medical system, practitioners find that they repeatedly face identical ethical dilemmas. The solution involves changing the rules, a process termed "proactive ethics," and requiring that all "stakeholders" (i.e. those with a vested interest in an equitable solution) find a compromise solution. Such groups will often include physicians, nurses, EMS personnel, lawyers, religious authorities, and representatives of affected groups. Armed with this agreement – often sample policy or legislation – it becomes relatively easy to change laws or administrative rules. One example of this process led to a landmark pre-hospital advance directive law that markedly lessened unwanted resuscitation attempts in the EMS, an extensive statutory surrogate list, and a simplified set of advance directives. (*Pirkei Avot*, 200–220 AD)

ETHICS TAKEOUT TIPS

- Bioethics theories, principles, and virtues stem from various philosophical schools.
- Clinical applications based on case-based reasoning usually give most weight to patients' autonomy and values while also being aware of other relevant bioethical principles.
- Emergency clinicians must be able to recognize bioethical dilemmas, formulate action plans based on their readings and discussions, and learn methods, such as the rapid decision-making model, through which to apply ethical principles in clinical settings.

FOR FURTHER READING

American College of Emergency Physicians Ethics Committee. (1997). *Code of Ethics for Emergency Physicians*. Dallas, TX: ACEP. Revised April 2011. www. acep.org/content.aspx?id=29144.

Arras, J. (2011). Theory and bioethics. *Stanford encyclopedia of philosophy*. Spring 2011 edition. www.science.uva.nl/~seop/archives/spr2011/entries/theory-bioethics/.

Arras, J. D. (2001). A method in search of a purpose: The internal morality of medicine. *Journal of Medical Philosophy*, 26(6), 643–662.

Beauchamp, T. L., & Childress, J. F. (1989). *Principles of biomedical ethics*, 3rd ed. (pp. 6–9). New York: Oxford University Press.

Iserson, K. V. (1993). A simplified prehospital advance directive law: Arizona's approach. *Annals of Emergency Medicine, 22,* 1703–1710.

Iserson, K. V. (2000). Telemedicine: A proposal for an ethical code. *Cambridge Quarterly of Healthcare Ethics, 9*(3), 404–406.

Iserson, K. V. (2006). Ethical principles – emergency medicine. In Schears R. M., Marco C. A. (Eds.), Ethical Issues in Emergency Medicine. *Emergency Clinics of North America, 24*(3), 513–545.

Iserson, K. V. (2011). The Rapid Ethical Decision-Making Model: Critical medical interventions in resource-poor environments. *Cambridge Quarterly of Healthcare Ethics, 20*(1), 108–114.

Iserson, K. V., Biros, M., & Holliman, C. J. (2012). Ethics of international emergency medicine. *Academy of Emergency Medicine, 19,* 683–692.

Iserson, K. V., & Heine, C. (2013). Bioethics. In J. A. Marx, R. S. Hockberger, & R. M. Walls (Eds.), *Rosen's emergency medicine: Concepts and clinical practice,* 7th ed. (pp. e33–e46). Philadelphia: Mosby.

Iserson, K. V., Heine, C. E., Larkin, G. L., Moskop, J. C., Baruch, J., & Aswegan, A. L. (2008). Fight or flight: The ethics of emergency physician disaster response. *Annals of Emergency Medicine, 51*(4), 345–353.

Jonsen, A. R. (2007). How to appropriate appropriately: A comment on Baker and McCullough. *Kennedy Institute of Ethics Journal, 17*(1), 43–54.

Kuczewski, M. (1998). Methods of bioethics: The four principles approach, casuistry, communitarianism. www-hsc.usc.edu/~mbernste/tae.methods.kuczewski.html.

Larkin, G. L. L., Iserson, K. V., Kassutto, Z., Freas, G., Delaney, K., Krimm, J., . . . Adams, J. (2009). Virtue in emergency medicine. *Academy of Emergency Medicine, 16,* 51–55.

Moskop, J. C., & Iserson, K. V. (2007). Triage in medicine, part II: Underlying values and principles. *Annals of Emergency Medicine, 49*(3), 282–287.

Pirkei Avot (The Book of Principles). (200–220 AD). 2:5.

2

Law and Ethics

ARTHUR R. DERSE, MD, JD, FACEP

OVERVIEW

Emergency physicians who confront difficult ethical dilemmas in their practice must consider not only how to resolve these cases utilizing principles of ethics but also the legal implications of possible choices. In the United States, emergency physicians may have a heightened awareness of legal factors because of the relatively high frequency of medical malpractice suits, as well as the frequent interactions of the emergency physicians with law enforcement and the court system. Emergency physicians also share anecdotal information about cases in which they have been sued and in some cases held liable. Thus, the U.S. legal system plays a considerable role as the societal backdrop against which ethical decisions must be made in emergency medicine.

U.S. LEGAL SYSTEM

The U.S. legal system can be considered in three subdivisions: federal/state law, legislative/judicial/administrative law, and civil/criminal law. The first differentiation is between federal and state law. In the federal system, laws passed by Congress or cases decided by the Supreme Court have jurisdiction over all of the United States. An example of a federal law that applies to all emergency physicians is the Emergency Medical Treatment and Active Labor Act (EMTALA). As well, each state has its own set of laws that are determined by the state's legislatures and court systems. Sometimes these state laws are variations along a general theme that may be fairly consistent throughout the country; for example, all states in the United States have some form of Good Samaritan protection for emergency physicians. Conversely, states may have vastly different legal approaches to a particular ethical problem. For instance, in several states, assistance by physicians in suicide under regulated circumstances may be permitted, whereas in the rest of the country physician-assisted suicide is illegal and may have associated criminal penalties. In general, federal jurisdiction takes precedence over state laws (e.g. the Health Insurance Portability and Accountability Act [HIPAA] supersedes state privacy laws, although states may give more protection than federal law requires).

U.S. law can also be differentiated by the three branches of government in both the federal and state systems. Legislatures pass laws that are enacted into statutes. Courts use prior cases as precedent for deciding on subsequent cases in the jurisdiction in which the court sits. The executive branch promulgates regulations based on legislation under its administrative law authority. Thus, emergency physicians are subject to a state legislature's determination of the statute of limitations, which spells out the period for which an emergency physician can be held liable for negligence. Emergency physicians are also subject to the common law (or judge-made law) of medical malpractice, which varies in each state depending on the cases that have been decided by the courts. As well, emergency physicians are regulated by the state's administrative licensing authority, which grants emergency physicians their ability to practice in their state.

The third way that U.S. law can be viewed is by the differentiation between civil law and criminal law. Under civil law, both intentional and unintentional wrongs (such as negligence) are redressed through a jury's or court's determination of liability and payment of damages or fines. In contrast, under the criminal system, used for more egregious wrongs, the penalties are fines and imprisonment.

Most of the ethical dilemmas that emergency physicians face entail federal and state laws and encompass legislative, judicial, or administrative law. In most circumstances, these ethical dilemmas concern civil law rather than criminal law.

RELATIONSHIP BETWEEN LAW AND ETHICS

The relationship between law and ethics is dependent on their roles in society. Both set standards of conduct to which individuals are expected to adhere. However, the law sets a minimal consensus that the state is willing to enforce through either litigation or prosecution. Ethical standards commonly exceed legal obligations. For instance, the emergency physician merely needs to provide the standard of care that the average prudent emergency physician would provide. In many cases, the law does not address many ethical issues. An example of this is error disclosure. In many cases, there may be no legal obligation to disclose an error to the patient; however, there may be an ethical obligation to disclose that error.

Many other areas of conduct by emergency physicians are not regulated by law. For instance, even though ethical standards would exhort emergency physicians to act with compassion and to engender trust in the doctor–patient relationship, the law does not mandate these. A suit that claimed damages for an uncompassionate physician who otherwise met the standard of competent treatment would be unlikely to be successful as a cause of action.

The law has been described as an inapt tool for resolving the difficult issues that arise in a doctor–patient relationship. The law's emphasis on rights and individual autonomy has been thought to be less helpful than the consideration of responsibilities to others (Schneider, 1994). In general, the law tends to look at the doctor–patient relationship as a dyad in which the individual is given the right to make decisions without consideration of the effects on others, such as family members, unless there is the danger of harm to others.

The generally recognized principles of bioethics may have a correlate in these legal duties that are set by the common (judge-made) laws of the fiduciary obligations of professionals toward their patients and clients. For instance, the principle of beneficence – that is, acting for the benefit of the patient – has a legal correlate in the fiduciary duty to act in the patient's best interests. That fiduciary duty is derived from the doctor–patient relationship and sets out a specific type of legal standard of conduct toward patients. These professional obligations are legally enforceable. The fiduciary duty includes the duty of nonabandonment. This is a strong legally enforceable obligation that requires emergency physicians to provide adequate treatment and follow-up for patients' emergency medical problems.

Another example of a legally enforceable professional duty is that of confidentiality, and a third example is the principle of nonmaleficence; that is, avoiding harm to patients. The bioethical principle of autonomy, the principle by which patients who have decision-making capacity can choose to accept or refuse offered medical treatment, has a correlation with the law of informed consent.

Not all bioethical principles have correlates in the law. For instance, the bioethical principle of justice, which includes a mandate for the fair distribution of resources, does not have a strong correlation in American law. Instead, health care resources are commonly distributed among those who have the ability to pay, those who have merited the resources (e.g. veterans), or those who are involuntarily confined (such as those in mental health institutions or prisons).

When confronted with a difficult ethical dilemma, emergency physicians often turn to the law for answers. However, in many cases, the law does not give specific guidance, and, in any particular case, the law is one factor among many to consider along with the ethical issues and other factors that the case involves. Rarely, the legal obligation in a case may be contrary to what may be the ethically best option. For instance, a state may require mandatory reporting of domestic partner abuse, but the emergency physician may not feel that this is the best course if the partner is unwilling to have this reported. In situations where the law conflicts with what the emergency physician determines to be the best ethical outcome, the emergency physician is faced with a difficult dilemma and should carefully consider the consequences. Although the law is an important factor in consideration, a good test of the ethically appropriate course of action is whether the physician can explain and defend openly the action chosen as the best ethical choice under the circumstances.

Emergency physicians should be aware of not only the laws that apply to their practices but also the policies of the health care institution that apply. For instance, besides the ethical obligation of informed consent and the legal statute or case law that may specify the elements of informed consent, the health care facility may also have its own policy on patient consent and refusal.

EXAMPLES OF SPECIFIC INTERACTIONS OF LAW AND ETHICS

Good Samaritans

Normally, the duty of an emergency physician to treat is only established after the doctor–patient relationship is formed. Merely the patient presenting to the emergency department (ED) for treatment can form that relationship. In general, an emergency physician has no legal obligation to provide emergency care in a situation in which the emergency physician is not on duty or on call. Nonetheless, emergency physicians have an ethical obligation to assist in an accident or an emergency if they are able to do so (see Appendix 1). The duty to assist in an accident or an emergency or disaster is based on the professional obligation to help as well as the social contract in which society expects emergency physicians to help, even in situations in which they are not legally obligated to do so.

The person who voluntarily offers him- or herself for an undertaking whose actions are not founded under any legal obligation to do so is a volunteer. In general, there is no legal duty to aid an individual unless there is a special relationship such as a parent–child relationship or the doctor–patient relationship. In most states, there is no obligation for a physician to assist at the scene of an accident or emergency although a few states view this as a legal obligation of the profession (e.g. Vermont and Minnesota).

Good Samaritan laws are laws based on the parable of the Good Samaritan, in which assistance was rendered when it was not required. Before these statutes, if physicians did assist at an accident or emergency, they were obligated to provide the standard of care and could be held liable for breach of that duty. Good Samaritan laws in all states allow an affirmative defense to a claim of professional negligence. Most of these laws give protection to a person who renders emergency care at the scene of any emergency or accident in good faith by providing immunity from civil liability for the acts or omissions in rendering such emergency care. Generally, this immunity does not extend when individuals trained in health care render emergency care for compensation and within the scope of their usual and customary employment or practice. There is also a federal law that protects individuals who provide assistance in the case of an in-flight medical emergency. Generally, gross negligence or willful misconduct is not covered by the Good Samaritan protection.

To be covered under the Good Samaritan statutes, emergency physicians should make clear when rendering assistance that they are a volunteer and should refuse any offer of compensation or remuneration for assistance. In the case of volunteers in disasters, a number of states have adopted the Emergency Volunteer Protection Act, which protects volunteers with immunity from liability when acting for a nonprofit organization or government entity in which they are acting within the scope of the responsibilities within the organization and are properly licensed, certified, or authorized by authorities to practice in the state where the harm occurred. There is no coverage for willful or criminal misconduct, gross negligence, reckless misconduct, or a conscious flagrant indifference to the rights or safety of the individual (42 USC 139).

Confidentiality

Confidentiality has been defined as the prohibition of disclosure of information gained in certain relationships to third parties without consent. There are consequentialist principles (e.g. utilitarianism), which support full disclosure of personal information for accuracy of diagnosis and treatment as well as the ability to seek help without stigma. As well, there are duty-based (i.e. deontological) principles of ethics that justify keeping confidentiality, which include respect for autonomy. Confidentiality is a long-standing professional requirement reaching back to the Hippocratic Oath. It is also enforced legally by the fiduciary duty of the doctor–patient relationship to keep confidences of patients. Confidentiality also has legal correlates, such as long-standing civil and criminal penalties for unauthorized access to medical records; these have generally been state laws with similar protections for mental health records and particularly sensitive diagnoses such as HIV/AIDS.

The electronic medical record gave rise to new issues concerning privacy because of the efficiency of the collection, storage, classification, and transmission of medical information that allowed breaches of sensitive information that could be disseminated widely. As a result, HIPAA, a federal privacy rule, applies to electronically transmitted or stored protected health information (PHI) and to any person or organization that stores or transmits individually identifiable health information through electronic means. The penalties can range from civil damages to $250,000 in criminal damages. HIPAA specifies PHI, which includes identifiers that must be removed for health information to be considered de-identified (i.e. not personal data).

The duty of confidentiality is constrained by ethical and legal exceptions, which generally fall into two categories: (1) public health concerns where reporting is mandatory for entities like infectious diseases, such as tuberculosis and sexually transmitted infections, to protect third parties who may be endangered by the affected individual (even though the endangerment is not intentional) and (2) mandatory reporting of alleged crimes including gunshot wounds or other suspicious wounds as well as suspicion of child abuse, elder abuse, and, in some states, partner abuse. These two exceptions are most often spelled out in statutes requiring emergency physicians to report these alleged crimes in the interests of protecting third parties and preventing further harm to individuals.

Although the duty to report infectious diseases was established in the early twentieth century, it was toward the end of that century that the duty was establish to warn third parties of potentially dangerous patients due to psychological impairment or mental health diseases. The Tarasoff case (California, 1976) established that physicians and therapists have a duty to third parties who are at significant risk of substantial harm from a patient. This duty ran counter to generally established mental health practice that maintained that confidentiality was essential to the therapeutic relationship necessary for successful treatment. The Tarasoff case holding was adopted in many other states. That duty might be discharged in some cases by warning the individual or taking measures to protect the person at risk of harm, such as asking authorities to detain the individual for evaluation and treatment.

The alignment between ethics and law is best exemplified by the duty – in all fifty states – to report suspicion of child abuse based on the policy decision that it is better to err in good faith in suspecting child abuse than to underreport potential abuse when, in retrospect, a child's life could have been saved. The same reasoning applies to the vast majority of states that protect an emergency physician's reporting of elder abuse. More controversial is the duty to report domestic partner abuse. States vary in their approach, and there is not a consensus as to the policy effectiveness of mandatory reporting of suspected abuse when the patient is unwilling to cooperate in the prosecution of abuse.

Emergency physicians often confront this tension between the ethics of keeping confidences and both the legal mandate and ethical goal of preventing harm to society and identified third parties. When considering a duty to warn an individual, factors the emergency physician should consider include the likelihood of harm, the legal requirement of disclosure, and what protection the emergency physician has for disclosure (e.g. immunity for good faith reporting). In addition, there may be situations in which disclosure is prohibited. For instance, a state may prohibit an emergency physician from warning a person who is at risk of transmission of HIV/AIDS from his or her partner but may require that information to be disclosed to the state Department of Public Health, which may be authorized to inform the patient.

A more recent phenomenon with challenges to traditional confidentiality is the emergence of social media. Emergency physicians and trainees, who generally are enthusiastic about sharing the interesting and challenging cases of their chosen profession, must be wary of posting any identifiable information about their patients.

Informed Consent and Refusal

Emergency medicine has long been predicated on the need for rapid diagnosis and treatment of medical emergencies. Given the ethical principle of beneficence and the corresponding bioethical principle of nonmaleficence, it is generally in the best interests of the individual presenting to the ED with an emergent medical condition to be treated. This was in accord with the general presumption that if a physician has determined that the patient should be treated, then the physician is authorized to treat. The fiduciary duty to treat the patient and the physician's superior knowledge of the medical situation logically meant that the patient should defer to the physician's decision about what needed to be done. In fact, the Hippocratic tradition considered the patient's participation in decision-making as unprofessional and undesirable. More than a century ago, a landmark U.S. legal case concerning the complications of an operation that was done without the permission of the patient resulted in the proclamation that "every human being of adult years and sound mind has a right to determine what shall be done with his own body" (*Schloendorff*, 1914). This case established a right of the individual to make decisions about health care and would be used as a buttress to the development of the bioethical principle of autonomy – that is, individual self-determination – with respect to health care matters.

Even in the Schloendorff case decision, it was also recognized that there was in the law an emergency exception or "privilege" for emergency treatment without consent. This emergency privilege applied when the patient lacked decisional capacity, no one was available who was legally authorized to speak for the patient, time was of the essence, there was a serious risk of bodily injury or death, and a reasonable person would consent to treatment under the circumstances (Prosser, Keeton, Dobbs, Keeton, & Owen, 1984). This emergency exception allows emergency physicians to treat a wide variety of patients under emergency circumstances without obtaining consent. However, if any of the requirements of the emergency exception were not present, then the consent of the patient was required. Since the vast majority of patients in the ED do not fit into the category where all of the requirements of the emergency privilege are, for most ED patients, consent for treatment is required.

In 1957, the legal requirement of consent was expanded in that consent must not only be voluntary but also informed. This was established in a case in which a patient who consented to a procedure had complications that were not disclosed as a possibility (*Salgo*, Cal. App., 1957). The case held that the physician should not only obtain consent, but must also disclose the nature of the procedure, the risks of the procedure, the alternatives available, and the possibility of what might happen if no treatment was provided. Courts in other states soon adopted the holding of this landmark case, and informed consent has become a standard of the doctor–patient relationship in the United States, applying to procedures, treatment, testing, and research.

The obligation to tell the patient the truth about his or her medical situation, including dire or life-threatening diagnoses, is also a more recent ethical mandate. Traditional medical ethics texts supported the use of deceit when necessary for the greater good of the patient. For instance, up until the middle of the twentieth century, physicians routinely did not inform a patient of a serious diagnosis such as cancer so that the patient would not be alarmed or lose hope in the effectiveness of treatment. With the rise both of informed consent as a legal principle and the establishment of patient autonomy as a bioethical principle (with the corresponding need for the patient to have information in order to make a medical decision), truth telling has become the ethical and legal norm in medical care.

Once it was established that the patient should be informed of risks, benefits, alternatives, and the option of no treatment, the next issue became whether the information that should be disclosed should be what the reasonable physician would disclose (the professional standard) or what the reasonable patient would find material to making the decision (the objective patient standard). The practical effect in states that have adopted the reasonable patient standard is that no expert testimony is needed to establish what the objective patient would want to know. It is, instead, a jury (or, in rare cases, judicial) determination. About half of the states in the United States use the professional standard and others the reasonable patient standard.

Informed consent has also been of interest to plaintiffs' attorneys, who recognized that even if an outcome was the result of a side effect or untoward effect that was a known complication of the procedure, if the bad outcome could not be litigated successfully as falling below the standard of care, instead the attorney could use the lack of the patient's knowledge of this possible complication when making a decision to consent to treatment as evidence of inadequately informing the patient when obtaining consent. Thus they could litigate consent rather than negligence.

Because of the relative lack of time for a robust discussion of proposed procedures, as well as the lack of a prior established doctor–patient relationship, emergency physicians are particularly vulnerable to suits concerning informed consent. Informed consent litigation has been used effectively by plaintiffs' attorneys against emergency physicians. Good communication and careful documentation are necessary to meet the legal standards for informed consent.

Informed consent also becomes more complex when considering the ability of adolescents to make medical decisions. In general, parents or guardians are the decision-makers for their young children who cannot make medical decisions. However, there are exceptions to the general rule that consent for tests and treatment of a minor must be obtained from the guardian of the minor (usually a parent). These exceptions include the emergency exception to informed consent, as well as minors who fulfill the legal requirements to be considered emancipated, minors who have been adjudicated as mature, and other exceptions authorized by state statute. Emancipation is defined as legal independence of the child from parents to make decisions and is presumed at the state's determined age of majority. Approximately half of the states designate emancipation by statutes and the others by common law in response to petitions of emancipation. Common emancipation landmarks include marriage, military enlistment, independent support in having a separate domicile, and, in some cases, completion of secondary education or giving birth to or fathering a child. However, it must be emphasized that the latter two are not true in all states, and that, paradoxically, an unemancipated minor who is a parent may be able to make decisions as a parent of his or her child but may not be able to make decisions as an unemancipated minor for him- or herself. In some cases, a court may give a minor emancipation for a specific purpose. However, courts more often will determine that a minor is mature and able to make any medical decision. A mature minor status may also be used to protect the confidentiality of the doctor–patient relationship for the adolescent.

Adolescents may also be able to make their own medical decisions if there is an age of consent that is established by statute. For instance, many states have a statutory age at which an adolescent may seek treatment for sexually transmitted infections, HIV/AIDS, mental health problems, and alcohol or other drug abuse treatment. As well, many state statutes also provide an age by which the minor may seek contraception or may be able to consent to an abortion without parental agreement.

In making ethical decisions about the treatment of adolescents, it is important for the emergency physician to become familiar with the statutes on mature and emancipated minors as well as the statutory exceptions that allow adolescents to be treated without parental permission.

There are two other exceptions to informed consent. One is the rarely used therapeutic privilege, which allows the interventionist to treat a patient when full disclosure of the information would have an extremely adverse effect on the patient. Even when this is justified, reasonable discretion must be used in the manner and extent of the disclosure, which should occur when feasible. This therapeutic exception is one whose acceptability by courts varies among states, and it should be rarely considered for use by the emergency physician. The other exception is that patients may also voluntarily waive their right to be informed. Patients who choose to waive their right to information should be informed that they always have the right to revoke that waiver to receive information.

End of Life

Withholding and Withdrawing Life-Sustaining Medical Treatment

Emergency physicians should become familiar with both the ethical and legal issues in end-of-life care, including the consensus of specific legal issues:

1. Patients have the right to refuse any intervention including resuscitation, ventilators, feeding tubes, and blood products.
2. All patients have the right to refuse life-sustaining treatment, and even incapacitated patients may have that right exercised through their guardians, agents of power of attorney for health care, or other surrogates or legal representatives.
3. Withholding or withdrawing life-sustaining medical treatment is not homicide or suicide, orders to do so are valid, and courts need not be involved. (Meisel, 1993)

Surrogate Decision-Making

Emergency physicians should also be aware of default surrogates for decision-making often authorized by state statute. The hierarchy of surrogates who are able to make medical decisions for nondecisional patients in order of priority may be spouse, adult child, parent, adult sibling, and, finally, close friend. Often with these statutes, if the decision concerns forgoing life-sustaining treatment, the patient must be in a terminal condition, permanently unconscious, or have an incurable irreversible condition.

Advance Directives

The issue of what a patient who is not decisional would want under the circumstances is very important for patients for emergency physicians. An advance directive is a direction by the patient in advance of his or her wishes should he or she become incapacitated. As a result of the Patient

Self-Determination Act (PSDA), every state has a form of an advanced directive that patients are able to complete. The most common types of written advance directives are (1) the *living will*, which is a direction to a physician that if the patient has a terminal condition (or, in some states, is in a persistent vegetative state), then the patient wishes to forgo life-sustaining treatment, and (2) the *power of attorney for health care*, which appoints an agent, often with some direction or description of the patient's wishes or values, and is activated with any incapacity that the patient experiences – whether or not the patient has a terminal condition. Initially, advance directives were thought to be ineffective in communicating patient wishes, and initial studies showed that, for seriously ill patients, these directives did not result in changes in treatment. However, recent studies show that patients who had prepared advance directives received care that was strongly associated with their preferences, whether they requested limited care or all care possible.

Emergency physicians may find advance directives to be very helpful for expressing the patient's preferences and values concerning life-sustaining medical treatment; however, advance directives may not be readily available, and they may be activated only when two physicians (or in some cases a physician and psychologist) determine the patient to be nondecisional. The mere presence of a power of attorney for health care does not imply a particular preference. It may direct either to provide or forgo life-sustaining medical treatment. Thus, an advance directive should be read by the emergency physician before acting on it.

DNR and POLST Orders

Emergency physicians should carefully distinguish advance directives, which are patient-written preferences about treatment, from Do Not Resuscitate (DNR) orders (also known as Do Not Attempt Resuscitation [DNAR] orders), which are physicians' orders to forgo resuscitation and that may be based on the patient's wishes or on medical ineffectiveness of resuscitation. There are programs in many states that allow for an out-of-hospital DNR order that reflects the implementation of the patient's wishes through an order by a physician. More comprehensive out-of-hospital order sets are the Physician's Orders on Life-Sustaining Treatment (POLST) that translate patient preferences into portable pre-hospital physician orders and address such issues as resuscitation, intubation, artificial nutrition and hydration, and other life-sustaining measures. These are known by different acronyms depending on the state in which they are adopted, and they allow the emergency medical services (EMS) system to differentiate between circumstances in which it is appropriate to begin a cascade of treatment and resuscitation and when it is appropriate to provide comfort care measures instead. Studies show that patient wishes (both forgoing and requesting treatment) are more likely to be honored if a POLST document is completed than if the patient does not have a POLST. POLST orders have been enacted through legislation that generally gives immunity to physicians who act in good faith according to the POLST order. The POLST legislation often comes with a proviso that a physician may conduct an evaluation of the individual and, based on the clinical circumstances, may issue a new order consistent with the most current information available about the individual's health status and goals of care. In general, emergency physicians should look upon the issuance of a POLST order by a physician as a documentation of an order that has been entered after a considered discussion with the patient or his or her representative. Emergency physicians may wish to confirm that the POLST order is appropriate but should, in general, not open a new conversation about goals of end-of-life care unless the emergency physician is prepared to have an extensive and thorough discussion.

Most studies show that if patients have a terminal condition, they would prefer to die at home under some comfort care protocol. The emergency medical system should be able to differentiate those patients for whom resuscitation is appropriate and those for whom the patient and a representative and the patient's physician have determined that resuscitation is not appropriate and that comfort care is the appropriate intervention.

Futility
The law of informed consent and refusal includes withholding or withdrawing treatment if the patient or surrogate expresses that the patient does not want or would not want that treatment. In addition, there is no legal obligation to offer treatment that will not work or is no longer working. Whether to offer and perform an emergency medical treatment or procedure in a given situation is a professional medical determination. "Physicians are under no ethical obligation to render treatments that they judge to have no realistic likelihood of medical benefit to the patient. Emergency physicians' judgments in these matters should be unbiased and should be based on available scientific evidence and societal and professional standards" (ACEP, 1998). The most common situation for this determination in emergency medicine is cardiac arrest. "For patients in cardiac arrest who have no realistic likelihood of survival" emergency physicians should consider withholding or discontinuing resuscitative efforts, in both the pre-hospital and hospital settings (ACEP, 2008).

There is a dearth of reported cases for malpractice or EMTALA violations for not providing treatment that the emergency physician determined to be futile. Several comprehensive studies have reported court cases that show that health care providers are overwhelmingly successful in lawsuits brought against them for not providing treatment that they deemed futile. Careful clinical determination of ineffectiveness as a standard for futility has the greatest ethical consensus. Even if there is no effective treatment for cure, emergency physicians still have the expertise and obligation to determine a prognosis and communicate bad news, to assist in advance care planning where possible, and, when appropriate, to withhold or withdraw life-sustaining medical treatment while still providing palliative care. Emergency physicians should be aware of standards and statements about futility, including those issued by professional medical organizations. Emergency physicians should also be aware of any policies at their medical facility that pertain to futility or other issues concerning appropriateness of resuscitation.

Physician-Assisted Suicide

There is no constitutional right to physician-assisted suicide in the United States. States are free to develop laws concerning physician-assisted suicide, and several states have laws that allow physician-assisted suicide under regulated circumstances. Physician-assisted suicide remains an extremely rare cause of death in those states in which this practice has been implemented and documented. Emergency physicians should consider how to respond if a patient who has attempted suicide comes to the ED. In general, emergency physicians should counter the medical consequences of the suicide attempt unless such measures would only prolong the dying process or would be ineffective. In states in which physician-assisted suicide is legal and where the law has been followed, emergency physicians rarely may be presented with patients who attempt suicide with a physician's assistance. In those circumstances, it would be appropriate for the emergency physician to provide palliative care unless the patient or legal decision-maker decides otherwise. Emergency physicians who see this as material participation in the suicide may need to ask another emergency provider to attend to the patient.

Error Disclosure

Error disclosure is another example where legal and ethical analyses may have different approaches. Errors are common in medicine, and patients' preferences about physicians' mistakes are that physicians acknowledge and disclose even minor errors. However, even though there may be no legal obligation to disclose an error that is undiscovered by the patient or family, there may be an ethical obligation to do so, both because of the ethical obligation to respect the patient and act in the patient's best interest and the ethical obligation to improve the system of health care delivery.

Emergency physicians have an ethical duty to be truthful with patients about errors. Patients and families wish disclosure of errors, and there are benefits to disclosure with an apology using appropriate steps to ethically disclose the error. Not all errors need be disclosed; for instance, if the physician is not responsible for the error or its oversight or if the disclosure would harm the patient.

There are recommended methods for maximizing a compassionate disclosure of error. However, emergency physicians should be careful to distinguish between unanticipated adverse events or outcomes and an acceptance of legal responsibility for an injury. Medical malpractice requires a deviation from the standard of care and a proximate cause of an injury to the patient within the context of the doctor–patient relationship. In the case of a bad outcome, it may be that not all of the factors of causation and responsibility are yet determined. A conversation with the emergency physician's insurer or risk manager should occur before the emergency physician accepts legal responsibility for the error.

In disclosing errors to patients, is important to take the lead on disclosure and not wait for the patient to ask and to outline a plan of care to rectify the harm and prevent a reoccurrence, all with careful documentation. Apologies and expressions of sorrow can convey empathy and dedication to determining whether there was an error for which an admission of fault and compensation is appropriate or if, instead, a bad outcome occurred without causation by an error. In some states, an apology may not be used as evidence of the physician's culpability; in other states, it may be used as evidence, but, in either case, an expression of sorrow may be the most appropriate sentiment by the emergency physician.

CONCLUSION

Ethical issues in emergency medicine are framed, in part, by the societal consensus of the law that may apply. Emergency physicians should be knowledgeable about the implications of federal and state law that should be taken into consideration when considering ethical factors and in choosing the best course of action. As noted earlier, the law is an important factor in consideration, but, ultimately, a good test of the ethically appropriate course of action is whether the emergency physician can explain and defend openly the action chosen as the best ethical choice under the circumstances.

ETHICS TAKEOUT TIPS

- Emergency physicians should be knowledgeable about the implications of federal and state law that should be taken into consideration when considering ethical factors and in choosing the best course of action.
- A good test of the ethically appropriate course of action is whether the physician can explain and defend openly the action chosen as the best ethical choice under the circumstances.
- Good Samaritan laws in all states allow an affirmative defense to a claim of professional negligence.
- When considering a duty to warn an individual, factors the emergency physician should consider include the likelihood of harm, the legal requirement of disclosure, and what protection the emergency physician has for disclosure (e.g. immunity for good-faith reporting). In addition, there may be situations in which disclosure is prohibited.
- The emergency exception or "privilege" for emergency treatment in the law without consent applies when the patient lacks decisional capacity, no one is available who is legally authorized to speak for the patient, time is of the essence (in that action needs to be taken quickly), there is a serious risk of bodily injury or death, and a reasonable person would consent to treatment under the circumstances.
- All patients have the right to refuse life-sustaining treatment, including resuscitation, ventilators, feeding tubes, and blood products, and even incapacitated patients may have that right exercised through their guardians, agents of power of attorney for health care, or other surrogates or legal representatives.
- Advance directives, if available, may be helpful to emergency physicians, but the mere presence of a power of attorney for health care does not imply a particular preference. To find out if an advance

directive is applicable to the situation, the emergency physician should read the provisions of the document.

- Emergency physicians should look on the issuance of a DNR or POLST order by a physician as documentation of an order that has been entered after a considered discussion with the patient or representative.
- Emergency physicians are under no ethical obligation to render treatments that they judge to have no realistic likelihood of medical benefit to the patient. Emergency physicians' judgments in these matters should be unbiased and should be based on available scientific evidence and societal and professional standards.
- In those states in which physician-assisted suicide is legal, emergency physicians should consider how to respond if a patient who has attempted suicide with the aid of a physician comes to the ED.
- Emergency physicians have an ethical duty to be truthful with patients about errors. There are benefits to disclosure with an apology, using appropriate steps to ethically disclose an error.

FOR FURTHER READING

American College of Emergency Physicians. (1998). Non-benefical ("futile") emergency medical interventions. Policy approved March 1998. www.acep.org/policy/PO400198.HTM

Derse, A. R. (2005). What part of "no" don't you understand? Patient refusal of recommended treatment in the emergency department. *Mt. Sinai Journal of Medicine*, 72, 221–227.

Derse, A. R. (2012). Futility in emergency medicine. In J. Jesus, S. A. Grossman, A. R. Derse, J. G. Adams, R. Wolf, & P. Rosen (Eds.), *Ethical problems in emergency medicine: A discussion based review* (pp. 117–125). New York: Wiley-Blackwell.

Jesus, J. E., Geiderman, J. M., Venkat, A., Limehouse, W. E., Derse, A. R., Larkin, G. L., & Henrichs III, C. W. (2014). Physician orders for life-sustaining treatment (POLST) and emergency medicine: Ethical considerations, legal issues, and emerging trends. *Annals of Emergency Medicine*, 64, 140–144.

Limehouse, W., Feeser, V. R., Bookman, K., & Derse, A. R. (2012a). A model for emergency department end-of-life communications after acute devastating events – part I: Decision-making capacity, surrogates, & advance directives. *Academic Emergency Medicine*, 19, 1068–1072.

Limehouse, W., Feeser, V. R., Bookman, K., & Derse, A. R. (2012b). A model for emergency department end-of-life communications after acute devastating events – part II: Moving from resuscitative to end of life or palliative treatment. *Academic Emergency Medicine*, 19, 1300–1308.

Meisel, A. (1993). The consensus about forgoing life-sustaining treatment: Its status and prospects. *Kennedy Institute of Ethics Journal*, 2, 309–345.

Moskop, J. C., Geiderman, J. M., Hobgood C. D., & Larkin, G. L. (2006). Emergency physicians and disclosure of medical errors. *Annals of Emergency Medicine*, 48, 523–531.

Moskop, J. C., & Iserson, K. V. (2001). Emergency physicians and physician-assisted suicide, part II: Emergency care for patients who have attempted physician-assisted suicide. *Annals of Emergency Medicine*, 38, 576–582.

Moskop, J. C., Marco, C. A., Larkin, G. L., Geiderman, J. M., & Derse, A. R. (2005). From Hippocrates to HIPAA: Privacy and confidentiality in emergency medicine – part I: Conceptual, moral, and legal foundations. *Annals of Emergency Medicine*, 45, 53–59.

Moskop, J. C., Marco, C. A., Larkin, G. L., Geiderman, J. M., & Derse, A. R. (2005). From Hippocrates to HIPAA: Privacy and confidentiality in emergency medicine – part II: Challenges in the emergency department. *Annals of Emergency Medicine*, 45, 60–67.

Prosser, W. L., Keeton, W. P., Dobbs, D. B., Keeton, R. E., & Owen, D. G. (1984). *Prosser and Keeton on torts* (5th edn., p. 113). St. Paul, MN: West Publishing.

Salgo v. Leland Stanford etc. Bd. Trustees, 154 Cal.App.2d 560, 317 P.2d 170 (1957).

Schloendorff v. Society of New York Hospital, 211 N.Y. 125, 105 N.E. 92 (1914).

Schneider, C. E. (1994). Bioethics in the language of the law. *Hastings Center Report*, 24(4), 16–22.

Stewart, P. H., Agin, W. S., & Douglas, S. P. (2013). What does the law say to Good Samaritans?: A review of Good Samaritan statutes in 50 states and on US airlines. *Chest*, 143(6), 1774–1783.

Tarasoff v. Regents of the University of California, 17 Cal. 3d 425, 551 P.2d 334, 131 Cal. Rptr. 14 (Cal. 1976).

3

Triage in Emergency Medicine

JOEL MARTIN GEIDERMAN, MD, SAM S. TORBATI, MD,
AND RAQUEL M. SCHEARS, MD, MPH, FACEP

Trier (French): to sort, sift, pick over
   Il faut trier les pommes de terre selon leur grosseur – We need to sort
the potatoes by size.
   La moitié des cerises sont pourries, il faut trier – Half of the cherries
are rotten, you have to sort through them.

The word "triage" is derived from the French language. In clinical practice, the verb *trier* refers to the rapid sorting and prioritizing of patients, not languidly picking through piles of them, as may be alluded to in the produce examples above. But, in keeping with its French heritage, the birth of modern triage can be traced back to nineteenth-century military medicine and the dire circumstances of the battlefield, whereby advancing the charge inescapably produced wounded soldiers. This predicament of war casualties in mortal combat was taken very seriously by Baron Dominique Jean Larrey, surgeon general to Napoleon's Army of the Rhine. Larrey is credited for being the first to implement a system in which the wounded were prioritized for care based on medical need rather than military rank. Moreover, initial care of the wounded took place on the battlefield, before evacuation elsewhere for definitive care.

Subsequently, in 1846, John Wilson, a British naval surgeon, would come to the conclusion that, in order for medical care (in scarce supply) to be truly life-saving in wartime, it must be provided to the wounded in most need of it. As a consequence, care was withheld from those who constituted a waste of resources, including those soldiers fatally wounded and expected to die soon or lucky enough to have sustained only minor injuries that could wait to be treated. Further refinement of this concept in casualty care, with the term "triage" anchored on, was introduced to U.S. physicians serving in Europe during World War I. By that time, categories were first established as to whom would be removed from the battle theater and treated first, thereby forming the first tiered triage system. A quote from a handbook of that era, cited by Winslow, also applied the following utilitarian principle:

> A hospital with 300 or 400 beds may suddenly be overwhelmed by 1000 or more cases. It is often, therefore, physically impossible to give speedy and thorough treatment to all. A single case, even if it urgently requires attention – if this will absorb a long time – will have to wait, for in that same time a dozen others, almost equally exigent, but requiring less time might be cared for. The greatest good for the greatest number of people must be the rule.

Remarkably, today's mass casualty triage strategy is based on the basic principle of the greatest good for the greatest number. However, the utilitarian intent is to maximize casualty survival and therefore benefit society as a whole, at times at the expense of individual needs. Regardless of the intention, it is actionable that no outcome data have ever shown that this triage system actually improves outcome for individuals or society at large. No prospective study has ever validated the stated goal of mass casualty triage, namely, that of saving more lives at either the individual or societal level. Retrospective data evaluate only the ability of the system to detect severity of injury. Clearly, mass casualty triage results remain unacceptably variable, considering the lack of scientific rigor and the consequences of societally imposed life-and-death end points and given international humanitarian law, which requires that triage provide the best opportunity to survive.

Meanwhile, the term "triage" has been incorporated into Western medicine and is now part of the everyday vernacular, surely known to many of the 130 million annual visitors to U.S. emergency departments and their families. To some it means, "how long do I have to wait?" and to others "check in here." Surely, as the demand for emergency services grows and the supply of hospitals shrink, as emergency department (ED) crowding increases, as the population expands and ages, as concierge medicine grows, and as EDs increasingly become the portal of choice for entering the medical system, the issue of who will be treated first – or, for large numbers of patients, in which order – will become increasingly important.

There is an ethical dimension rooted in justice and beneficence as well as other moral concepts attached to the forgoing issues. This chapter will examine those ethical challenges involved in routine triage as commonly practiced in U.S. EDs. Although the ethics of battlefield triage and civilian catastrophe is fascinating (see Chapter 17 for further discussion), it is also a distinctly different meeting place and agenda that aims to save lives where not all lives can be saved and, as such, calls for public dialog and further debate. Instead, here, we focus on daily triage using case studies to illustrate clinical ethical decision-making points occurring commonly within the ED itself and one step beyond. From an emergency perspective, this represents the prioritization of patient care during periods of the day when ED resources (beds) are scarce. Nonetheless, increasingly, EDs rely on triage acuity systems to aid in sifting through the plethora of patients' illnesses and injuries that are conditional and range from nonurgencies to life-threatening. The aim is to find and speed care to those patients in most need of it. Therein, the sickest few of the ill and injured gain the highest level of care, even if they have the lowest probability of survival and even if others have arrived earlier. Briefly, we will also return to the subject of disaster triage as it relates to the emergency medicine subspecialty of emergency medical services (EMS). Finally, we will argue that no single ethical principle/concept prevails in all scenarios involving emergency medicine triage.

CASE SCENARIOS

Scenario 1

The emergency physician at a base station is called to the radio to assist the nurse. An elderly man has had a syncopal episode. He is borderline hypotensive (BP 90/60) but otherwise stable and without symptoms. The nearest hospital, his hospital of choice, is on diversion, with waiting room times of up to 3 hours. When told he can't be transported to his hospital of choice, he wants to sign out against medical advice and stay home. If he is transported, other patients awaiting triage in the waiting room will be delayed. What should the physician and nurse do?

Scenario 2

You are the director of an ED that sees 65,000 patients a year in 30 treatment bays. Patients with higher acuity triage codes (which are numerically lower) are brought to a bed first. Patients triaged as level 4 (i.e. lower acuity, including many children with minor illnesses or injuries) wait for many hours to be seen along with many other sicker patients. Is it ethical to add a section that will not have monitors but will be used exclusively for lower acuity patients? Or should extra space be added and used only for the highest acuity patients?

Scenario 3

The ED is full, with 30 patients waiting to be seen in the waiting room with up to 4-hour waits, and the ED is on diversion. The department chair and nursing director receive a call from the hospital CEO that the chairman of the board of directors (who has devoted countless hours and has given or raised millions of dollars) has taken a fall. She is on her way to the ED with a possible fractured wrist and some cuts and bruises. How should this person be triaged?

Scenario 4

A 32-year-old man presents with shortness of breath. He has a history of end-stage renal disease and is dialysis dependent. He also has a history of drug abuse and noncompliance with dialysis and medical therapy. He was recently banned from the institution's ambulatory care network and "fired" from dialysis for theft and disorderly conduct, not to mention medical noncompliance. He has not been dialyzed in 10 days, and he has recently used IV heroin and cocaine. Should treatment of noncompliant patients be delayed? Should noncompliant patients receive a different level of care?

BASIC CONCEPTS OF ED TRIAGE

The ED is subject to demands that are predictable and based on probability but not on possibility; nor can every permutation and combination of patient presentations at a particular moment be predicted in advance. Even in rare EDs with plenty of physical capacity, staffing will usually be adjusted for probability and not possibility in such a way that a treatment space and providers may not always be available immediately. But, theoretically, it must be noted that if there is no resource limitation, then no form of triage is needed. In actuality, even if the only scarce resource in patient management is time, a process must be in place to prioritize who is brought to a bed first. Assessment by the triage nurse involves clinical judgment often in combination with the chief complaint, vital signs, and general appearance of the patient; this defines the *gestalt* of an experienced practitioner. Assessed patients are placed in a queue that reflects the spectrum of minor to severe disease or injury. Beyond trying to sort through who absolutely needs to be seen immediately or almost immediately, patients are generally prioritized according to time of arrival as well as matching the needs of the patient with the type of treatment space that becomes available.

Several different triage schemes are used in various parts of the world and within the United States to manage patient flow safely when clinical needs exceed capacity; some are based on national models and norms, and some are based on acuity levels with different features or number of categories applied to assign a group level of acuity or priority to a given patient presenting for treatment. Although a full discussion of all of these schemas is not relevant to this chapter, the requirement of three conditions for triage in emergency practice articulated by Iserson and Moskop are listed for review purposes: (1) at least modest scarcity of resources exists, (2) a health care worker assesses each patient's medical needs based on a brief examination, and (3) the health care worker uses an established system or plan, usually based on an algorithm or set of criteria, to determine a specific treatment or treatment priority for each patient. From an ethical perspective, all schema are trying to achieve the best outcome for patients based on the principles of beneficence, nonmaleficence, justice, and utilitarianism as outlined in the next sections.

ETHICAL PRINCIPLES AND CONCEPTS

Beneficence

The concept of beneficence dictates that physicians (and some would argue other health professionals) have a positive duty based in tradition to bring benefit to patients, to promote their welfare, and to do good. Nowhere is this obligation expressed more strongly than in emergency medicine. Triage aims to ensure these goals by having the sickest patients seen first, but doing so may also produce some harms. As Aacharya (2011) points out, overtriage (assigning a higher priority than is actually warranted) is often employed in order to err on the side of caution but may actually result in a higher cost of care and worse outcomes. It may also disadvantage other patients who are made to wait longer and who perhaps may leave. Nevertheless, the primary goal of triage is to confer benefit to those most in need as well as to prevent harm from waiting.

Nonmaleficence

As referenced earlier, triage schemes and the practitioners who perform the function have a duty to prevent harm from coming to patients – the essence of nonmaleficence, as sometimes summed up in the Hippocratic concept of to "do no harm" (note that those exact words never appear in the Hippocratic Oath, despite the common belief that they do). Because triage is based on rapid assessments, signs and symptom complexes, and *gestalt*, it is imprecise. As a result, there may be a tendency to overtriage in order to protect oneself from judgment or punishment and to prevent harm to the index patient. If taken to an extreme, this could theoretically harm another patient, whether it is a physical harm or the harm of waiting, which includes the loss of personal time or income. However, as long as triage is carried out in good faith and acts to ensure nonmaleficence toward the patient, it is the morally correct approach.

Justice

The principle of justice or the more narrowly drawn concept of distributive justice seeks to assure that goods and services are distributed in a fair but not necessarily equal way. As discussed herein, what is fair may be deduced from ethical precepts and principles or sometimes not because there are cases involving limited resources distribution that can be subject to judgment and other factors. In general, distributive justice dictates that the benefits (of immediate or timely care) and the burdens (of waiting) are distributed fairly to all members of society regardless of race, creed, color, gender preference, and the like. In the United States, this extends to insurance coverage and economic status as well, as enshrined in Emergency Treatment and Active Labor Act (EMTALA).

There are three relevant categories (equality, utility, and the priority of the worst- off) of ethical theories that are applied to problems of justice and among which a balance must be created in justifying the triage approach applied to patients in the ED context.

Equality and Fairness

First, equality and fairness are important components of justice. Daily triage succeeds in part because of a lottery principle, thus providing a natural chance ("first-come, first served") element to need-based triage. Everyone should have an equal chance to receive necessary care. Each person's life is of equal worth: thus, there is a duty to prevent the death/

disability of an identified individual if means are available, regardless of cost or resource use. The latter is referred to as the "Rule of Rescue" and is commonly used to justify heroic life-saving efforts in the ED.

Utility and Consequences

Second, whether we are "fighting the good fight" or just playing along with hypothetical tabletop exercises that may result in a "truth or dare" type game, the discussion of moral rules that underlie ED triage can hardly turn off all utility considerations (as befits a blind-eyed judge in a timeless courtroom setting). Utilitarianism is a concept first espoused by Hutcheson. Bentham, Mill, Hume, and others who aver that *when choosing the most moral (course of) action, virtue is in proportion to the number of people a particular action brings happiness to. In the same way, moral evil, or vice, is proportionate to the number of people made to suffer. The best action (therefore) is the one that procures the greatest happiness (or benefit) for the greatest numbers – and the worst is the one that causes the most misery (or harm).* Utilitarianism is cited and popularized as "doing good for the most people" by Beauchamp and Childress, but their rendition amounts to a boilerplate version of *consequentialism*, which holds that actions are right or wrong according to the *balance* of their good and bad consequences *and in proportion* to their tendency to promote the greatest total happiness or the most worst misery, respectively. Thus, the most just decisions aim to increase net usefulness to society by both maximizing societal benefit and minimizing harm. This ethical theory may be found in medical term correlates of quality-adjusted life years or public health initiatives supported in the ED context, such as vaccination programs, which value the common good above individual freedoms.

The Priority of the Worst-Off

The third theory of justice attempts to pick up those who may have fallen through the cracks of the other two categories. It may encompass the poor or needy, the disenfranchised, and/or ED frequent visitors (lacking access to primary care); those with the worst possible outcome or in the dying process; and those with no prospects for cure. Anybody down and out may make his or her case for membership in the most disadvantaged group. The basic theory, with respect to medical ethics, agrees with Aristotle that, in matters of formal justice, the equals should be treated equally and the unequals unequally. Rawls advanced the *maxmin ideology* that says inequalities are acceptable in an egalitarian society so long as they max-imize the benefit to those worst-off or until it is no longer possible to improve the lot of those worst-off. However, a triage system guided by this theory may be highly inefficient, if maximizing the benefits of this group implies investing a disproportionate share of limited resources into a group of patients who may be defined as those least likely to survive.

Autonomy

Autonomy is the concept that patients (or, in the case of incapacity, surrogates) have the right to make their own choices over their own health care within agreed upon limits (such as suicide or assisted suicide in most states). Surely, except for the occasional altruistic person, most patients presenting to an ED, if given the choice, would want to go first or nearly first (think of what happens on Black Friday post-Thanksgiving Day sales in the United States). Clearly, a system of allowing unrestricted autonomy would not work. Since not all patients can be accommodated in their desire to go first, autonomous decision-making is relegated to the choice of waiting, going elsewhere, or not being seen at all. For patients seeking convenience care or nonessential treatment, this appears to be a fair balance. If, however, patients' welfare is being put at risk, institutions and governments have a moral obligation to ensure that individuals do not die or suffer physical harm as a result of triage decisions. Patients and families who insist that their family members need to be seen immediately are often right. Family or friend advocacy can then be seen as another form of autonomous expression. Nevertheless, it cannot always be accommodated.

One example of autonomy being severely restricted is in the case of ambulance diversion, in which case, population decisions and facility/provider considerations will generally but not always countermand individual choice.

AMBULANCE DIVERSION AS A FORM OF TRIAGE

As stated, ED triage systems aim to ensure adequate and optimal treatment with priority given to those in greatest need. As noted by Geiderman et al. (2015), this often is more of a challenge logistically and practically as EDs fill up and become crowded with patients, including those that are being held pending admission (boarding) and those that continue to arrive via ambulance and private conveyance. Ambulance diversion ("diversion") is a common method used by EDs and regional EMS systems to reduce stress on individual departments, physicians, and nurses and to relieve mismatches in supply and demand. As such, it is a pre-hospital triage system one step removed from the actual ED waiting room or ambulance entrance. Under this strategy, ambulances that would otherwise transport patients to a particular hospital are redirected to a different hospital, usually according to policies or protocols approved by regional or state-wide EMS systems.

Often, and ideally, there are medical exceptions to patients being diverted, for instance when a patient with a ST-elevation myocardial infarction (STEMI) is transported to a STEMI receiving center that is on diversion rather than being sent to a hospital without a catheterization lab or interventional cardiologist available. A similar rerouting agenda may take the polytrauma patient or left ventricular assist device patient to specialized treatment locations. Such exceptions are for the purpose of fulfilling the duties implied in beneficence and nonmaleficence – that is, to produce maximal benefit and to prevent harm from lack of timely and appropriate treatment.

Diversion is not equally just or fair because it affects only those patients seeking care at a hospital via the public EMS system and not those arriving via private ambulances or other private conveyance. However, when it does involve the publicly operated EMS system, it should apply equally to all patients, and preference should not be granted to one group of patients over others except for medical reasons, as noted earlier.

Autonomy is often not considered during diversion decisions because patients who are unconscious or in extremis are not consulted about their transport preference and are typically taken to the closest facility able to treat their condition out of the duty to provide maximal benefit in the timeliest manner. Alert patients who would otherwise be taken to the closest hospital sometimes request to be taken to another hospital where they may have an established relationship. These have been termed *special consideration diversions* and impose a form of self-triage into the system when possible. Of course, these patients may need to be retriaged and wait nonetheless if transported to a crowded facility with sicker patients waiting.

A final consideration with regard to the field triage that occurs during diversion is the instance of the patient who the EMS system wishes to divert but refuses diversion and wishes to stay home against medical device. In such a case, if there is any chance the patient may be harmed by not honoring his or her request, autonomy should be – respected. Once again, secondary triage according to need may still occur at the receiving facility.

SPECIAL POPULATIONS

The VIP

VIP: A person of great importance or influence, especially a dignitary who commands special treatment.

There is very little published in the medical literature on the issue of the care of VIPs in EDs, perhaps because it is an issue that is swept under the rug. Every locale has them: athletes (college or professional); board of trustee members, directors, and administrators; actors or musicians; politicians, movie producers, senior physicians, business tycoons, major donors, and more. In all of these situations, contributions one way or the other, past, present, or future, or, in some cases, merely social status or familiarity, produce expectations that may challenge our moral sensibilities but must be faced and adjudicated. In a letter published in *Annals of Emergency Medicine*, Dr. A. J. Smalley reported that half of the thirty-three ED directors in his home state of Connecticut said they routinely reported expedited care to influential people (and, as the old joke goes, the other half are lying). MSNBC's "Truth on Call" conducted a survey of 100 emergency physicians, and 84 reported that they had given or would give extra attention to a VIP. Such VIP care often involves some special dispensation in the triage area.

A subheading to the issue of VIPs is that group of individuals who enjoy celebrity status. This group has needs that are similar to other VIPs but that include other considerations; namely, the need to protect their privacy over and above the norms established by Health Insurance Portability and Accountability Act (HIPAA) legislation for other patients. For celebrities, sitting in a waiting room or other public area may result in harm to them and therefore violate the principle of nonmaleficence simply by their presence in these areas. For this reason, these patients, who often arrive with entourages (small or large), are often whisked out of the waiting room into either a treatment space or at least to a more private place to wait. Undoubtedly, there will be pressure to get these patients into a treatment room.

No one denies that VIPs, both celebrities and others, will often be given priority to some extent. From an ethical point of view, this can be justified as long as other patients are not harmed. Often, these patients have been supporters of the hospital, contributing their time and talents to the institution, and they may continue to do so again in the future.

Politicians, for example, may be able to provide great benefit (or produce great harm) to a hospital. Sometimes, but not always, these patients have provided great value to other members of society and thus have an expectation of reciprocity. Many health care workers will object to giving VIPs priority, but staff members should be reassured that the medical care each patient receives will be equal and fair, even if social or economic pressures allow some patients triage priority. It might be helpful to point out to staff that if their close family members or they themselves needed care in the ED, they would probably be given priority and not simply wait their turn in line. Philosophically, once it is assured that no one will be harmed, the principle of *consequentialism* can be invoked to justify such practices; that is, that actions are right or wrong according to the balance of their good and bad consequences.

Children and the Elderly

Children, especially infants, are often given triage priority even if they are not the sickest patients. This may be to prevent harm coming to them via infectious vectors, to shield them from exposure to traumatic injuries or profanities, to help assure confinement, or to avoid annoyance to other waiting patients or visitors. Some EDs provide sub-waiting rooms for these purposes, but others allow priority access to available treatment spaces. Similar consideration may be given to the elderly who may not be able to tolerate long waits due to frailty, caregiver limitations, transportation options, or for other reasons.

Other Special Populations

At the opposite end of the social spectrum from VIPs may be patients who have voluntarily jeopardized their health, patients such as the chronic alcoholic, the intoxicated, the homeless, the disheveled, the schizophrenic, or others who may not be able to tolerate a long wait in the waiting room and may in fact influence other people to leave, thus exposing them to potential harm. Their presence in close proximity to other waiting patients (including, potentially, children if they cannot be otherwise accommodated as described earlier) may also be viewed as harmful. For these reasons, they may be given priority access to a room even when not the sickest.

Patients may also need to be prioritized for other reasons, such as the behaviorally dyscontrolled patient in the assisted care setting, for religious accommodations (e.g. the arrival of Sabbath for Orthodox Jews), or for overseas travellers with airplane reservations.

In all of these situations, as long as no one with a life- or limb-threatening presentation is harmed, triage prioritization must be viewed as relative and fluid, under which consequentialism can be invoked in rendering a triage judgment, rather than basing every decision on medical acuity and time of presentation. Under no circumstances should any group of people be discriminated against.

"TRIAGE AWAY" AND EMTALA

The U.S. Federal mandate, EMTALA stipulates that patients who "come to the hospital" be given a medical screening exam and are not turned away or transferred while they have an unstabilized emergency medical condition except under certain specific conditions, such as for a higher level of care than can be provided at the transferring hospital. As such, for patients with very minor complaints, such as an upper respiratory infection or someone seeking a prescription refill, it would be legally permissible for a specially trained nurse to perform vital signs, compare the chief complaint to a list of fifty minor diagnoses, rule out an unstabilized emergency medical condition, and refer away from the ED for further care to other potential community locations.

In the early 1990s, Derlet and others at the University of California Davis (UCD) in Sacramento advocated such a strategy, termed "triage away," as a mechanism to reduce the demand on overburdened EDs and to reduce crowding. In their original study, it was found that no actual harm could be proved as a result of this practice, which they described as "refusal of care" in the title of the publication. Subsequent studies by Lowe and others (1994) failed to reproduce the original results, and thus "triage away" (also sometimes called *triage out*) has become a discredited notion by the mid-1990s. Iserson and other prominent ethicists deplored the misnomer of refusing care attributed to patients because it failed to satisfy the principles of autonomy, beneficence, nonmaleficence, and social justice, all at the same time. It also failed on utilitarian grounds because it was never shown to increase happiness or benefit to anyone.

RISKS TO PROVIDERS IN TRIAGE

The triage station itself poses a risk of harm to health care workers. Patients are often dissatisfied and may be violent. They may suffer from mental illness or substance abuse, and they may carry an infectious disease or a concealed weapon. Hospital administrators and others in positions of authority must make every effort to assure that health care workers or other patients are not harmed in the triage station. Measures taken might include proper design and equipment, provision of adequate security, and training in and enforcement of the proper use of personal protective equipment. Notably, a practical application of the three-part "run, hide, fight protocol" was recently put forward by the U.S. Department of Health and Human Services (DHHS) in recognition of active shooter incidents as an extant threat to health care facilities. It appears that the frequency of hospital-based active shooter incidents has evolved to constitute at least a monthly occurrence by 2015. Preparatory drills of the emergency operation plans must be routinely pursued to safeguard health professionals and limit hospital liability in the wake of active-shooter incidents.

DISASTER TRIAGE

Disaster triage is clearly and unequivocally based on the utilitarian principle of the most good for the most people. When resources are truly over-whelmed, heroic measures that might be undertaken to save an individual life might be set aside if the effort is unlikely to yield a positive result and the next most injured patients might suffer from delays. Fortunately, this situation rarely occurs in civilian life. In smaller mass casualty incidents (e.g. a local railroad accident), incident commanders in the field will attempt to distribute victims to multiple hospitals capable of caring for polytrauma patients. The goals of such triage are (1) to provide maximum benefit to all patients, (2) to prevent avoidable harm, and (3) to distribute patients fairly so that all hospitals and providers share the burden of caring for these patients (regardless of insurance status or other status) and so that all such patients enjoy the benefits of the (often publicly funded) trauma system.

SCENARIO RESOLUTIONS

Scenario Case 1

This elderly patient is a borderline hypotensive who has suffered syncope and refuses transfer to a hospital other than his preferred hospital that is on diversion because of long wait times for patients in the waiting room. In these authors' opinions, diversion should be overridden because this patient may suffer severe harm if not transferred. Diversion had been described as "an advisory condition, not an absolute constraint." The primary interest in a case like this is the welfare of the index patient, barring any evidence that such attention would specifically harm another patient.

Scenario Case 2

Is it ethical to add space that is designed to treat other than the sickest? In any health care system, decisions must be made prospectively as to how to allocate resources among the population. If resources went only to the oldest and sickest, others would suffer. Many hospitals build within their EDs a "fast track" or other such space to care for minor-complaint patients in parallel with other potentially sicker patients. In hospitals with a large number of visitors and a short supply of beds, if not for a fast track "lane," patients with lower acuity complaints would wait inordinately long times to be seen. Therefore, assuming all patients with life-threatening conditions will be seen immediately, it is ethical to build space dedicated to treating patients with lower level complaints.

Scenario Case 3

The hospital's chairman of the board is on her way to the ED with seemingly minor injuries. Some theorists argue that making this person or a high-level administer or politician wait for 3 hours might force them to focus on addressing the needs of the institution and bring in needed resources. Of course, it might have the opposite effect. A consequentialist would probably opt to treat such a person as soon as possible, as long as it doesn't bring harm to others.

Scenario Case 4

The 32-year-old man presents with shortness of breath that is likely attributable to volume overload, since he is dialysis-dependent and presenting with his usual symptoms of hypertensive headache and weight gain consistent with his previous episodes of medical noncompliance and chronic renal failure with anuria.

He is intoxicated and demands to be dialyzed in the ED observation unit. He refuses a chest x-ray and any blood draw. His electrocardiogram shows peaked t waves, and a lung examination reveals crackles throughout. Moreover, he refuses to be admitted to the medical intensive care unit

(MICU) for emergent dialysis. Medical documentation review confirms that he was legally "fired" by the entire nephrology practice group and is banned from the institution's outpatient dialysis center.

Should treatment of noncompliant patients be delayed? All ED patients deserve prompt and appropriate medical care. The patient has signs and symptoms and physical findings of volume overload, which qualify as a medical emergency. Despite the nephrologists' desire not to provide ongoing care any longer for this patient being both reasonable and ethically acceptable, refusing to provide dialysis for him in an emergency situation is ethically unacceptable. The ethical justification for triage to the ED observation unit for dialysis (scarce medical resource allocation) could be sustained on the priority of the worst-off only in terms of distributive justice. The principle of nonmaleficence would also push to dialyze emergently. It seems of some benefit to avoid overtriage to the MICU or upscaling care to transfer to an outside facility if the system can arrange for an ED observation unit dialysis session. Finally, the best way to honor the patient's autonomy is to acquiesce to his request, if possible. Legal obligations under EMTALA would not likely support the alternative to transfer for emergent dialysis, unless the treatment to stabilize his condition was not available at the index hospital, thus providing the rationale to move him to higher care.

Should noncompliant patients receive a different level of care? Noncompliant patients may benefit from additional resources, such as social services, case management, and care plans in consultation with the primary care physician.

In summary, routine daily triage works in part on a lottery principle, providing a natural chance (first-come, first-served) element to need-based triage. Screening patients in triage is a necessary function in all EDs to sort out the subset of the sickest patients seeking care. The purpose of daily triage is to identify the life-threatening presentations, to rapidly expedite care for those most in acute need. The highest level of care is provided to these patients, even if they have a low probability of survival. In this way, daily triage refers to a system that occurs when available resources are sufficient to provide for the needs of few patients. Ethical challenges arise when ED demand exceeds its resources for short or sustained periods of time. All special cases require triage prioritization to be viewed as relative and fluid. Threats to life and limb supervene all other considerations. In contrast to daily triage, disaster triage refers to a system that occurs when available resources are insufficient to provide for the needs of all patients.

ETHICS TAKEOUT TIPS

- Triage may be viewed as the means by which scarce medical resources are allocated; it is relative and fluid rather than absolute.
- Major ethical underpinnings for daily routine triage are nonmaleficence, beneficence, and distributive justice.
- Ambulance diversion is a form of triage that is unjust because it only applies to patients being transported in publicly operated statewide EMS vehicles.
- VIPs should not get better medical care but may need special accommodation to avoid the public spectacle their presence may bring to a waiting room of sick patients. Since this occurs commonly, we should be honest about it.
- Children, the elderly, and others may also need special accommodation, meaning that they are triaged to a treatment bed ahead of other patients.
- "Triage away" refers to the practice of performing a medical screening exam without providing subsequent definitive care, and it does not satisfy any ethical interest.
- Nurses and others performing ED triage may be exposed to physical harm and workplace violence, and all episodes should be reported to authorities to prevent future recurrence.
- Disaster triage reorders ethical priorities, and, by concentrating on the utility of societal good, it may place a burden of unacceptable sacrifices on individuals.

FOR FURTHER READING

Aacharya, R. P., Gastmans, C., & Denier, Y. (2011). Emergency department triage: An ethical analysis. *BMC Emergency Medicine*, 11, 16–18 [16-22X11-16].

Beachamp, T. L., & Childress, J. F. (1994). Types of ethical theory. In T. L. Beauchamp & J. F. Childress (Eds.), *Principals of Biomedical Ethics*, 4th edn. (pp. 44–119). New York: Oxford University Press.

Bullard, M. J., Unger, B., Spence, J., & Grafstein, E. (2008). CTA National Working Group: Revisions to the Canadian Emergency Department Triage and Acuity Scale (CTAS) adult guidelines. *Canadian Journal of Emergency Medicine*, 10(2), 136–151.

Celebrities in the ED: Managers often face both ethical and operational challenges. (2006, December). *ED Management*, 18(12), 133–144.

Derlet, R. W., & Nishio, D. A. (1990, March). Refusing care to patients who present to an emergency department. *Annals of Emergency Medicine*, 19(3), 262–275.

Docs Admit Hospital VIPS Get Faster Care. www.nbcnews.com/id/4472339/ns/
   health_care/t/docs-admit-hotpital-vips-get-faster-care-er/#.UINM5tKshNc
Gatter, R. A., & Moskop, J. C. (1995). From futility to triage. *Journal of Medical Philosophy*, 995(20), 191–205.
Geiderman, J. M., Marco, C. A., Moskop, J. C., Adams, J., & Derse, A. (2015, March). Ethics of ambulance diversion. *American Journal of Emergency Medicine*, 33(3), 455–460.
Iserson, K. V. (1992, May). Assessing values: Rationing emergency department care. *American Journal of Emergency Medicine*, 10(3), 263–264.
Iserson, K. V., & Moskop, J. C. (2007). Triage in medicine, part I: Concept, history and types. *Annals of Emergency Medicine*, 49, 275–281.
Iserson, K., & Moskop, J. C. (2007). Triage in medicine, part I: Concept, history, and types. *Health Policy and Clinical Practice/Concepts*, 49(3), 275–281.
Iserson, K., & Moskop, J. C. (2007). Triage in medicine, part II: Concept, history, and types. *Health Policy and Clinical Practice/Concepts*, 49(3), 282–287.
Lowe, R. A., Bindman, A. B., Ulrich, S. K., Norman, G., Scaletta, T. A., Keane, D., . . . Grumbach, K. (1994, February). Refusing care to emergency department of patients: Evaluation of published triage guidelines. *Annals of Emergency Medicine*, 23(2), 286–293.
Schmidt, T. A., Iserson, K. V., Freas, G. C., et al. (1995, November). Ethics of emergency department triage: SAEM position statement. *Academy of Emergency Medicine*, 2(11), 990–995.
Winslow, G. R. (1982). *Triage and justice* (p. 169). Berkeley: University of California Press.
Zimmermann, P. G. (2001). The case for universal, valid, reliable 5-tier triage acuity scale for U.S. emergency departments. *Journal of Emergency Nursing*, 27(3), 24

4

Privacy, Confidentiality, and Public Health Reporting

JOY HARDISON, MD, MPH

As emergency physicians, we all experience the trust patients place in us every day in the emergency department (ED). Patients freely disclose sensitive information to us that allows us to deliver the best care possible, and patients allow themselves to become vulnerable to us during examinations and procedures. The American College of Emergency Physicians (ACEP) Principles of Ethics for Emergency Physicians states, "Respect patient privacy and disclose confidential information only with consent of the patient or when required by an overriding duty such as the duty to protect others or to obey the law" (ACEP, n.d.; see Appendix 1). The duty to protect the privacy and confidentiality of the patient is in line with the principle of beneficence, and we must never take this duty lightly. However, there are many circumstances in the practice of emergency medicine that challenge our ability to protect the privacy and confidentiality of our patients.

The nature of working in the ED presents dilemmas with respect to privacy and confidentiality on a daily basis. Emergency medicine physicians care for vulnerable populations, including victims of violent crimes, victims of abuse, patients under investigation, children, prisoners, homeless, undocumented immigrants, patients with mental illness, intoxicated patients, patients who are incapacitated or unable to communicate, patients who are cognitively impaired, and patients at the end of life. Many times, the emergency physician is medically working up and treating the patient while an investigation is being conducted by law enforcement or child protective services. Emergency physicians are often confronted with questions from law officers, prison staff, state agencies, the media, and organ procurement organizations, as well as the family and friends of the patient. We also must often emergently make decisions on behalf of our patients when they are incapacitated by their medical condition and no loved one is available to speak on the patient's behalf. Navigating this unique landscape of care delivery in the ED can at times feel like an ethical landmine. Success requires a mindful approach that balances the physician's duty to protect the patient's privacy and confidentiality while still complying with mandatory reporting and the physician's responsibility to protect the public at large.

Breaches in confidentiality and privacy have been shown to be fairly common in the ED environment (ACEP, 2007a). Often, these breaches have less to do with negligence and more to do with the environmental and patient limitations that are inherent to emergency medicine. The need to communicate in a timely and effective manner to care for the patient in a potentially life-threatening situation, the limitations of spatial layout in the ED, and the need to speak loudly to patients who are hard of hearing or have an altered level of consciousness are just a few of the factors that can make it difficult to adhere to the privacy and confidentiality standards that would be easy to follow under more ideal conditions.

Emergency medicine physicians are also challenged by their unique, frontline role in responding to the medical needs of patients during natural disasters, mass casualty events, infectious disease outbreaks, terrorist attacks, and other chaotic situations in which patient volume and acuity is high and resources and information are relatively scarce. These situations are rife with ethical dilemmas, as emergency physicians must decide when safety (of an individual patient or of the public at large) should trump privacy and confidentiality.

The good news is that the Health Insurance Portability and Accountability Act (HIPAA), the Joint Commission on Accreditation of Healthcare Organizations (JCAHO), and the American College of Emergency Physicians (ACEP) policies and standards regarding privacy and confidentiality are written to hold physicians to a high standard of protecting the privacy and confidentiality of patients while also allowing for the flexibility to override the protection of privacy and confidentiality when danger to the patient or the public health justifies deviation from the standard.

DEFINITIONS OF PRIVACY AND CONFIDENTIALITY

Privacy in health care is typically defined according to two different applications of the concept: physical privacy and informational privacy. Physical privacy refers to freedom from bodily exposure to others, whereas informational privacy pertains to freedom from disclosure of personal information (ACEP, 2007b). In clinical environments, physical privacy may be compromised at times when the medical needs of the patient take precedence, such as during physical examinations, procedures, or surgeries. In these circumstances, the physician must protect the patient's privacy from unnecessary exposure, such as making sure curtains are drawn and covering parts of the patient's body that are not medically necessary to expose during an examination. When medical necessity requires bodily exposure, the patient or their representative gives verbal or written consent. If the patient is incapacitated and no representative is available, then the physician must make the decision based on medical necessity in the interest of saving the patient's life or protecting the patient from harm.

When the term "confidentiality" is used in health care, it typically refers to informational privacy or the need to protect patient health information from leaking to individuals who are not directly involved with the patient's care and thus do not need to know the patient's private health information. Confidentiality is a frequent theme in the ED. Concerns regarding confidentiality must be considered when health care providers are communicating face-to-face, telephonically, or through digital means; documenting medical findings in electronic or paper form; handling physical records such as a medical chart; requesting or sending records via fax or other means; accessing historical records; displaying information on dashboards; and addressing questions from the patient's loved ones. Private health information is entrusted to us by our patients so that we may provide the best care possible. Physicians are stewards of private health information, which is often sensitive in nature, and, as good stewards of this information, we must ensure that we share it only when medically necessary in the best interest of the patient.

HIPAA PRIVACY RULE AND CONFIDENTIALITY

The HIPAA Privacy Rule was created to protect all "individually identifiable health information held or transmitted by a covered entity or its business associate, in any form or media, whether electronic, paper, or oral" (ACEP, 2009). The intent of the HIPAA Privacy Rule is to regulate the way health information must be handled in the interest of protecting the patient's informational privacy. According to HIPAA, individually identifiable health information is considered protected. The HIPAA Privacy Rule describes the way that protected health information (PHI) can be used in the context of patient care without explicit consent of the patient. All other uses or disclosures of PHI that fall outside of the uses permitted by the HIPAA Privacy Rule must be authorized in writing by the patient or the patient's representative. Tables 4.1 and 4.2 describe more specifically how the HIPAA Privacy Rule defines PHI, which

TABLE 4.1. *HIPAA: Definition of protected health information*

Identifies the individual (or reasonable basis to believe it can be used to identify the individual)
AND
Contains information about one or more of the following:

1. Past, present, or future physical or mental health or condition
2. Provision of health care to the individual
3. Past, present, or future payment for the provision of health care to the individual

---

From ACEP Board of Directors. (2009). *Filming in the emergency department.* ACEP policy statements on ethical issues.

TABLE 4.2. *Protected health information defined by HIPAA*

---

1. Names;
2. All geographic subdivisions smaller than a state, including street address, city, county, precinct, zip code, and their equivalent geocodes, except for the initial three digits of a zip code;
3. All elements of dates (except year) for dates directly related to an individual, including birth date, admission date, discharge date, and date of death; and all ages over 89 and all elements of dates (including year) indicative of such age, except that such ages and elements may be aggregated into a single category of age 90 or older;
4. Telephone numbers;
5. Fax numbers;
6. Electronic mail addresses;
7. Social security numbers;
8. Medical record numbers;
9. Health plan beneficiary numbers;
10. Account numbers;
11. Certificate/license numbers;
12. Vehicle identifiers and serial numbers, including license plate numbers;
13. Device identifiers and serial numbers;
14. Web Universal Resource Locators (URLs);
15. Internet Protocol (IP) address numbers;
16. Biometric identifiers, including finger and voice prints;
17. Full face photographic images and any comparable images; and
18. Any other unique identifying number, characteristic, or code, except as permitted by paragraph (c) of this section;

From 45 CFR 160.103.

TABLE 4.3. *HIPAA: Permitted uses and disclosures of protected health information*

1. To the individual patient who is the subject of the information
2. For the purpose of treatment, payment, and health care operations activities
3. When the patient has the opportunity to agree or object
4. Incident to an otherwise permitted use and disclosure
5. Public interest and benefit activities
6. Limited dataset for the purposes of research, public health or health care operations

Covered entities may rely on professional ethics and best judgments in deciding which of these permissive uses and disclosures to make.

includes information not only about the patient's medical condition, but also encompasses information about payment for health services and health care utilization.

The HIPAA Privacy Rule describes in detail the uses and disclosures of PHI that are permitted without formal authorization from the patient. However, the HIPAA Privacy Rule also states that providers should "rely on professional ethics and best judgments in deciding which of these permissive uses and disclosures to make" (ACEP, 2009). Although the HIPAA Privacy Rule may technically allow sharing of PHI under the circumstances described in Table 4.3, the rule compels us to be judicious and conscious of our professional obligation to act in the patient's best interest as we make choices about how and when to disclose information. From an organizational standpoint, ACEP publishes a Code of Ethics for Emergency Physicians (see Appendix 1) that includes further guidance regarding patient privacy and confidentiality as it pertains to the practice of emergency medicine. As emergency physicians, we are faced with choices every day regarding how and when we disclose PHI, and familiarity with the HIPAA Privacy Rule and the ACEP Code of Ethics policies and standards regarding patient privacy and confidentiality provide foundational guidance. Still, the nature of our profession will present many and varied circumstances pertaining to patient privacy and confidentiality that could never be fully encompassed in text, and, ultimately, we must rely on our professional ethical compass to help us make decisions that balance the often competing duties and responsibilities that we carry as emergency medicine physicians.

A NOTE ABOUT TERMINOLOGY

The HIPAA Privacy Rule uses the general term "privacy" to refer to informational privacy (synonymous with confidentiality). For purposes of clarity, in this chapter, the term "privacy" will here be used to refer to physical privacy, while the term "confidentiality" will be used to describe informational privacy.

PRIVACY AND CONFIDENTIALITY DILEMMAS IN EMERGENCY MEDICINE

Emergency Department Design

EDs historically were not designed for patient privacy; instead, they were designed for efficient triage and rapid stabilization of many patients simultaneously. EDs also need the ability to flex space in response to patient volume. Thus, many EDs have rooms separated by curtains rather than walls. In some cases, there may be common treatment areas. In cases of ED overcrowding (including in EDs that have been remodeled with private rooms), makeshift care areas are created on the fly, such as lining up patient beds down a hallway. It is often easy for conversations between physicians and patients to be overheard by other patients, visitors, and staff. Sometimes it may be necessary to examine a patient in an open hallway, although triage nurses try to limit the types of patients roomed in hallway beds or common areas to those requiring focused, not full-body examination.

The issue of privacy breaches in the ED is not insignificant. One study reported that ED breaches in privacy and confidentiality occurred 3–24 times per hour (1.5–3.4 times per patient hour) in one university hospital (ACEP, 2007a). In the ED, the high level of acuity and need for urgent treatment often trumps the concern for patient privacy when it comes to space utilization. Emergency medicine physicians are faced with the dilemma of trying to protect patient privacy despite the fact that the spatial layout of the department does not lend itself well to privacy.

In the redesign and remodeling of EDs, an attempt to improve patient privacy has been endeavored by many institutions. There has been a substantial improvement in patient privacy with ED remodels that replace curtains with walls and also with increasing the total square footage of treatment space (ACEP, 2011). One study reported that the number of patients who overheard conversations about themselves or other patients was cut almost in half, from 36 percent down to 14 percent, after remodeling the department (Allen, 1995). ACEP's Policy Statement on Emergency Department Planning and Resource Guidelines states "The ED should be designed to protect, to the maximum extent reasonably possible consistent with medical necessity, the right of the patient to visual and auditory privacy" (Barlas, Sama, Ward, & Lesser, 2001). Although challenges to patient privacy exist in the ED, bringing a hallway bed patient into a private room for physical examination, putting up temporary privacy screens in a shared treatment area, being mindful of the volume of conversations in common areas, and other temporizing measures can help to support maintaining patient privacy in crowded EDs with less than ideal spatial design.

Observers and Learners, Visitors, and Other Personnel

There are many members of the ED care team for any individual patient. Members of the care team may include attending physicians, residents, nurses, mid-level providers, technicians, transporters, paramedics, and other first responders. These individuals typically do not come into contact with the patient unless they are truly needed in order to provide a specific clinical service. However, there are other individuals who may participate in the patient's care as observers or learners. These individuals are not typically playing an essential role in the patient's care, but rather they are there for their own educational benefit.

Generic consent forms signed by the patient during the registration process are usually designed to include acknowledgment of the presence of and possible administration of care by students under supervision (U.S. Department of Health and Human Services, 2003). Although these students are participating appropriately, some patients may not feel comfortable exposing their bodies or intimate details regarding their medical condition to additional people who are not essential members of the care team. When possible, observers and learners should identify themselves and their role, and many patients will agree to allow students to observe and learn through participation in their care (especially if under direct supervision) (Geiderman, Moskop, & Derse, 2006). If a patient prefers to not have students participate in his or her care, this request should be honored unless there is a compelling reason why the student should continue to participate (such as in a mass casualty event when staff are spread thin and the student may be assisting the physician in a critical role in place of a nurse).

Visitors, especially family members and close friends, can contribute positively to the patient's comfort, sense of security, and mood. Still, it is important to be sensitive to the fact that not all visitors may be welcome by the patient. Before allowing a visitor to come back to the patient's room, the patient should be asked if he or she would like to see that visitor. If a patient presents in the ED with a loved one, it is commonly assumed that the patient feels comfortable with that person being around (U.S. Department of Health and Human Services, 2003). If a patient is unconscious or incapacitated, it is generally acceptable to allow "next of kin" to be present at the bedside and to be the patient's surrogate decision-maker. If a patient has an advanced directive, the surrogate decision-maker will likely be identified explicitly in the paperwork.

Before performing physical examinations or procedures that would expose the patient's body (and also when a sensitive history must be obtained from the patient, such as questions regarding sexuality, sexual practices, risk-taking behaviors), visitors should be asked to step out of the room unless the patient explicitly requests the visitor to stay. When visitors must step out of the room, it is important to make sure that they do not linger in the acute treatment areas because the privacy of other patients undergoing assessments may be compromised. Therefore, returning to the general waiting area until the patient is ready to receive visitors again is most appropriate.

At times, other types of personnel are required to be present during patient care. Security guards, prison guards, and sometimes law enforcement officers may be required at the bedside to protect the physician and other medical staff from being harmed by the patient. In general, the need to protect the safety of providers outweighs the patient's right to privacy. If there is no threat to the safety of providers, the exposure of these types of individuals to patients should be limited. Law enforcement officials may be under court order or other legal mandate to investigate a crime, although they should not do so in a way that interferes with patient care (Geiderman et al., 2006). Also, certain individuals may transport patients even though they are not involved in their medical care (such as border patrol or other law enforcement officers who bring patients in for treatment).

Recording Devices

The recent rise in reality television shows depicting actual cases in the ED, particularly involving critically ill patients who are unable to consent at the time of filming, has raised privacy concerns. "The American College of Emergency Physicians (ACEP) opposes the filming for public viewing of emergency department patients or staff members except when they can give fully informed consent prior to their participation" (10). Video recording using departmental equipment for internal quality improvement activities or research may be acceptable from an ethical standpoint depending on the intended use and internal review board (IRB) considerations. The legal implications of video recording in the ED for internal use are outside the scope of this chapter.

The ubiquity of smartphones with built-in cameras and video-recording capability has created new privacy challenges in emergency medicine. Whether it is a patient or loved one wanting to take photographs or video during the patient encounter, a clinical staff member desiring to take a photograph of a wound for either teaching purposes or care continuity, or, in rare cases, a staff member who inappropriately is tempted to take a photo or video of a patient and post it on a social media website for recreational purposes, digital recording devices are in the hands or pockets of almost everyone who passes through the ED. A policy statement was released by ACEP in 2011 stating that "The use of recording devices, including cell phone cameras, in the emergency department for the purpose of capturing photographic, video, or audio media poses significant risks to the privacy and confidentiality of patients and staff. ACEP encourages EDs to adopt policies regulating the use of such devices" (ACEP policy statement, http://acep.org). What many clinicians may not realize is that not only do smartphones pose a risk to patient privacy because of inappropriate use, but even if a physician desires to snap a photo on a smartphone for the purpose of providing better clinical care, such as taking an image of rash to show a dermatology consultant who is off site, the sending of that image using usual methods is itself a HIPAA violation. HIPAA has very strict requirements regarding the use of mobile devices and email for sending and receiving data. PHI must be encrypted when being transmitted electronically, and there must be similar protections for the data once it is received at the other end of the transmission as well (Olsen, Cutcliffe, & O'Brien, 2008). Mobile devices for personal use that are not password-protected or that are shared among family members do not adequately protect PHI. Although physicians are anxious to use efficient technology to provide better care, we must be careful that we take proper precautions to protect patient privacy. HIPAA-compliant secure messaging and secure email services, as well as dedicated mobile devices for institutional use only, are some of the solutions that have emerged to facilitate the use of modern technology in health care.

Public Health Reporting and the "Duty to Warn"

According to the HIPAA Privacy Rule, "Providers can share patient information with anyone as necessary to prevent or lessen a serious and

imminent threat to the health and safety of a person or the public –
consistent with applicable law and the provider's standards of ethical
conduct" (Purdy et al., 2000). This concept is synonymous with the "duty
to warn," a concept that has been upheld many times in federal court cases
(U.S. Department of Health and Human Services, 2003). Also, public
health reporting of PHI can be ethically justified if it meets the criteria of
preventing or lessening the threat to the health and safety of the population
(similar to the earlier discussion). The type of information that falls under
public health reporting includes certain infectious diseases, driving impairment, abuse and other acts of violence, accidental deaths, suicide, and
information about hazards and natural disasters.

The Centers for Disease Control (CDC) maintains an active list of
National Notifiable Infectious Conditions (see Table 4.4). In some cases,
the hospital laboratory automates the reporting of these conditions to the
CDC, whereas in other cases providers must report manually. Also, if the
patient meets the definition of illness based on clinical criteria, the physician may be mandated to report to the CDC prior to completing con-
firmatory testing (such is the case with Ebola, listed in Table 4.4, under viral
hemorrhagic fever).

Mandatory reporting reaches far beyond infectious disease reporting to
public health officials. Most states require mandatory reporting to the state
motor vehicle department of conditions that affect a patient's ability to
safely operate a motor vehicle, such as seizures or vision impairment.
Injuries suspected to be from child abuse are mandatory to report to
child protective services in all states, whereas most states have similar
statutes regarding reporting of suspected elder abuse. The mandatory
reporting of violent injuries to law enforcement also varies by state regarding what types of injuries are mandatory to report. In the case of wrongful
death (or suspected wrongful death), emergency physicians may be
required by law to report PHI that informs law enforcement officials
regarding the circumstances and nature of the death as a component of
the investigation (U.S. Department of Health and Human Services, 2003).

Some states have mandatory reporting of domestic violence to law
enforcement, although ACEP has authored a policy opposing the mandatory reporting of domestic violence to the criminal justice system, prefer-
ring that the victim retain that decision. However, ACEP does encourage
reporting of domestic violence to other agencies, such as victims' services
organizations, local social services, or any other agency where the victim
can obtain confidential counseling and assistance (U.S. Department of
Health and Human Services, 2005).

TABLE 4.4. *CDC 2014 national notifiable infectious conditions*

Anthrax
Arboviral diseases, neuroinvasive and non-neuroinvasive
Babesiosis
Botulism
Brucellosis
Chancroid
Chlamydia trachomatis infection
Cholera
Coccidioidomycosis
Congenital syphilis
Cryptosporidiosis
Cyclosporiasis
Dengue virus infections
Diphtheria
Ehrlichiosis and anaplasmosis
Giardiasis
Gonorrhea
Haemophilus influenzae, invasive disease
Hansen's disease
Hantavirus pulmonary syndrome
Hemolytic uremic syndrome, post-diarrheal
Hepatitis A, acute
Hepatitis B, acute
Hepatitis B, chronic
Hepatitis B, perinatal infection
Hepatitis C, acute
Hepatitis C, past or present
HIV Infection (AIDS has been reclassified as HIV Stage III)
Influenza-associated pediatric mortality
Invasive pneumococcal disease
Legionellosis
Leptospirosis
Listeriosis
Lyme disease
Malaria
Measles
Meningococcal disease
Mumps
Novel influenza A virus infections
Pertussis
Plague
Poliomyelitis, paralytic
Poliovirus infection, nonparalytic

TABLE 4.4. *(continued)*

Psittacosis
Q fever
Rabies, animal
Rabies, human
Rubella
Rubella, congenital syndrome
Salmonellosis
Severe acute respiratory syndrome-associated coronavirus disease
Shiga toxin-producing *Escherichia coli*
Shigellosis
Smallpox
Spotted fever rickettsiosis
Streptococcal toxic-shock syndrome
Syphilis
Tetanus
Toxic shock syndrome (other than streptococcal)
Trichinellosis
Tuberculosis
Tularemia
Typhoid fever
Vancomycin-intermediate *Staphylococcus aureus* and
    Vancomycin-resistant *S. aureus*
Varicella
Varicella deaths
Vibriosis
Viral hemorrhagic fever
Yellow fever

From Centers for Disease Control and Prevention (n.d.).

In the wake of a natural disaster such as Hurricane Katrina in 2005 on the Gulf Coast, 1,836 people died in the hurricane and millions were displaced from their homes. An estimated 80 percent of New Orleans was flooded for weeks (U.S. Department of Health and Human Services, 2005). According to the HIPAA Privacy Policy, "when necessary, the hospital may notify the police, the press, or the public at large to the extent necessary to help locate, identify or otherwise notify family members and others as to the location and general condition of their loved ones" (Purdy et al., 2000). Health care providers are encouraged to obtain verbal permission when possible, but often this may not be feasible if the patient is incapacitated.

Communication of Patient Information

Requests for information about patients are often made in the ED. Loved ones may be calling to find out how a patient is doing. Before releasing information, ideally, the patient should verbally consent to sharing information about his or her health status, and an effort must be made to confirm the identity of the requestor. If the patient is unable to consent due to being unconscious or incapacitated, the next of kin should be identified (or advance directive reviewed if available), and the next of kin or person listed in the advance directive should assume the role of deciding on the patient's behalf who is allowed to receive updates (U.S. Department of Health and Human Services, 2003). As mentioned previously, registries noting patient presence in a facility and general health status can be maintained on an opt-out basis in hospitals, and, in the case of a natural disaster or mass casualty event, it may be appropriate to publish lists of patients and their general status to help locate people who have gone missing.

Communication between providers about patients is an essential function in the ED. Communication between providers may be verbal (in person or over the phone) or written (in the form of notes attached to the chart or entered into the electronic health record). Discussion of patient information in order to provide the required care to the patient is one of the HIPAA-permitted disclosures, and disclosures that occur inadvertently and incident to the primary disclosure (such as a consultant overhearing a conversation between two physicians regarding a patient that the consultant is not responsible for) are permitted as long as the inadvertent disclosure took place despite best efforts to speak in low voices and avoid public areas when patient information was being discussed (ACEP, 2009). Even though incident disclosures are permitted under HIPAA, clinicians have an ethical obligation to try their best to avoid incident disclosures by being mindful of where discussions about patient information are taking place and who may be within hearing range. If it would not interfere with patient care to take the conversation to a more private location, then that should be the course of action, although it is not always possible to do so in the busy ED. Privacy and confidentiality should not trump patient safety.

Also, at times, providers may need to communicate by fax if a consultant is not present in the hospital facility and does not have access to the electronic health record maintained where the patient is being treated. Care must be taken to not leave PHI in the fax machine after transmission in order to avoid inadvertent disclosures, and fax machines should be kept in an area without public access. Similarly, clinicians should take care to password-lock their workstations when they are not physically present at the computer, and they should secure paper charts to avoid inadvertent exposure of PHI.

With the rise of mobile devices, HIPAA specifically regulates the restrictions placed on digital transmission of data via text, email, and video (see section 4.3 on recording devices), and the use of these devices to digitally transmit patient data is not advised unless through a specific protocol developed by administrators that complies with HIPAA regulations.

Patient dashboards are another way that providers convey information to each other. Patient dashboards should not contain information about patient identity if they are to be displayed in areas where visitors or other patients may see them.

PRIVACY AND CONFIDENTIALITY CASE EXAMPLES

The cases introduced here were selected to provide a few real-world examples that illuminate some of the ethical dilemmas surrounding privacy and confidentiality that emergency physicians may face. The cases are inspired by many real-life scenarios experienced by emergency physicians, but the cases are fictional.

Privacy and Confidentiality: Case 1

You are one of several emergency medicine attending physicians working in a level one trauma center. You suddenly get a text page on your phone, which is connected to the hospital's internal phone network as part of the trauma response system. The message reads, "MASS SHOOTING, MANY DEAD ON SCENE, MULTIPLE CRITICAL VICTIMS EN ROUTE, ETA UNKNOWN."

The page has activated the trauma team, as well as all staff on back-up. Working with the charge nurse, you call all boots on deck to the trauma resuscitation area. Within 10 minutes, approximately thirty or more staff, including nurses, technicians, pharmacists, attending physicians and surgeons, medical students, and residents, have congregated in the trauma resuscitation bay. Many of the staff are not typically part of the trauma care team, but they have responded to offer assistance in anticipation of receiving numerous critical or "Red" level trauma patients simultaneously. Another text page comes through stating, "10+ CRITICAL PATIENTS EN ROUTE, ETA 1–2 MINUTES."

Seconds later, you hear sirens rapidly approaching, and then the double doors of the trauma bay burst open. Pairs of paramedics pushing gurneys come flying down the hallway, one after the other. You have been appointed to direct traffic and assign care teams, so you start guiding the arrivals into separate resuscitation rooms within the trauma bay, ensuring that each room is adequately staffed with appropriate combinations of providers.

Each resuscitation room is the same. They are comprised of three solid walls, with the fourth wall (the wall facing the hallway) being made of floor-to-ceiling transparent glass with large glass sliding doors that can break away if needed. As you are guiding the victims into rooms, you realize that you recognize several of the victims – not because you know them personally, but because they are well-known public figures. Several other staff also recognize the victims, and soon there is a buzz going through the trauma bay about the high-profile identities of some of the victims.

Soon you realize that you are running out of rooms. More new ambulances are stacking up outside, and there are two patients who have not yet been assigned to a room because the rooms in the trauma bay are full. You also notice that a crowd of ten or more people, mostly hospital staff and paramedics, as well as several law enforcement officers, are peering into the resuscitation scene that is taking place on the other side of the glass where one of the high-profile victims has been roomed.

You start to triage the patients lining up in the hallway of the trauma bay. The charge nurse comes up to you and asks, "Where would you like to room these new patients?" She adds, "By the way, someone from the local news called and is holding, wanting to confirm whether or not certain victims are alive or dead."

Discussion Questions for Case 1

1. What is your responsibility to protect the physical and informational privacy of the patients who are victims of this mass casualty event?
2. How does the setting and environment in the trauma bay affect your ability to protect patient privacy?
3. Which HIPAA-permitted disclosures of PHI are relevant in this scenario? Is there PHI that would fall under the permitted disclosures but that you would choose to refrain from disclosing due to your professional ethics and best judgment?
4. Does your duty to protect public safety conflict with your duty to protect individual patient privacy and confidentiality in this scenario? Describe why or why not.

Discussion Points for Case 1

EM physicians must make reasonable attempts to protect patient privacy and confidentiality, even in chaotic situations, to the extent that it does not negatively impact patient care. When possible, curtains should be drawn or temporary screens should be placed in common treatment areas or when space must be flexed due to unexpected increase in patient volume. The HIPAA Privacy Rule allows for flexibility, so when time-sensitive communication must take place in tight quarters and shared treatment areas to provide appropriate patient care, inadvertent disclosures are permitted. In general, it is best to defer to the hospital public relations team regarding disclosure of patient information to the media. Disclosure of PHI to law enforcement may be appropriate to protect the public from further harm by a deadly perpetrator.

Privacy and Confidentiality: Case 2

You are an emergency physician working in a community hospital with moderate patient volume. Your institution is not a tertiary care center, and many patients requiring emergent specialty care must be transferred to another facility for a higher level of care. Your hospital has partnership agreements with these outside facilities to provide certain services that you are not able to provide at your location. The electronic health record system you use at your hospital does not communicate with outside hospitals by any mechanism such as a health information exchange, so records must be faxed or printed and sent with the patient by ambulance.

It's Friday night at 8 p.m. An overweight 39-year-old man is brought in by EMS for severe chest pain, onset 20 minutes ago. As the nurse connects him to the monitor and supplemental oxygen, he is clenching his chest and moaning in pain. He is pale, diaphoretic, blood pressure is 185/100, heart rate is 104, respiratory rate is 20, and pulse oximetry reads 96 percent. Bedside glucose is 105. He denies any medical history, but admits that he has not seen a doctor for 20 years and smokes one pack of cigarettes per day. He denies drug use. The paramedics have already given him aspirin, nitro (which brought the pain down from 10/10 to 8/10), and morphine. One of the paramedics mentions that she thinks she saw ST segment elevation on the monitor, but they were unable to get a formal electrocardiogram (EKG) during their short transit time.

You order repeat doses of nitro and morphine and blood tests, as well as a bedside chest x-ray as the nurse collects a twelve-lead EKG. She hands you the tracing, and you instantly recognize an ST-elevation myocardial infarction (STEMI). You note ST elevation in leads V1 through V4, suggesting anteroseptal infarction. Your hospital's STEMI protocol for activating the cardiac catheterization team starts with a call to the interventional cardiologist on-call at the outside facility to relay the case information. The on-call cardiologist is the only person with the authority to activate the cardiac catheterization team. The transport time to the cardiac catheterization lab is 20 minutes with lights and sirens, so time is of the essence. You page the cardiologist on-call.

Within 5 minutes, he calls back. You succinctly describe the case to him, including a verbal description of the EKG, noting the ST segment elevation in V1 through V4. You are expecting that the cardiologist is going to give the OK to send the patient (as has been the case every other time you have called with a STEMI case), but instead he challenges you. He expresses his concern that the patient is only 39 years old with no medical history, and the cardiologist is dubious about whether or not the patient is actually having a STEMI. He refuses to activate the cardiac catheterization team without first seeing the EKG himself. You offer to fax him the EKG, but he explains he is out to dinner with his family and nowhere near a fax machine. He asks you to take a picture of the EKG with your smartphone and send it to him in a text message. You express your hesitance to send the EKG using your smartphone. The cardiologist reiterates that he will refuse to accept the patient unless you send him a text message with a photo of the patient's EKG, proving that the patient really does have a STEMI. He claims that other emergency physicians from your hospital send him photos of EKGs all the time. He also offers that if you are concerned about protecting the patient's confidentiality that you should just fold over the patient's name at the top of the EKG so there is no personally identifying information in the text message.

Discussion Questions for Case 2

1. Does this case represent an ethical dilemma of physical privacy or confidentiality (informational privacy)?
2. How has the evolution of modern technology created challenges with respect to privacy and confidentiality in the clinical environment?
3. What can be done to mitigate breaches of privacy associated with modern technology such as smartphones?
4. Are there ethical or legal considerations beyond privacy and confidentiality that should be considered in this case?

Discussion Points for Case 2
Sending PHI via personal smartphones or other personal mobile devices puts patient physical privacy (in the case of a photo or video of the patient's body) and confidentiality (in the case of test results, reports, notes, etc.) at risk. The ubiquity of smartphones, which all include built-in digital cameras and video recorders, makes protecting patient privacy and confidentiality more difficult than ever before. The use of mobile devices to communicate about patients via text or email is tempting because it is an efficient way of sharing information that cannot be easily conveyed verbally. Institutional programs implementing HIPAA-compliant mobile device technology are required to ensure that patient privacy and confidentiality is protected. In general, physicians should not refuse appropriate requests for transfer to a higher level of care because this represents violation of EMTALA.

Privacy and Confidentiality: Case 3

You are an emergency physician working for a large tertiary care center in the ED. It's November, and there have been quite a few cases of influenza lately. As you are about to see your next patient, you review the triage notes:

> *37-year-old male with 2 days of fever, headache, fatigue, "achy muscles," nausea*
> *Temp 39 C, BP 105/70, HR 121, RR 16, O2 Sat 97% on room air*
> *No medications, no allergies, no reported medical history*
> *Tylenol 1,000 mg given in triage*

You walk into the room and see a Caucasian man sitting upright in the bed. He appears fatigued but is able to carry a conversation. He is not short of breath. He shows no signs of acute distress. He has bilateral conjunctival hemorrhages. No meningismus is noted. His abdomen is mildly tender in all four quadrants. His temperature and heart rate have come down after the acetaminophen to 37°C and 89 beats per minute, respectively, and the remainder of his exam is unremarkable. He reports receiving a flu shot this year.

As you ask him more about his medical and social history, he confides in you that he is a nurse and that he just returned 1 week ago from a medical mission trip to Sierra Leone where he and his wife (also a nurse) cared for many patients known to be infected with the Ebola virus. He reports that they were very careful to always wear proper personal protective equipment; however, when he developed a fever, he became concerned. He asks you to keep this information confidential because he is afraid of becoming stigmatized like some of the other health care workers who have recently returned from West Africa and have been treated poorly by health care institutions, the media, and the government.

Discussion Questions for Case 3

1. Would this case be subject to mandatory public health reporting?
2. In this case, how is your duty to protect the patient in conflict with your duty to protect the public?
3. How can you best balance your duty to the public with the patient's request to keep his information confidential?

Discussion Points for Case 3

Ebola virus is listed by the CDC as one of the infectious diseases subject to mandatory public health reporting. Mandatory reporting must occur prior to laboratory confirmation of Ebola because the patient meets the clinical case definition. When the duty to protect the public outweighs the duty to protect patient privacy and confidentiality, the physician should explain to the patient that this private health information is subject to mandatory reporting due to the great risk to society if the information is not reported. The physician can try to protect patient privacy and confidentiality by limiting unnecessary disclosures to the extent possible while still complying with mandatory reporting to protect public safety. In cases where patients feel their rights are being violated, calling for an ethics consultation can be a helpful resource.

CONCLUSION

As emergency physicians, we have a duty to protect our patient's privacy and confidentiality despite the often chaotic environment of the ED, and environment that does not lend itself well to this task. HIPAA and the ACEP Code of Ethics have provided a framework that guides us in our efforts to protect patient privacy and confidentiality, but some flexibility has been built into the language of these policies to allow clinicians to use their professional ethical judgment when unique circumstances arise with competing duties, such as the duty to protect patient privacy versus the duty to protect public safety.

Every day, our patients come to us in their moments of greatest need, filled with faith in our professional judgment and skillset; they expose their bodies to us and share with us personal information that they may not even disclose to their closest friends or family. Our patients trust that we will be good stewards of their privacy and confidentiality and that we will only use the information we obtain in order to act in their best interest. As professionals, we are compelled to always conduct ourselves in a way that honors the trust our patients place in us.

ETHICS TAKEOUT TIPS

- Breaches of privacy and confidentiality are common in the ED.
- Crowded conditions, patient acuity, and department design are unique aspects of the ED environment that create challenges to privacy and confidentiality.
- Emergency physicians must strive to protect patient privacy and confidentiality despite these challenges, as long as doing so does not compromise patient care.
- Privacy should not trump safety (of individual patients or the public).
- Certain kinds of public health reporting or mandatory reporting are ethically justifiable.
- HIPAA and the ACEP Code of Ethics provide a framework for best practices regarding patient privacy and confidentiality, but certain circumstances may require emergency physicians to use their professional ethical judgment when competing duties arise.

FOR FURTHER READING

ACEP Board of Directors. (n.d.). Code of ethics for emergency physicians. *American College of Emergency Physicians policy statements on ethical issues.* www.acep.org/Clinical-Practice-Management/Code-of-Ethics-for-Emergency-Physicians/
ACEP Board of Directors. (2007a). Domestic family violence. American College of Emergency Physicians policy statements on ethical issues. www.emergencycareforyou.org/Health-Tips/Prevention/Domestic-Violence; also see, www.acep.org/Clinical-Practice-Management/List-of-Key-Elements-of-Family-Violence-Protocols
ACEP Board of Directors. (2007b). Emergency department planning and resource guidelines. American College of Emergency Physicians policy statement. www.acep.org/Clinical-practice-management/from-hippocrates-to-hipaa--privacy-and-confidentiality-in-emergency-medicinedpart-ii--challenges-in-the-emergency-department
ACEP Board of Directors. (2009). Filming in the emergency department. American College of Emergency Physicians policy statements on ethical issues. www.acep.org/Clinical---Practice-Management/Filming-in-the-Emergency-Department
ACEP Board of Directors. (2011). Recording devices in the emergency department. American College of Emergency Physicians policy statements on ethical issues.

www.acep.org/Clinical---Practice-Management/Recording-Devices-in-the-Emergency-Department

Allen, A. L. (1995). Privacy in healthcare. In E. Warren & T. Reich (Eds.), *Encyclopedia of bioethics* (vol. 4, pp. 2064–2073). New York: Macmillan.

Barlas, D., Sama, A. E., Ward, M. F., & Lesser, M. L. Comparison of the auditory and visual privacy of emergency department treatment areas with curtains versus those with solid walls. *Annals of Emergency Medicine*, 38(2), 135–139.

Centers for Disease Control and Prevention. (n.d.). National Notifiable Diseases Surveillance System (NNDSS). *NNDSS notifiable condition list.* wwwn.cdc.gov/nndss/script/conditionlist.aspx?type=0&yr=2014

Geiderman, J. M., Moskop, J. C., & Derse, A. R. (2006). Privacy and confidentiality in emergency medicine: Obligations and challenges. *Emergency Medicine Clinics of North America*, 24(3), 633–656.

Mlinek, E. J., & Pierce, J. (1997). Confidentiality and privacy breaches in a university hospital emergency department. *Academic Emergency Medicine*, 4(12), 1142–1146.

Olsen, J. C., Cutcliffe, B., & O'Brien, B. C. (2008). Emergency department design and patient perceptions of privacy and confidentiality. *Journal of Emergency Medicine*, 35(3), 317–320.

Purdy, S., Plasso, A., Finkelstein, J., Fletcher, R., Christiansen, C., & Inui, T. (2000). Enrollees' perceptions of participating in the education of medical students at an academically affiliated HMO. *Academic Medicine*, 75(10), 1003–1009.

U.S. Department of Health and Human Services. (n.d.). Summary of the HIPAA Privacy Rule. www.hhs.gov/ocr/privacy/hipaa/understanding/summary/

U.S. Department of Health and Human Services. (2003). Security standards – final rule. The HIPAA Security Rule. *Federal Register*, February 20. www.hhs.gov/ocr/privacy/hipaa/administrative/securityrule/securityrulepdf.pdf

U.S. Department of Health and Human Services Office for Civil Rights. (2005). Hurricane Katrina bulletin: HIPAA privacy and disclosures in emergency situations. www.hhs.gov/ocr/privacy/hipaa/understanding/special/emergency/katrinanhipaa.pdf

Zimmermann, K. A. (2012). Hurricane Katrina: Facts, damage & aftermath. *LiveScience*. TechMedia Network, 20 August. www.livescience.com/22522-hurricane-katrina-facts.html

5

Social Media and Electronic Communications

JILLIAN MCGRATH, MD, DIANE GORGAS, MD,
AND LYDIA SAHLANI, MD

DEFINING SOCIAL MEDIA AND ELECTRONIC COMMUNICATION

Social media (SM) and electronic communication (EC) have changed the landscape of the health care industry by impacting exchanges among and between patients and health care professionals. As consumers of health care and their providers have become increasingly connected via mobile phones, tablets, and computers, it is inevitable that the health care industry becomes comfortable with the use of social media. Many ethical considerations have arisen from the widespread adoption of SM and EC into health care. Historically, emergency medicine (EM) providers have led the medical community in both quantity and quality of SM-related endeavors, including websites, blogs, and microblogs devoted to the discussion of the practice of medicine.

Terminology

To effectively utilize SM and EC, it is important to understand some basic terminology. The early World Wide Web was much different from the current Web we have become accustomed to. The early Internet, dubbed Web 1.0, has transformed into the current Web 2.0. During Web 1.0, very few creators of information existed. Users mainly acted as consumers of content that had already been created. In contrast, Web 2.0 refers to "the social web" that has evolved to allow users to interact in a more collaborative environment. Users now routinely generate content in virtual communities, such as social networks, blogs, wikis, and other media-sharing sites. In this new Web, users are experts in sharing perspectives, opinions, thoughts, and experiences. Some

74

platforms that allow this sharing include podcasting, blogging, tagging, and social networking.

In the most basic sense, SM refers to web-based and mobile communication technologies and tools. It is commonly defined as a group of web-based applications that allow for the creation and exchange of user-generated content. SM has the ability to impact how we find, share, and discuss information. It emphasizes interactive, user-driven communication through use of text, audio, photo, and video communication platforms.

The popularity of SM and EC use among health care professionals has influenced current methods of communication, time management, patient access to information, health care provider routine, and practice management. Within Web 2.0, Health 2.0 refers to the use of technology in the collaboration between health care professionals and their patients through a variety of modalities discussed herein. The current generation of health care professionals is connected to the Web through a myriad of Internet-accessible devices, including mobile phones, tablets (iPad, Android, reader devices), and computers (laptops, desktops). As a result, the widespread use of SM and EC has created unique opportunities and challenges for the health care community. Understanding the basic terminologies associated with SM and EC is important in defining the subject in order to maximize its most effective use.

Modalities

Social Networks

Facebook. Facebook is the most commonly used form of SM and the largest social network in the world with approximately 1.2 billion users worldwide. Facebook focuses on building social relationships between individuals and has a multilingual platform. The network consists of individual user profiles and personal timelines as well as business or professional "pages." Profiles consist of basic personal, employment, and contact information, as well as user uploaded photos/videos, status updates, and memorable life events. Users can "like" and comment on information shared through the site. There is also a chat functionality and the ability to create and join groups or events. The newsfeed function allows users to browse through recent picture additions, status updates, and advertisements on the site. Users are able to apply some privacy settings to limit viewership of information.

LinkedIn. LinkedIn is a business-oriented social professional networking site. There are currently more than 300 million users of this multilingual site. The site has features that may act as a user's "resume." Users maintain a profile and upload a photo as well as information representative of experiences, education, skills and expertise, and summary and contact information. Connections the user makes can endorse the skills and expertise of the user. The site can be utilized to find jobs, collaborators, and business opportunities. The user may also join interest groups where discussions can take place. Users can "like" or "congratulate" other users on updates and new employment.

Secure Social Networking Sites
Doximity. Doximity is a professional social networking site for physicians. It offers physicians the ability to earn continuing medical education (CME) credits, connect with other physicians, search a directory of more than 700,000 physicians, and network with colleagues and employers. The site also allows for secure collaboration regarding patient treatment.

Blogs
Blog. The word "blog" was created from the words "web log." It refers to a discussion or informational site that consists of posts, with the most recent appearing first (reverse chronological order). Blogs may include commentary on a particular subject or represent a personal online diary. Most blogs are interactive and allow users to leave comments and to message one another. Blogs consist mostly of text content, but can include photos, videos, audio, and links to other blogs, websites, and social media modalities. "Blog" can also be used as a verb, in reference to adding content to a blog.

RSS Feed. RSS or Really Simple Syndication or Rich Site Summary utilizes webfeed formats to publish frequently updated information, such as blogs, videos, or news headlines. By subscribing to a feed, the user does not have to manually check the site for updates, but receives updates automatically. Specific software presents the feed data to users.

Twitter. Twitter is a social networking and microblogging site with approximately 255 million active users (https://about.twitter.com/company). It allows users to send and read messages of 140 characters or less, called "tweets." Users can follow or subscribe to others and send direct messages to other users (via @username). Hashtags (#) are utilized to annotate messages and link to important events, conferences, or ideas. Tweets are public by default but can be restricted so that only followers can see them.

Visual Media
Instagram. Instagram is an online, mobile photo and video sharing application that allows users to take photos or videos, apply filters, add

locations, and share on the Instagram network or other social networks such as Facebook and Twitter. It currently has about 200 million users.

YouTube. YouTube is a video sharing website where users can upload, share, and view videos. Media corporations upload some content to YouTube, but most of the content is individual user-driven. Most videos enable users to leave comments. Currently, more than 1 billion unique users visit YouTube each month.

Although this discussion has used specific sites as an example of broader platforms of SM, it should not be viewed as an all-inclusive list of available platforms. The complexity of the social networks (illustrated in Figure 5.1) is rapidly evolving.

Electronic Communication

Text messages, media messaging services (MMS). MMS is the exchange of text as well as multimedia content to and from mobile devices over a network. Photos, videos, and hyperlinks can be sent over MMS.

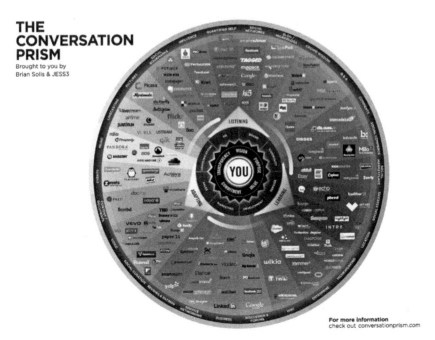

FIGURE 5.1. *The conversation prism* illustrates the vast array of social media platforms. (Reprinted with permission).

Email. Email, or "electronic mail" refers to the exchange of digital messages from an author to one or more recipients that includes a message header followed by the body of the message. Attachments such as hyperlinks, photos, videos, and audio can be added to the message. Email operates using many different platforms (e.g. Gmail, Hotmail, Outlook) and connects billions of users worldwide.

Digital Storage Devices
Cloud storage. Cloud storage devices allow the user to store, access, and manage digital data on variable infrastructure platforms that can span different servers and locations. These platforms are managed by a host, who is responsible for the access and protection of the data.

Summary

SM and EC are part of a complex electronic social web. They are continuously evolving entities, with new platforms consistently added, making it impossible to cover the topic comprehensively – only a sampling of SM modalities have been highlighted here. Generally, SM and EC platforms should be divided into unsecure and secure modalities, both of which have the ability to confer important personal, professional, and educational benefits onto users while presenting unique ethical dilemmas.

BENEFITS OF SOCIAL MEDIA AND ELECTRONIC COMMUNICATION

Despite the ethical dilemmas surrounding health care professional use of EC and SM, there are personal, professional, and educational advantages of these platforms within medicine.

Personal Benefits

There is clear evidence that a strong interpersonal support system can decrease stress levels and improve physical and psychological well-being. This sense of support has been positively correlated with the absolute number of Facebook friends. A strong positive relation of online support to coping mechanisms and psychological well-being has yet to be proved. However, the penetration of this technology globally speaks for itself in popularity, and many tout the downstream effect of improved connectivity. Despite the concerns of potential patient access to SM sources, health care professionals' use of SM outlets including Facebook is roughly that of the general population. SM and EC use among physicians has increased from 41 percent in 2010 to 90 percent in 2011, and is greater than 90 percent among medical students. The implication is that health care professionals tend to reap the same personal rewards of SM as the general population.

Social isolationism has been studied as a factor contributing to burnout. SM and EC can be used as platforms to encourage peer support and maintain connectivity with friends, family, and peers in an at-risk time of social isolationism, given the focus on work productivity. Therefore, these systems may promote learner wellness.

Professional Benefits

The professional advantages of SM utilization include its use in finding employment and in health care professionals marketing themselves. SM can be successfully utilized to develop a patient base and to market a practice. These platforms can facilitate the exchange of ideas involving professional areas of interest and career strategies.

Within an academic environment, social platforms can be used for personal career development. SM can engage a large community, which can aid in mentoring for both faculty seeking career mentorship and mentorship to students and residents. This can be particularly advantageous to students and faculty at smaller training programs or at medical schools without an associated specialty training program. It can also be used to connect health care professionals and trainees with diverse backgrounds to those nationwide who may share their perspectives, thus allowing gender-specific mentorship and mentorship of underrepresented minorities. In addition, topic-specific mentorship helps align career, clinical, and research goals. Examples of SM being utilized for professional career development are entering into the literature. These include topics related to time and resource management, academic productivity, or conflict resolution.

A distinctive advantage of SM and EC for professional development is that it is often free and asynchronous. This minimizes the barriers of expense and distance that have been challenging to health care professionals. SM can also enhance and encourage life-long learning initiatives, including the opportunities for health care professionals to learn from one another, discuss clinical issues, and even coordinate health care team interactions.

Opportunities for health care research and collaboration can be driven forward by SM and result in improved outcomes across health systems. SM provides a myriad of pathways to stay connected with remote collaborators and professional societies and for individuals to actively participate in advancing the causes and goals of a specialty. These platforms can be effective tools to influence health policy as well.

In supervising trainees and direct reports, SM can give clues to the onset of wellness issues and be an early-warning system for monitoring depression or signs of burnout. Unfortunately, this includes a growing number of anecdotal cases of SM being used to broadcast suicidal intent.

Educational Benefits

Many applications of SM and EC can be used in the educational setting, including:

- *Blog websites.* Topics are generally selected by the author periodically, and additional content is supplied by bloggers. *Wikis* are a subset of blogs that can be edited by third-party users.
- *Twitter.* Twitter is enhanced for medical providers via the use of health care hashtags that keep pertinent interest groups aware of topics. Twitter comments are now showing up on PowerPoint discussions within the more traditional classroom lecture format to engage lecture attendees.
- *Podcasting.* In podcasting, audiovisual files are available online. Media sharing is a type of podcasting (most notably www.youtube.com). This allows for the preservation of procedurally based videos for asynchronous viewing across either time or distance.
- *Collaborative environments* like editing drop boxes and venues for online meetings can allow for distance access to medical experts and promote collaboration.
- *Immersive learning environments,* such as Second Life or Unity, provide an opportunity for virtual and remote simulation.

Of note are some specific examples of SM and its penetrance into medical education. A number of institutions are now using Twitter to administer successful journal clubs. This can broaden the reach of a discussion and allow for remote and asynchronous access to the discussion. Twitter can be used not only as a means of access to medical information, but also can be used to "push" information to its users. One such program established a daily "tweet" based on a teaching point in emergency ultrasound; the resulting surveys of satisfaction regarding user friendliness and educational content were both greater than 80 percent.

Another educational example is the use of a secure SM platform to encourage reflection in an EM residency training program. The access-restricted blog was well accepted by both residents and faculty alike and heavily utilized for discussions of everything from specific clinical case questions to social planning to general ethical questions about the practice of medicine.

Immersive learning environments have been used for virtual simulation (e.g. an EM oral board simulation of a patient case encounter), and these eliminate the need for face-to-face interaction. Distinct advantages are that learners can feel more integrated into the simulation experience and be able to access simulations remotely.

Free Open Access Meducation (FOAMed), created by and for emergency and critical care (EMCC) physicians is touted as a "personalized, continuously expanding medical curriculum that embraces an individual's attention deficits, evolves as one learns, encourages active learning, and pushes the bounds of what one 'ought' to know." FOAMed is not a single modality, but rather a route for accessing and managing medical information. This includes contact streams and search platforms for EMCC. Although there have been no studies that correlate online collaboration with improved learning, the FOAMed network and others like it espouse increased engagement, input, and access to EM with a global perspective.

Patient Education and Care

EC and SM have become the new "word of mouth" for patients when it comes to seeking a health care professional. Patients frequently use EC and SM to find a local health care provider, and many choose to rate health care professionals or write reviews of them. Likewise, physicians exploit SM to recruit patients to their practices. Once established as a patient, many health care professionals are using online technologies to improve patient interaction, enhance patient motivation, and raise timely issues with their patients. This frequently results in improved patient satisfaction and can result in improved patient outcomes given the real-time collaborative advantages of SM. EC and SM have become a booming source of connectivity and support for patients. From disease-specific online support groups to increased patient awareness and access to clinical trials, SM has made a significant impact on patient's online lives, and many practices have chosen to use SM as a vehicle for promoting healthy lifestyles among their patients. Furthermore, the practice of *crowdsourcing* interesting cases via health care professional-specific and often specialty-specific SM platforms is rising in popularity and has led to a proliferation of online communities especially designed for health care professionals to collaborate with respect to unique patient care or research interests.

Summary

One constant challenge for all online resources lies in the ability and efforts required of moderators to curate the content. The success of sites like Up to Date can be linked to continuous curating of posted material.

There are distinct benefits – personally, professionally, educationally, and related to patient care – to the adoption of EC and SM into practice, and innovations regarding the use of these platforms are beginning to be seen in education and specialty-specific literature.

CONTROVERSIES AND ETHICAL DILEMMAS IN SOCIAL MEDIA AND ELECTRONIC COMMUNICATION

Despite the many educational and collaborative benefits of SM and EC, health care professionals must consider the ethical dilemmas posed by such forms of exchange.

Personal Dilemmas

Personal wellness and a sense of connection among health care professionals must be balanced with professional responsibility and codes of ethics. The concept of separation of online professional and personal identities is thought to be imperative to maintaining medical professionalism online. This differentiation is operationally challenging and places psychological and physical burdens on health care providers to maintain two identities. However, health care providers should proactively manage professional and personal profiles in order to maintain as much control over their online presence as possible. This is best accomplished by using advanced privacy settings that allow for more deliberate sharing of information online. Despite this recommendation, health care professionals should always assume that posted content online is both public and permanent. Privacy settings can be circumvented, and even deleted content may remain archived and accessible.

Online presence and participation in EC may be misinterpreted by both health care professionals and patients as an expectation for immediate, real-time responsiveness. The notion that "the doctor is always in" can be detrimental to physician wellness and balance. This can also lead to discord if appropriate temporal expectations are not negotiated and communicated ahead of time with patients and colleagues. Health care professionals should designate specific times for EC to avoid the fatigue or burnout associated with lack of "electronic downtime."

Another consideration regarding SM for health care professionals and trainees is its potentially negative psychological effect. Deemed in the media as "Facebook Depression," studies have suggested that there may be a correlation between time dedicated to social networking and a worsening subjective sense of well-being. This could be related to feelings of inadequacy or "fear of missing out," as well as to the pressure of online social interaction.

Professional Dilemmas

Translation/Context
Electronic and online communication poses unique challenges in regard to professionalism and may result in unintended outcomes or consequences. First, translation is difficult in any form of communication that involves written words without the context of body language, facial expression, and tone or voice inflection. Furthermore, the ease of use, rapidity of data exchange, and immediate availability of electronic media and social networks may preclude careful consideration and thoughtful distribution of content or responses. Many users may not even be aware of the potential abuses of electronic media. Furthermore, rapid dissemination allows a larger audience than may be initially intended, and information may be made quickly public. It is particularly challenging for health care professionals to predict the way that the general public may perceive seemingly harmless medical banter or humor. Therefore, significant consideration and reflection is required to avoid misinterpretation and translational or context errors in the use of EC.

Appropriateness of Social Interactions with Patients
Whom health care professionals choose to interact with in an online setting requires careful consideration of both intentions and appropriate boundaries. Although electronic communication may be used to supplement the clinical relationship with a patient, health care professionals should use

extreme caution when extending patient interaction to an online setting. Specifically, an established clinical relationship must already exist, and the patient should consent to EC with documentation of his or her awareness of security measures in place to protect confidentiality.

Standards consistent with professional relationships in the clinical setting must be maintained online. In a survey of state medical boards, most respondents had received reports of online violations of medical professionalism. "Inappropriate patient communication online" was the most common violation cited (e.g. sexual misconduct), followed by use of the Internet for inappropriate practice (e.g. prescribing without an established clinical relationship). The Federation of State Medical Boards (FSMB) has specifically discouraged health care professionals from interacting with current or past patients on social networking sites. Health care professionals should not contact patients through personal SM.

Appropriateness of Social Interactions with Trainees, Staff, Colleagues
Relationships between physicians of varying levels of training, students, and other staff and allied health professionals should always be considered inequitable and should align with traditional ethical boundaries. When extended to the online setting, relationships should continue to serve the purpose of professional mentorship. Seemingly harmless interactions such as "friending" on Facebook's SM platform could be interpreted as intrusive or in violation of personal boundaries. Furthermore, a lack of consistency in such interactions may lead to the perception of "favoritism," and responses to prompts on SM platforms should be uniform. Unless it is imperative for educational or remediation purposes, individuals in a position of authority should never initiate a personal online relationship with an individual in a subordinate position.

Professionalism

When considering professionalism in EC, a guiding principle should be to maintain public trust in the medical profession and in patient–physician relationships. Health care professionals should be mindful of their affiliations and understand that they are representatives of both their institution and their profession. Derogatory or discriminatory language toward patients or populations of patients, trainees, or colleagues should routinely be avoided. Furthermore, lapses in professionalism in online behavior could suggest or imply physician impairment; whether real or perceived, this could be extremely detrimental in the role of health care provider.

Physicians should refrain from portraying any unprofessional depictions of themselves on SM and social networking websites. Additionally, they should monitor for unprofessional online posting initiated by others in reference to them (tagging practices) on SM platforms. The online behaviors of physicians and trainees could affect current and future employment opportunities, and some medical schools and residencies report routinely reviewing applicants' social networking sites – many reported that online unprofessionalism could affect an applicant's admission. State medical boards (SMB) have reported violations in online medical professionalism with regard to derogatory remarks or discriminatory language or practices, as well as online depictions of intoxication.

Legal

Confidentiality and Identifiable Information
Patients have a right to privacy, defined by both local and federal legal requirements including the Health Insurance Portability and Accountability Act (HIPAA). Health care professionals must follow appropriate protocols for secure storage and transfer of patient information to maintain patient confidentiality. Digital sharing of patient information requires a level of security superior to standard connections; encryption or proxy network connections should be utilized to ensure secure digital environments. Institution-based policies regarding remote access of protected health information on personal devices and mobile device management for tablets or smartphones should be consistently followed. Remote monitoring and remote disabling are necessary capabilities in the event that devices are misplaced or stolen. Online violations of patient confidentiality have been reported by many SMBs.

SM sites allow immediate online posting of digital imagery. The American College of Emergency Physicians (ACEP) believes that the use of recording devices, including cell phone cameras, in the emergency department for the purpose of capturing photographic, video, or audio media poses significant risks to the privacy and confidentiality of patients and staff (see Appendix A). The practices of obtaining formal written consent and de-identifying photographs and radiography must be extended to digital images and the sharing of digital media. Simple markers like tattoos, scars, or jewelry could be overlooked and serve as patient identifiers when producing digital images. Institutional policies should be developed and followed to maintain appropriate de-identification and sharing of digital media.

Informed Consent

The informed consent of patients must occur prior to initiation of EC. This should include security disclosures, a clarification of appropriate content and temporal expectations for EC (e.g. avoidance of time-sensitive or emergent medical concerns communicated by email), and an explanation of routine measures taken to authenticate patient identity. Licensing jurisdictions must be respected in online communication with patients.

e-Discovery

Litigation discovery increasingly focuses on EC, deemed e-discovery. Electronic records and communication may be required to be preserved and produced through this formal legal process. SM is not subject to any special privacy considerations regardless of security settings, and it is subject to the same legal treatment as other forms of EC.

Legal Ramifications

Legal ramifications for online violations of medical professionalism have been reported by many SMBs. Half of surveyed SMBs reported formal disciplinary hearings, and many reported issuance of consent orders with agreed sanctions or informal warnings. More than half of SMB respondents reported the occurrence of license restriction, suspension, or revocation related to online professionalism violations.

Educational

Academic Integrity

Health care professionals frequently employ EC and SM in the education of patients, colleagues, and trainees. These forms of communication do not preclude the employment of accepted academic principles of reliability and credibility. EC and SM are considered to be subjected to retrospective rather than prospective peer review. Therefore, it is necessary for health care professionals to be extremely mindful and respectful of copyrights and intellectual property when posting online. Content should be reviewed and monitored for academic reliability, and, whenever possible, references should be cited. A clear indication or disclaimer of whether posted information is based on scientific studies, expert consensus, professional or anecdotal experience, or personal opinion should accompany online content. Patients and trainees should be guided to peer-reviewed media or venues that are monitored for quality of disseminated information.

Health care professionals should be careful to represent credentials accurately and directly, and care should be taken to appropriately disclose potential conflicts of interest. Many SMBs have received reports of online violations of medical professionalism involving misrepresentation of credentials and failure to reveal conflicts of interest.

Oversight/Monitoring

Health care professionals have a duty to educate themselves as well as their trainees and ancillary staff regarding institutional policies relating to EC and SM. A content manager who is a permanent employee (not a trainee) should be designated to maintain and monitor posted content. Content managers should be proficient in the chosen platform and should monitor for violations in relation to professionalism, privacy, or academic integrity.

Health care professionals should monitor their own online presence and may consider using online reputation management services on a case-by-case basis.

Guiding Principles within Social Media and Electronic Communication

Guiding Principles

Health care professionals should be aware of institutional policies designed to guide EC and social networking behavior. If institutional policies do not exist, physicians and staff should work with their public relations, legal and privacy, information technology departments, and, if applicable, with their designated institutional officer (DIO) to develop institutional guidelines for health care professionals and ancillary staff. Many state medical associations offer guidelines for appropriate EC and SM practices as well.

Several national guidelines and policy statements from professional societies exist to direct health care provider use of EC and SM, including those from the American College of Physicians (ACP) and Federation of State Medical Boards (FSMB), the American Medical Association (AMA), American College of Emergency Physicians (ACEP), the Society for Academic Emergency Medicine (SAEM), and the Council of Residency Directors (CORD) in EM.

A summary of guiding principles for the use of EC and SM by health care physicians follows:

- Understand privacy settings and use them to the fullest extent to safeguard personal information on social networking sites. Consider separating personal and professional content.

- Routinely monitor personal and professional online presence to ensure that information is accurate, appropriate, and professional.
- Maintain boundaries of the patient–physician relationship and ensure patient privacy and confidentiality when interacting online.
- Be forthcoming about employment, credentials, and conflicts of interest.
- Posted information should be supported by current peer-reviewed literature whenever possible and should clearly indicate whether it is based on studies, consensus, experience, or personal opinion.
- Posted content may be available to anyone and may be misconstrued.
- Recognize that online behavior can negatively impact one's reputation among patients and colleagues, represents one's practice institution(s), and may have permanent consequences for medical careers.

Legal Ramifications

Patient confidentiality and privacy violations are typically enforced under specific legislation such as HIPAA. SMBs have the authority to discipline physicians for unprofessional behavior relating to inappropriate use of EC and SM. Disciplinary options range from a letter of reprimand to revocation of a board license. Such behaviors include:

- Inappropriate communication with patients online
- Use of the Internet for unprofessional behavior
- Online misrepresentation of credentials
- Online violations of patient confidentiality
- Failure to reveal conflicts of interest online
- Online derogatory remarks regarding a patient
- Online depiction of intoxication
- Discriminatory language or practices online

Summary

SM and EC are rapidly evolving tools in medicine and offer many benefits when used responsibly and judiciously. However, these are modalities that can engender significant ethical concerns, both in maintaining professionalism for a health care provider and in preserving the sanctity of the health worker–patient interaction. Professional guidelines have been developed to help safeguard the use of SM and EC in medicine. It is the responsibility of each and every health care provider to be aware of these overriding ethical guidelines and to operate within them.

ETHICS TAKEOUT TIPS

- Always assume all EC and SM postings are public and permanent.
- Use privacy settings liberally to limit others' access.
- Monitor and be aware of your online presence.
- Consider separating personal and professional content online.
- Maintain appropriate boundaries for patient interactions.
- There are many ever-changing modalities that have beneficial applications in medical careers, education, and patient care.

FOR FURTHER READING

Bahner, D. P., Adkins, E. Patel, N., Donley, C., Nagel, R., & Kman, N. E. (2012). How we use SM to supplement a novel curriculum in medical education. *Medical Teacher*, 34(6), 439–444.

Bernard, A. W., Kman, N. E., Bernard, R. H., Way, D. P., Khandelwal, S., & Gorgas, D. L. (2014). Use of a secure social media platform to facilitate reflection in a residency program. *Journal of Graduate Medical Education*, 6(2), 326–329.

Chretien, K. C., Farnan, J. M., Greysen, S. R., & Kind, T. (2011). To friend or not to friend? Social networking and faculty perceptions of online professionalism. *Academic Medicine*, 86, 1545–1550.

DeCamp, M., Koenig, T. W., & Chisholm, M. (2013). Social media and physicians online identity crisis. *Journal of the American Medical Association*, 310(6), 581–582.

Farnan, J. M., Snyder Sulmasy, L., Worster, B. K., Chaudhry, H. J., Rhyne, J. A., & Arora, V. M. (2013). Online medical professionalism Patient and public relationships Policy statement from the American College of Physicians and the Federation of State Medical Boards. *Annals of Internal Medicine*, 158(8), 620–627.

Greyson, S. R., Chretien, K. C., Kind, T., Young, A., & Gross, C. P. (2012). Physician violations of online professionalism and disciplinary actions: A national survey of State Medical Boards. *Journal of the American Medical Association*, 307(11), 1141–1142.

George, D. R., Rovniak, L. S., & Kraschnewski, J. L. (2013). Dangers and opportunities for social media in medicine. *Clinical Obstetrics and Gynecology*, 56(3), 453–462.

Hamm, M. P., Chisholm, A., Shulhan, J., Milne, A., Scott, S. D., Given, L. M., & Hartling, L. (2013, May 9). Social media use among patients and caregivers: A scoping review. *BMJ Open*, 3(5).

Modahl, M., Tompsett, L., & Moorhead, T. (2011). Doctors, patients & social media. www.quantiamd.com/q-qcp/DoctorsPatientSocialMedia.pdf

Nabi, R. L., Prestin, A., & So, J. (2013). Facebook friends with (health) benefits? Exploring social network site use and perceptions of social support, stress, and well-being. *Cyberpsychology Behavior and Social Networking*, 16(10), 721–727.

Pillow, M. T., Hopson, L., Bond, M., Cabrera, D., Patterson, L., Pearson, D., & Takenaka, K. (2014). Social media guidelines and best practices Recommendations from the Council of Residency Directors Social Media Task Force. *Western Journal of Emergency Medicine*, 15(1), 26–30.

Radecki, R. P., Rezaie, S. R., & Lin, M. (2014). Annals of Emergency Medicine Journal Club. Global Emergency Medicine Journal Club Social media responses to the November 2013 Annals of Emergency Medicine Journal Club. *Annals of Emergency Medicine*, 63(4), 490–494.

Schulman, C. I., Kuchkarian, F. M., Withum, K. F., Boecker, F. S., & Graygo, J. M. (2013). Influence of social networking websites on medical school and residency selection process. *Postgraduate Medical Journal*, 89, 126–130.

Schwaab (McGrath), J., Kman, N., Nagel, R., Bahner, D., Martin, D. R., Khandelwal, S., & Nelson, R. (2011). Using second life virtual simulation environment for mock oral emergency medicine examination. *Academic Emergency Medicine*, 18(5), 558–561.

Snyder, L. for the American College of Physicians Ethics, Professionalism, and Human Rights Committee. (2012). American College of Physicians Ethics Manual Sixth edition. *Annals of Internal Medicine*, 156, 73–104.

6

Multiculturalism and "Cultural Competency"

KELLY BOOKMAN, MD, FACEP

CASE

A young Asian mother brings her three-year-old son to the emergency department (ED) for evaluation of a fever and cough. The mother is quiet as you introduce yourself, and she maintains little eye contact. A family friend, who has accompanied the mother and son and who speaks very little English, says that "he is sick for long time." When you ask if they have given any medicine for the fever, the friend replies "yes, pills." Further history is limited.

ROS Fever and cough. No NVD.
PMH Immunizations UTD as reported by friend.
FH Noncontributory.
SH Lives at home with Mom, Dad, grandparents, and two younger brothers. Family arrived from Vietnam "a while ago." He does not attend school.
Meds/ALL Unknown.
PE
- Temp: VS: T – 100.1 F, HR – 90, BP – 100/70, R – 20, O2Sat 98% RA
- General: Alert male in NAD
- ENT: Mild rhinorrhea, MMM, TMs clear bilaterally, oropharynx erythematous without exudates, nonenlarged tonsils
- Neck: Supple, mild lymphadenopathy
- Cardiovascular: RRR, no M/G/R
- Lungs: CTA bilaterally
- Abdomen: Soft, + BS, NTND
- Extremities: No clubbing, cyanosis or edema

- Skin: *Multiple purpuric lesions on back in angular, descending pattern bilaterally encompassing entire back. No other rashes, petechiae, or bruising on extremities*
- Neuro: Alert and awake, motor/sensation grossly intact

SUPPORTING AND IMPROVING EFFECTIVE COMMUNICATION

What are the barriers to effective communication?

- The language barrier
- Certain cultural practices limit the effectiveness of a clinical interaction:
  – Asian culture emphasizes the avoidance of eye contact and politeness as a sign of compliance.

What can be done to promote better communication?

- Use interpreter services:
  – Do not use family or friends.
- Use a friendly tone, appropriate eye contact, and positive hand gestures to establish verbal and nonverbal trust and rapport.

How do you interpret the physical exam findings on the back?

- The lesions on the child's back are concerning for either intentional burns/rubs from child abuse or cultural practices such as coining, common in the Asian culture.

What would be your next appropriate step to take?

- Some physicians jump directly to child protective services in such cases. The proper procedure in this case would be to obtain a full historical account of the markings from both the parent and the child, separately if needed.

What could be done to facilitate mutual understanding?

- Ask the family for their opinions about what has caused this illness and how it is affecting them.
- Understand that many patients will not volunteer that they have sought alternative medical help for fear of offending a Western doctor or embarrassment.

CASE OUTCOME

With the aid of a trained interpreter, the provider is able to discern that the family arrived in the country 18 months ago and has visited a traditional Asian healer in their community who has practiced coining on the boy. (In coining, hot coins and warm oil are rubbed on the backs of the chronically ill to release the "bad wind.")

It is widely acknowledged that minorities receive worse health care and that individual providers often provide differential treatment that results in negative health outcomes. Many analyses over the years have shown that issues such as poor access to care, systematic misdiagnosis, variability in medication selection and dosing, patient absenteeism, and adherence problems are among the disparities in care. In 1978, Kleinman described that negative health consequences that result from ignoring culture lead to missed diagnoses due to lack of familiarity with the prevalence of conditions among certain cultural groups, failure to take into account differing responses to medication, lack of knowledge about traditional remedies leading to harmful drug interactions, and diagnostic errors resulting from miscommunication. The groups that tend to be affected the most by a lack of cultural awareness are at-risk groups (people with limited financial resources, the old, the young), ethnically and racially distinct groups, immigrants, migrants, refugees, gay men, lesbians, bisexuals, transgenders, and people with disabilities.

A landmark report in 2002 by the Institute of Medicine (IOM) entitled "Understanding and Eliminating Racial and Ethnic Disparities in Health Care" really brought this issue into the forefront by seeking to assess racial and ethnic differences in the quality of health care not related to access to care or ability to pay, to evaluate sources of disparities, and to provide recommendations to eliminate health care differences. The IOM committee found that racial and ethnic disparities in health care exist even when insurance status, income, age, and severity of conditions are comparable and that death rates from cancer, heart disease, and diabetes are significantly higher in racial and ethnic minorities than in whites. The paper declared that these disparities are unacceptable. The authors described that differences in health care occur in the context of broader historic and contemporary social and economic inequality and of persistent racial and ethnic discrimination. Furthermore, they said that bias, stereotyping, prejudice, and clinical uncertainty on the part of health care providers, health systems as a whole, patients, and health care plan managers are widespread.

The IOM put forth many recommendations including creating a "Patient's Bill of Rights" that should be accorded to publicly funded HMO enrollees, increasing the numbers of racial and ethnic minorities among U.S. health professionals, strengthening the Office of Civil Rights within the Department of Health and Human Services to evaluate civil rights violations, ensuring that clinical practices are uniform and based on the best available science, structuring payment systems to guarantee an adequate supply of services to minority patients and to limit provider incentives that may promote disparities, and providing financial incentives for practices that reduce barriers and encourage evidence-based decision-making. In addition, they recommended using language interpretation services, using community/nonmedical personnel to help patients navigate the health care system, and creating education programs for health professionals that integrate cross-cultural education, as well as promoting better patient education to increase patients' knowledge of how to best access care and participate in treatment decisions.

In 1996, the American College of Emergency Physicians (ACEP) and the Society of Academic Emergency Medicine (SAEM) both included "diversity" as a line item in their core content curriculum. A 2000 SAEM policy statement says that "SAEM encourages the development of didactic, educational, research, and other programs to assist academic emergency medicine departments to improve the diversity of their faculties and residencies." A Council of Emergency Medicine Residency Directors (CORD)/SAEM Diversity Task Force, also known as the Cultural Competency Curriculum Task Force (CCCTF) was created in 2003 with the primary objective to develop a curriculum to incorporate diversity awareness, cultural competency knowledge and skills, and to promote awareness and acceptance of differing cultures, as well as awareness about our own inherent biases toward those of different backgrounds. In 2008, the ACEP board of directors approved a cultural awareness policy that replaced its previous iteration that used the term "cultural competency." This policy asserts that cultural awareness is the ability of health care providers to understand and respond to the unique cultural needs brought by patients to the health care encounter. It further states that quality health care is based on not only scientific competence, but also on cultural awareness, and it describes the beliefs that cultural awareness should be a part of the training for all health care providers and that resources should be dedicated to assuring that all patients get their needs met regardless of their cultural background.

"Cultural competency" has become a popular approach to improving the provision of health care to minority groups with its goal of decreasing health disparities, and it has been consistently appearing in health care literature since the early 1990s. *Culture* is a pattern of learned beliefs, values, and behaviors that are shared within a group. It may include common language, communication styles, practices, customs, art, morals, educational class, laws, and views on roles, responses, and relationships. In essence, culture is the sum total of the way people live. *Multiculturalism* is the philosophy that several different cultures can coexist equitably. Cultural competency was originally conceived of as a way to help health care providers recognize the importance of understanding the impact of the history and culture of different minority populations on their health care outcomes. Guidelines have been created to aid providers in assessing cultural context and to promote awareness of and respect for cultural traditions without stereotyping individuals and making inappropriate assumptions about their beliefs. Approaches to cross-cultural training include not only gaining knowledge of specific cultural groups, but also developing general attitudes and skills. These general attributes include respecting the legitimacy of a patient's health beliefs and recognizing their role in effective health care delivery; shifting from viewing a patient's complaints as stemming from a disease occurring within their organ systems to viewing illness as occurring within a bio-psychosocial model; eliciting a patient's explanation of illness and its perceived causes; explaining the provider's understanding of illness and its etiology in layperson's language; and negotiating an understanding within which a safe, effective, and mutually agreed upon care plan can be established. Many models of cross-cultural communication and negotiation have been developed to assist health care providers in eliciting cultural information. Examples include the BELIEF and ETHNIC models and Kleinman's questions models (see Table 6.1). These models represent the critical skills needed to conduct a culturally successful patient interview.

It is important to recognize that both patients and providers bring cultural perspectives to each encounter. Inherently, physicians bring a "culture of medicine" to each patient interaction as well as their own personal cultural background. It is encouraged that providers engage in a process of self-reflection and critique, including considering those beliefs acquired through their medical training and even the power and privilege associated with their status as professionals. One can consider the term "cultural humility" as contrasted to "cultural competency" as a way to embrace this idea. Being humble in the face of diverse cultures as opposed

TABLE 6.1. *Various cultural belief systems*

- BELIEF
  - Beliefs about health (What caused your illness/problem?)
  - Explanation (Why did it happen at this time?)
  - Learn (Help me to understand your belief/opinion.)
  - Impact (How is this illness/problem impacting your life?)
  - Empathy (This must be very difficult for you.)
  - Feelings (How are you feeling about it?)

- ETHNIC
  - Explanation (How do you explain your illness?)
  - Treatment (What treatment have you tried?)
  - Healers (Have you sought any advice from folk healers?)
  - Negotiate (mutually acceptable options)
  - Intervention (agreed on)
  - Collaboration (with patient, family, healers)

- KLEINMAN'S QUESTIONS
  - What do you think caused your problem?
  - Why do you think it started when it did?
  - What do you think your sickness does to you?
  - How severe is your sickness? Will it have a long or short course?
  - What kind of treatment do you think you should receive?
  - What are the most important results you hope to receive from this treatment?
  - What are the chief problems your sickness has caused for you?
  - What do you fear most about your sickness?

to being competent in understanding other cultures reflects a paradigm shift from a provider-centric to a patient-centric approach. Cultural humility does not imply the mastery of beliefs and behaviors of others but rather the development of partnerships that focus on the similarities and differences between the provider's and the patient's values and priorities.

To try to address health care disparities in a universal way, the field of cultural competence has expanded to encompass not only specific provider–patient interactions but also to include health systems and communities. This is a direct and appropriate reaction to reports about minority health care disparities such as the IOM committee report described earlier. One outcome of this scope expansion has been incorporating broader issues into provider cross-cultural training, such as concepts of race and class and their impact on health care outcomes; the relevance of trust in provider–patient relationship; and historical reasons behind potential distrust – factors such as literacy and social support, as well as consideration of provider biases and prejudices. Disparities in health care are likely not only to be due to interpersonal barriers between providers and patients but also due to barriers between communities and health systems. Culturally competent systems have been described as valuing diversity, having the capacity for cultural self-assessment, being conscious of the dynamics inherent when cultures interact, having institutionalized cultural knowledge, and having developed adaptations to diversity. Recommendations that reflect systemic solutions include having providers and staff who are ethnically similar to the community, analyzing health quality measures stratified by race, and encouraging community participation in the design of health services.

The concept of "insurgent multiculturalism" further expands the concept of cultural competence by moving the focus away from studying nondominant groups and their culture to studying how unequal distributions of power allow some groups but not others to acquire and keep resources. These resources can be considered to include mainstream ritual perpetuation, national policies, and even hospital protocols. It has been suggested that studying multiculturalism should be an integral part of professional development. Using the dialectical presentation of opposing worldviews to highlight how these perspectives may operate in clinical situations allows the learner to see the issue in a multifaceted way. Thus, interactive, case-based sessions focused on clinical applications seem ideal for teaching multiculturalism or cultural competence. Good evidence based on systematic reviews suggests that cultural competence training improves the knowledge, skills, and attitudes of health care providers. However, it has not clearly been shown that this translates into improved health outcomes for ethnically diverse groups, and further research needs to focus on which training methods are most effective.

One issue that comes up is the question of whether respecting cultural diversity implies that all practices related to cultural beliefs must be respected and tolerated. Female genital mutilation represents an example of a ritual that brings out quite differing opinions based on cultural perspective. Multiculturalism describes multiple cultures living harmoniously. It implies that all cultural groups must be treated as equals, but it does not say that all cultural practices must be tolerated and respected. It would be unjust not to try to educate parents who may be exposing their children to health risks not borne by other children from the majority culture. Another example of beliefs that certain communities have and that might adversely effect medical treatment is the notion that bad magic (i.e. hexes, voodoo, witchcraft) causes illnesses (i.e. Ebola) as opposed to viruses or other scientifically held beliefs about etiology. This type of cultural belief may lead poor/uneducated individuals to avoid proven public health measures to control or eradicate contagious diseases. The skill needed here is to continue to recognize the impact of diverse cultures (both the provider's and the patient's) on perspectives of illness and disease and to come to the discussion with respect while trying to get to a mutual understanding of what the most patient-centered plan of care will be. It also becomes very important that providers are able to communicate the fallacy of certain nonscientific beliefs in a culturally respectful way so that fear of use of technology or other proven treatments can be alleviated. Ultimately, cultural sensitivity should never lead to unethical behavior; despite the challenges of ethical relativism as described by Macklin (1998) at the turn of the 21st century, modern multicultural society ought to be able to respect cultural diversity without having to accept every ritual or practice.

In addition to considering cultures that are well-integrated into Western communities such as Latino, Jewish, and African American, there are a number of examples of specific cultural contexts to which providers should be exposed during cultural education to help broaden the understanding of potentially unfamiliar community health practices. That said, it is very important to remember not to stereotype individuals when they present and to allow the awareness and knowledge of possible cultural differences to guide patient-centered interactions. There are many belief systems that are less commonly encountered but must be considered, such as Hmong, Navahoe, Arab, and Islander just to name a few. For instance, Arab communities are most often Muslim. In general, they do not hold superstitious beliefs about treatments but will turn first to family members or elders for advice that often include simple home remedies such as resting under heavy covers to keep warm, which is believed to bring rapid recovery from common childhood illnesses. Other remedies include drinking fluids to relieve abdominal pain, consuming sugar or citrus fruit to relieve sore throat, drinking boiled grain water to remove kidney stones, or burning of a body part to reduce sciatic/nerve pain. In this culture, sometimes amulets are worn to protect against illness or avoid harm. That said, members of this culture, with its emphasis on maintenance of good health, will not delay very long in seeking professional help. They usually bring a family member to an evaluation to help answer questions. Arab patients are typically very private, and the provider will need to establish trust in order to get all necessary information, especially if the discussion involves personal matters about sexual or mental health issues. Patients are often anxious to receive medications quickly, and they expect relief from pain and medication at the first visit. Regarding death, the belief is that it is the will of God. Family members will stay with the body until it can be removed from the hospital, and they prefer immediate burial.

The Hmong healing practices that include shamanistic healing as opposed to accepted Western interventions exemplify another specific instance of cultural "context." Differences include the idea that the *twix neeb* (Hmong healer) might visit a person's home for hours at a time, whereas Western physicians expect patients to come to the hospital and be seen for minutes at a time. In addition, *twix neebs* don't ask questions: they render an immediate diagnosis, they don't undress the patient or poke and prod the patient in private places, and they address the body and soul. In contrast, doctors are considered rude and ask intimate questions; they need labs, radiology studies, and sometimes days to render an opinion; they often disrobe the patient and may even perform a genital exam; and they never seem to mention the soul. When a patient fails to get better, for the Hmong, it is the "intransigence of the spirits," whereas in Western cultures, failure to heal is blamed on the science or on the failure of the healer herself.

In conclusion, the primary goal of teaching cultural competence is to promote quality and equity of health care for people of differing cultures. The goal is not to pretend to know or understand all the possible cultural practices but instead to develop awareness that culture, both the provider's and the patient's, has a dramatic impact on a provider's ability to deliver excellent health care. This education has predominantly been focused on improving care for disadvantaged minorities but can be broadened to encompass a patient-centered focus for all. Having providers come to all interactions with self-awareness and a respectful attitude toward diverse points of view should naturally create an overall more equitable distribution of health care resources.

ETHICS TAKEOUT TIPS

- Minorities receive worse health care, and individual providers often provide differential treatment resulting in negative health outcomes.
- Culture is a pattern of learned beliefs, values, and behaviors that are shared within a group.
- Remember that both patients and providers bring cultural perspectives to each encounter.
- Multiculturalism is the philosophy that several different cultures can coexist equitably.
- "Cultural competency" is a way to help health care providers recognize the importance of understanding the impact of the history

and culture of different minority populations on their health care outcomes.

- Respect the legitimacy of a patient's health beliefs.
- Elicit the patient's explanation of illness and its perceived causes.
- Explain the provider's understanding of illness and its etiology in layperson's language.
- Negotiate an understanding within which a safe, effective, and mutually agreed upon care plan can be established.

FOR FURTHER READING

Beach, M., Price, E. G., Gary, T. L., Robinson, K. A., Gozu, A., Palacio, A., & Cooper, L. A. (2005). Cultural competency: A systematic review of health care provider educational interventions. *Medical Care*, 43(4), 356–373.

Betancourt, J. (2004). Cultural competence-marginal or mainstream movement? *New England Journal of Medicine*, 351(10), 953–955.

Boylan, M. (2004). Culture and medical intervention. *Journal of Clinical Ethics*, 15(2), 188–200.

The Cross Cultural Health Care Program. www.xculture.org

Fadiman, A. (1997). *The spirit catches you and you fall down.* New York: Farrar, Strauss and Giroux.

Gregg, J., & Saha, S. (2006). Losing culture on the way to competence: The use and misuse of culture in medical education. *Academic Medicine*, 81(6), 542–547.

Heron, S., Stettner, E., & Haley, L. Racial and ethnic disparities in the emergency department: A public health perspective. *Emergency Medicine Clinics of North America*, 24, 905–923. www.med-ed.virginia.edu/courses/culture/index.cfm

Hobgood, C., Bowen, J., Sawning, S., & Savage, K. Educating students and residents to provide culturally competent care: A review of models, educational methods. www.med-ed.virginia.edu/courses/culture/index.cfm

Hunt, L. (2001). Beyond cultural competence: Applying humility to clinical settings. *Park Ridge Center Bulletin*, 2001(24), 3–4.

Kleinman, A., Eisenenberg, L., & Good, B. (1978). Culture, illness and care: Clinical lessons from anthropologic and cross-cultural research. *Annals of Internal Medicine*, 88(2), 251–258.

Macklin, R. (1998). Ethical relativism in a multicultural society. *Kennedy Institute of Ethics Journal*, 8(1), 1–22.

Ramalanjoaona, G., & Martin, M. EM faculty caring for multicultural patients. www.med-ed.virginia.edu/courses/culture/index.cfm

Scott, C., Martin, M., & Hamilton, G. (2003). Training of medical professionals and the delivery of health care as related to cultural identity groups. *Academic Emergency Medicine*, 10(11), 1149–1152.

Saha, S., Beach, M., & Cooper, L. (2008). Patient centeredness, cultural competence and healthcare quality. *Journal of the National Medical Association*, 100(11), 1275–1285.

Taylor, J. (2003). Confronting "culture" in medicine's "culture of no culture." *Academic Medicine*, 78, 555–559.

Truong, M., Paradies, Y., & Priest, N. (2014). Interventions to improve cultural competency in healthcare: A systematic review of reviews. *BMC Health Services Research*, 14, 99.

Wear, D. (2003). Insurgent multiculturalism: Rethinking how and why we teach culture in medical education. *Academic Medicine*, 78, 549–554.

7

Informed Consent

LESLIE R. VOJTA, MD, AND JAMES E. BROWN, MD, MMM

Informed consent is an ethical concept that emerged from legal doctrine and case law in 1957 but quickly captured the attention of the medical community. Rooted in patient autonomy, it gives each patient the authority to make decisions about what he will do with his own body. It legally protects patients from battery by medical providers. But perhaps its greatest value is to catapult patients into a more active role in making decisions about their health care, a role shared with their physicians. It means that a medical provider has discussed the indications, risks, and benefits of a procedure or course of therapy with a patient or his medical decision-maker. It requires that a patient has the capacity to make a decision given adequate information to make an informed decision and can freely communicate his choice after duly considering his options without coercion from the medical team or other parties. It holds a resonate level of responsibility for the participants in the physician–patient relationship, whereby the physician educates the patient (or his surrogate decision-maker) relevant to his medical condition, and the patient synthesizes this information to have the final say in choosing a treatment plan that aligns with his own values and goals.

Accomplishing this requires medical providers to spend time with patients to ensure that they fully understand their medical conditions and the possible treatment options. It also requires that providers discuss the expected outcomes and complications of different treatment options. This is a lofty goal when providing emergency medical care. In some circumstances, informed consent is not possible in the emergency setting. This has led some to erroneously believe that informed consent is not required in the emergency department (ED). To the contrary, informed consent is an essential element of emergency care when the patient is able to participate in the informed consent process.

Informed consent refers to a process, not merely a signature on a document. Furthermore, it is important to note that the majority of patients who present to the ED do not have truly emergent conditions. Most conditions are urgent or semi-urgent. In most situations, there is time to properly obtain informed consent for a proposed treatment plan before beginning the treatment.

EMERGENCY EXCEPTION TO INFORMED CONSENT

There are three proposed criteria (created by Dr. Heather Gert) that would make a situation an emergency: there must be an expectation of serious harm, there must be an expectation that someone can act to reduce that harm, and there must be a time-critical condition. If a patient's condition does not satisfy all three of these criteria, then it is not a true emergency, and informed consent should be obtained from the patient or his surrogate decision-maker.

The "emergency exception" to informed consent applies in true emergencies. Physicians should act according to the "reasonable patient" doctrine and presume that any person in that situation would consent to treatment to preserve their life or health if he or she were able to do so and if there were sufficient time to obtain that consent. For example, an unresponsive patient needs emergent interventions – intubations, central venous catheters, and diagnostic testing. There is no way to discuss options with this patient. Emergency medical providers may justifiably fear that this patient's unprotected airway is at high risk for aspiration and that, without immediate intubation, she will die. Emergency physicians presume that she would want action taken to preserve her life. If she were coherent on initial evaluation, one may feel compelled to ask her for permission ahead of performing the invasive procedure. Is this consent? No, not unless we take the time to discuss treatment options and the risks of all options. If she nods her head to our query, is this assent or implicit agreement? Yes, and communicating with the patient, even in limited circumstances, is valuable in allowing the patient to participate in medical decision-making. Likewise, it should be noted that any presumption that the patient would consent to treatment can be defeated by clear evidence to the contrary, such as a valid advance directive (AD) or Do Not Resuscitate/ Physicians Orders Life-Sustaining Treatment (DNR/POLST) form. The rationale is based on the assumption that the patient had decisional capacity when her AD was formalized. Any subsequent reversal of an explicit refusal of treatment would require a large burden of new proof.

By design, ADs are considered the capacitated patient's answer to what should be done in the event that she is incapacitated. Therefore, overturning a patient's wish to forgo resuscitation is disrespectful and inconsiderate and should be avoided.

INFORMED CONSENT IN EMERGENCY MEDICINE

An essential portion of the informed consent process is that a patient must have the mental capacity or competence to make the proposed medical decision. The term "competence" is determined by a legal authority to determine if an individual can make his own decisions. Physicians determine if a patient has decision-making capacity rather than if he is legally competent to make the decision.

Most patient encounters begin with the assumption that patient does have the decision-making capacity to express his wishes in health care. There are a few situations in which a patient is deemed not to have decision-making capacity. These can be straightforward judgments at times, as when a patient has limited mental capacity or an altered mental status (from a medical condition or from substance use), is being evaluated for mental health concerns, or has not reached the age of majority. Threats to decisional capacity may include any condition that impairs a patient's ability to understand and deliberate over his alternatives. Impaired cognition can be acutely precipitated by substances and situational factors such as medications, illicit drugs, alcohol, delirium, trauma, pain, or anxiety.

DETERMINATION OF DECISIONAL CAPACITY

Decisional capacity refers to the ability to make an authentic choice. Decisional capacity incorporates cognitive and affective functions. Appropriate decisional capacity requires the following elements:

1. The ability to receive information
2. The ability to process and understand information
3. The ability to deliberate
4. The ability to make and articulate a choice

Decisional capacity should be assessed for all ED patients, although a formal process may not be necessary for patients who are alert and of sound mind. Frequently, decisional capacity can be assessed during routine interactions with the patient who is alert and demonstrates appropriate speech and judgment. In many cases, however, the determination of adequate decisional capacity requires additional steps.

Decisional capacity may not be consistent over time, as the patient's mental status, psychological status, or environmental factors may change. Decisional capacity is a dynamic attribute and is also task-specific. Decisional capacity may be recognized as a spectrum of ability depending on the particular health care decision. An individualized assessment of capacity must be done for each patient. Standardized tests may be valuable in the determination of capacity when capacity is unclear. The Mini-Mental Status Examination is an example of a test easily administered in the ED. Another available evaluation is the formulation by the President's Commission for the Study of Ethical Problems in Medicine and Biomedical and Behavioral Research.

Numerous conditions and circumstances may present a threat to decisional capacity, some of which are reversible. Some examples of clinical conditions that may result in impaired capacity include dementia, intoxication, psychiatric conditions, language impairment, cultural issues, physical communication impairments, severe pain, organic disease states, and numerous other conditions. Reversible etiologies of impaired capacity should be addressed if possible. Even in cases of some impaired capacity, patients may demonstrate sufficient understanding of the decision to make an appropriate informed choice.

DISCLOSURE OF INFORMATION

Informed consent requires the provider to disclose the proposed intervention and expected risks and benefits. This discussion should include the most likely risks, as well as the most severe, even though they might be unlikely to occur. This can be as simple as itching after administration of intravenous morphine or pain at the site of venipuncture. It can also be a more complex discussion, such as when obtaining consent before performing a lumbar puncture: although the most likely risk is a severe postdural puncture headache, a patient will likely want to know the risks of nerve injury or meningitis because these are severe and feared complications. It should include precautions that will be taken to mitigate the risks of the procedure. For most procedures, this will include minimizing pain with analgesics or equipment adjuncts and patient positioning, as well as reducing the potential for postprocedural infection through employing sterile technique and potentially limiting the number of procedural attempts.

A provider should also delineate the consequences of refusing to consent to the proposed intervention. While some may erroneously paint a picture of gloom and doom, an objective discussion of the expected consequences is warranted. A patient deserves to understand the reasonable alternatives for refusing a procedure, even when it is harder on the medical staff. If a patient refuses intravenous fluid hydration, for example, he can be offered oral rehydration. Although possibly slower and perhaps more difficult to track, this may be a safe and reasonable alternative that may be preferred by some patients.

DISCLOSURE OF TRAINING STATUS

Disclosure of a provider's level of experience or training may be controversial. Many patients lack an understanding of the hierarchy among health care providers and the differences in the levels of training between professional groups caring for them during their ED visit. A study published in 2010 by Larkin and Hooker compared patients' willingness to see mid-level providers or residents and provided detailed explanations of the level of training for each defined category (nurse practitioner, physician assistant, resident). For a serious injury or complaint (defined as chest pain or accidental amputation), less than 1 percent of patients surveyed were willing to see a mid-level provider. For the same situation, only 22.7 percent of patients were willing to be treated by a resident.

Patients in the ED have a reasonable expectation to know who provides their care. As discussed earlier, patients with perceived emergencies give implied consent to an evaluation and physical examination in the ED. By presenting in an emergency setting, the patient does not have the expectation of being evaluated by his primary provider. All members of the health care team should wear photo identification that includes credentials, and each member should introduce him- or herself to the patient, including his or her role in health care.

> *Case: A forty-two-year-old woman presents to the ED with a headache and fever. She appears ill, and you suspect bacterial meningitis. You recommend a lumbar puncture to evaluate her cerebrospinal fluid for infection. She asks "how many of these have you done?"*

This case demonstrates an important issue regarding disclosure of expertise and experience. Should a resident disclose his actual experience with the proposed procedure, as the case may be, or identify his lack of experience for patient consideration? Most experts agree that a provider does not need to inform the patient that this is his first lumbar puncture. However, he should be ready to discuss his practice experience if asked. It is permissible for a resident to discuss his relevant experience and to specify the level of supervision that will be present during the procedure to reassure the patient.

DOCUMENTATION OF INFORMED CONSENT

Some ethicists assert that every patient who voluntarily presents to the ED for evaluation implicitly consents to minimally invasive monitoring and testing aimed at diagnosing the emergency condition that occasioned their ED visit. Because venipuncture and laboratory analysis fit into this category, providers typically interpret patient cooperation with interventions as implied consent. However, consent for treatment does not automatically confer specific consent for venipuncture, administration of medications, laboratory and radiologic evaluations, or disposition decisions.

Case: A twenty-five-year-old man presents to the ED with his wife. They report that he has a new penile lesion that is non-tender. They noticed the lesion that day. They both deny a history of sexually transmitted infections. They have been married for four years and deny marital infidelity. When suggested that the lesion could be a genital wart due to the human papillomavirus, the wife becomes irate and insists that it is from "something else." The patient refuses any further testing for possible sexually transmitted infections.

Common sense argues that all providers should inform their patients when ordering tests and what is expected with the results from those tests. If the tests ordered could give a socially incendiary result, such as a new diagnosis of sexually transmitted infection, HIV, or the like, the patient should be informed. Hospitals vary regarding requirements for HIV screening, but some require a signed consent form beforehand. The social stigma of HIV is unique, but the bystander ramifications (spouse) and public health reportability can be extrapolated to other sexually transmitted infections. Although it is rarely necessary to obtain written consent for laboratory evaluations, a patient should be informed that he or she will be tested for sexually transmitted infections and, in turn, that a positive test will require a report to the local health department with notifications to any sexual partners determined to be at risk.

Recently, there have been increased discussions in the medical literature about overuse of radiologic testing and the long-term ramifications to patients. Risks of radiographics may include radiation exposure and/or the risks of administration of intravenous contrast. Most departments routinely obtain informed consent from pregnant women undergoing radiologic imaging procedures but do not have a required conversation with other patients. Some have argued that because computed tomography (CT) scans are becoming ubiquitous, the cumulative dangers of radiation and the immediate effects of the intravenous contrast on kidney function should be disclosed to patients for their informed consent prior to performing the imaging.

VULNERABLE POPULATIONS

Pediatric Patients

Laws in individual states vary, but most recognize emancipated and mature minors. An emancipated minor typically includes patients who are married, in the military, or living independently. Many states recognize a minor's right to consent to issues related to reproductive health (pregnancy, sexually transmitted diseases), mental health, substance abuse treatment, or when she is a parent providing consent for her child. In all circumstances, the pediatric patient should be respected as an autonomous agent when possible and should be included in the informed consent process with parents.

What should be done when parents refuse to give consent for a medically necessary procedure for their child? Every attempt should be made to understand the perspective of the parents and to involve both the parents and mature minor, if possible, in the decision. If parents or guardians refuse a life-saving intervention, the physician should seek a court order to treat the pediatric patient appropriately.

Prisoners

Case: A man is brought to the ED by the local police. They report that he was arrested for possession of illegal drugs. They assert that he swallowed a plastic bag filled with suspected drugs. The police request a cavity search for the object. The patient refuses any further examinations or procedures. He denies that he swallowed anything and denies that he uses or is involved with drugs.

Prisoners represent a specific vulnerable population. Special attention should be made to advocate for patient autonomy when appropriate. In most cases, we presume implied consent for basic physical examinations because a patient has voluntarily presented to the ED. Prisoners in the custody of law enforcement are not free to navigate any potential treatment options. Assuming this patient has capacity to refuse bodily invasion, his wishes should be honored. A physician should tread carefully when attempting to facilitate law enforcement-guided examinations. Physicians have each pledged to *do no harm*, and this applies to every patient seen, regardless of their legal circumstances. It is not uncommon for law enforcement personnel to ask the emergency provider to perform a certain examination to ensure that a patient is safe to go to prison. A provider should always provide the appropriate medical screening to exclude an emergency medical condition, but is not required to act unless a life-threatening situation is uncovered or evolves while the patient is in the ED. Interventions that are not medically indicated are tantamount to harming patients, and providers should refuse to cross any such line.

Mental Illness

Case: A man is brought to the ED by his sister for evaluation of mental health problems. He has a history of schizophrenia and has been hospitalized in the past. She suspects that he has stopped taking his medication. He insists that he does not need medication anymore because he "feels great." When approached about repeat hospitalization, he becomes agitated and paces around the examination room. He begins yelling at his provider and his sister. You call for help and a nurse offers to medicate the patient for you.

This case begs the question, is it appropriate to medicate a patient without his consent? Most emergency providers can relate to this scenario. Each likely has his own preferred method of administering medications to the acutely agitated and possibly dangerous patient. It is easy to rationalize administering intramuscular sedating medication in a dangerous patient.

Impaired Decisional Capacity

Case: A sixty-five-year-old man with metastatic cancer is brought to the ED from his skilled nursing facility for altered mental status. During his initial evaluation, he becomes pulseless. He has a Do Not Resuscitate order on his chart that was signed by him and his wife. His wife becomes distraught and asks you to start chest compressions on her husband.

By signing a DNR order, the patient or his next of kin has given informed consent *not* to perform procedures – namely chest compressions, airway management, or other invasive life-sustaining interventions. How should the emergency provider navigate a conflict between a patient's wishes and a family member who wants to reverse his or her previous decisions? The patient's wishes should be honored, regardless of the patient's ability to express them at that time. If family members disagree, it is important to discuss the patient's wishes, rather than family wishes.

Procedures on the Newly Deceased

After the pronouncement of death in the ED, some instructors recommend that their trainees practice procedures on the deceased's body. This can range from diagnostic laryngoscopy to invasive procedures such as central venous catheter placement or thoracotomies. Although this practice is perhaps less common than in years past, the ethical considerations have not changed. It is not appropriate to perform procedures on a patient who has been declared dead without the express permission of the next of kin. While a resuscitation is ongoing, it is acceptable to perform procedures that could contribute to a better outcome, such as intubation, central venous access, pericardiocentesis, or resuscitative thoracotomies in the appropriate clinical circumstances. When the prognosis is poor during a resuscitation, it is not acceptable to escalate care that is not expected to succeed solely for educational purposes.

Some advocates of this practice have argued that patients who present to a training facility are giving consent for teaching-related activities. This argument is flawed because it suggests that a patient was informed of the training affiliation of a hospital before presenting at that particular medical facility. It also suggests that performing invasive procedures on newly dead patients is a standard practice at all teaching facilities. Using the bodies of deceased patients' for education is not an avant garde practice, but the newness of the death makes unconsented procedures on it seem disrespectful and more akin to bodily harm than anything else (including deceased donation pathways that still must also be primed with informed consent by the surviving family). It is now recognized that there needs to be a discussion of intent and consent given before proceeding.

In 2005, researchers in Brooklyn and Oslo surveyed patents and family members to determine if, hypothetically, they could anticipate granting permission to perform procedures on their newly deceased relatives. Nearly half of the survey respondents said that, hypothetically, they would give permission to perform procedures on their newly dead infant or child. Most respondents felt that it was acceptable to perform procedures on the newly dead if the family gives consent. The literature has demonstrated that many families are willing to consent to invasive procedures in their newly deceased loved one. It reminds providers to simply ask for permission before using this training opportunity.

CONCLUSION

The principle of informed consent is essential to the practice of emergency medicine. Practicing informed consent in the emergency setting can be challenging. One must first determine if an emergency exists. Applying Dr. Gert's criteria, there must be a time-critical condition that could create serious harm and the ability to reduce harm if emergent action is taken. If there is no emergent condition, providers must determine if a patient has the capacity to consent. Then, a provider must provide essential information about the proposed intervention and ensure that the patient understands the proposed treatments, risks, and benefits of agreeing to or refusing the treatment and likely outcome. Finally, the emergency provider must recognize the intricate relationships between patients and family members and the high level of stress to all of these when faced with emergencies. understanding that informed consent is a process demonstrates that physicians respect their patients enough to give them the final say in their health care decisions. Informed consent improves the physician–patient relationship and ensures active participation in medical decision-making.

ETHICS TAKEOUT TIPS

- Informed consent is a process designed to respect patient autonomy. It is not simply legal paperwork.
- Patients must have decision-making capacity before they can participate meaningfully in their own medical decision-making.
- Some special populations are not able to give informed consent – minors, intoxicated patients, acute mental health emergencies. These patients can still be included in medical care decisions.
- The emergency physician's duty is to fully explain the proposed intervention, risks and benefits, and alternatives.

- Providers in training should be prepared to discuss their experience and level of supervision with a patient, if asked.
- Procedures should not be performed on the newly dead without permission from the next of kin.

FOR FURTHER READING

Derse, A. R. (2005). What part of "no" don't you understand? *Mount Sinai Journal of Medicine, 72*(4), 221–227.

Easton, R. B., Graber, M. A., Monnahan, J., & Hughes, J. (2007). Defining the scope of implied consent in the emergency department. *American Journal of Bioethics, 7*(12), 35–38.

Gert, H. J. (2005). How are emergencies different from other medical situations? *Mount Sinai Journal of Medicine, 72*(4), 216–221.

Hartman, K. M., & Liang, B. A. (1999). Exceptions to informed consent in emergency medicine. *Hospital Physician, 35*, 53–59.

Jones, J. W., & McCullough, L. B. (2011). Ethics of rehearsing procedures on a corpse. *Journal of Vascular Surgery, 54*(3), 879–880.

Larkin, G. L., & Hooker, R. S. (2010). Patient willingness to be seen by physician assistants, nurse practitioners, and residents in the emergency department: Does the presumption of assent have an empirical basis? *American Journal of Bioethics, 10*(8), 1–10.

Lewin, M. R., Montauk, L., Shalit, M., & Nobay, F. (2006). An unusual case of subterfuge in the emergency department: Covert administration of antipsychotic and anxiolytic medications to control an agitated patient. *Annals of Emergency Medicine, 47*, 75–78.

Morag, R. M., DeSouza, S., Steen, P. A., Salem, A., Harris, M., Ohnstad, O., & Brenner, B. E. (2005). Performing procedures on the newly deceased for teaching purposes: what if we were to ask? *Archives of Internal Medicine, 165*(1), 92–96.

Moskop, J. C. (2006). Informed consent and refusal of treatment: Challenges for emergency physicians. *Emergency Medicine Clinics of North America, 24*, 605–618.

Sirbaugh, P. E., & Diekema, D. S. (2011). Policy statement – Consent for emergency services for children and adolescents. *Pediatrics, 128*(2), 427–433.

Veatch, R. M. (2007). Implied, presumed and waived consent: The relative moral wrongs of under- and over-informing. *American Journal of Bioethics, 7*(12), 39–54.

Zuraw, J. M. (2010). Doctors, patients, and the ED: The resident's role. *American Journal of Bioethics, 10*(8), 17–18.

Zutlevics, T. L, & Henning, P. H. (2005). Obligation of clinicians to treat unwilling children and young people: An ethical discussion. *Journal of Pediatric Child Health, 41*, 677–681.

8

Against Medical Advice, Refusal of Care, and Informed Consent

JEREMY R. SIMON, MD, PHD, FACEP

Patients who refuse to accept their physicians' advice and ask to leave the emergency department (ED) against medical advice (AMA) create difficult, challenging situations for their physicians, both ethically and emotionally – ethically, because physicians in this situation may feel unable to fulfill their duty to care for their patient, and emotionally, because the request to leave AMA may be rooted in conflicts between the patient and physician, may cause conflicts (within the care team and with the patient), and may cause physicians to question their professional role and ability. Leaving AMA is also potentially problematic for the patient. Those who leave the hospital AMA have a significantly increased risk of ED visits and readmission to the hospital within thirty days.

Such potentially troubling encounters with patients are not uncommon. One study estimates that 2.7 percent of ED patients leave AMA, which is comparable to the numbers found for hospital inpatients, which range up to 2 percent. However, significant as these numbers are, they mask the problem's true extent. Patients who leave AMA are only a subcategory – albeit an extreme one – of the much wider phenomenon of patients who refuse at least some of the care their doctors recommend. Thus, to understand the ethics of AMA, we must understand the ethics of refusal of care.

INFORMED CONSENT

Background

The right to refuse care is simply the flip side of the requirement that patients provide informed consent to care. Beginning with the Schloendorff case and continuing with the Salgo case, U.S. law has recognized that patients have the right to decide what is done to their bodies and to have relevant information when making these decisions. What is the underlying rationale for thus respecting patients' decisions?

There are two presumptions that give rise to this approach. The first is that medicine's goal is to maximize the patient's good, and, in general, when there is any question in the matter, the patient is the one best suited to judge how to do this. Second, one of the four principles of bioethics is respect for patient autonomy. Allowing patients to decide how their medical care will proceed is one of the primary ways we can respect this autonomy. Furthermore, this respect for patients' right to make autonomous decisions outweighs our desire and obligation to help patients and protect them from harm. Therefore, with exceptions to be noted later, without informed consent, we cannot treat patients regardless of the consequences.

What Is Informed Consent?

If consent is ethically mandatory, information is equally so. One cannot reasonably make a decision without the relevant information that bears on it. In the medical situation, the following information is generally considered relevant:

1. *Diagnosis.* What does the team believe is going on?
2. *Nature and purpose of proposed treatment.* What does the team recommend and why? Why is it better than the alternatives?
3. *Risks and consequences of this plan.* What downsides should the patient be aware of?
4. *Probability of success.* If the patient follows the team's recommendations, how likely is the plan to achieve it goals?
5. *Feasible alternatives.* If any, even if they are not team's first choice of treatment.
6. *Prognosis otherwise.* What does the team believe will happen if the patient does not take their advice, and how likely is this outcome?

Each of these six points can be communicated in varying degrees of detail, from cryptic half-sentences to hour-long lectures. Clearly, the former is inappropriate because it would communicate very little information to the patient, but what of the latter? Are we required to convey to the patient all of the detail a professional in the field might be interested in?

American courts have adopted two different standards in deciding how much information a patient must receive. Initially, they adopted the "professional standard," which requires physicians to disclose what other physicians would disclose in similar circumstances. This is a provider-centered standard. More recently, others courts have adopted the patient-centered "reasonable person standard," which asks what information a reasonable person would feel he or she needs to make a good decision in the situation at hand. Although somewhat subjective and vague, this standard usually provides adequate guidance. Thus, the molecular biology or mechanism of action of a given therapy is unlikely to be relevant to an informed decision about the therapy, but a clear understanding of exactly what is entailed in undergoing the therapy and how long it will last is (e.g. will the antibiotics being recommended be one pill a day for 3 days or intravenous via a PICC line twice a day for 6 weeks?). An important corollary of this standard is that the information must be presented in a manner the patient can understand. In particular, there should be no medical jargon, and a translator should be used when appropriate. Furthermore, although the reasonable person standard is based on a generic person, the information provided to the patient should also be sensitive to the needs of the particular patient. Although the legal standard in the United States is still not unequivocal, from an ethical perspective, it is most appropriate to adopt the patient's perspective in providing information. This best allows us to facilitate the patient's own decision-making, which is the purpose of the informed consent process. Such disclosure should also likely meet either legal standard. It is also important that the information be accurate. Facts should not be underplayed or exaggerated to influence a patient's decision.

Another important feature of informed consent is that it must be voluntary; that is, free from coercion. In the ED, such coercion is frequently the result of other parties, such as family members who are present and pressuring the patient to make a particular decision. If there is any concern that this is happening, efforts must be made to remove or reduce this coercion, at the least by talking to the patient alone. Of course, physicians should be careful not to exert their own coercion either.

Obtaining informed consent prior to performing any invasive procedures accomplishes two purposes. Most importantly, it assures that we are not violating patients' ethical right to determine what happens to their bodies. It also provides certain legal protection to the physician. Without consent, any touching of another person, let alone cutting with a scalpel or stabbing with a needle, is battery, for which the physician can be held criminally and civilly liable. Obtaining consent from a patient before performing a procedure eliminates this problem.

Exceptions

Although obtaining informed consent before beginning treatment is a fundamental ethical principle of medical practice, there are several exceptions to at
least part of the process just described. The one most commonly encountered
in the ED is "implicit consent." Formal written consent is often not obtained,
or even explicitly discussed, for many of the minor, routine encounters in the
ED, such as physical exam, phlebotomy, or IV placement, even though,
technically, patients must consent to even these minor invasions of their
bodies. The reason we are allowed to do this is that by not objecting to the
exam, by extending an arm for an IV catheter, the patient implicitly consents
to the exam or needle. If the patient does object to the exam or needle, we
would not be allowed to proceed. We can rely on implicit consent in these
cases only because the risks are so low or so minor that they are likely evident
to the patient, and the procedures are so commonplace in the ED that we
assume patients who present to the ED expect to undergo them.

Emergencies create a second exception to the need to obtain consent. If,
due to the emergent need for an intervention, there is no time to obtain
consent, treatment can and should proceed under the concept of presumed
consent. In the absence of evidence to the contrary (such as a documented
"do not intubate" request), we presume that the patient would want the
necessary treatment. We do not allow obtaining consent to endanger the
patient. On the other hand, it is important to realize that this only applies to
true emergencies. Most situations in the ED, even many involving significant procedures such as a chest tube for a large simple pneumothorax, do
not fit this definition of emergency. If the procedure or treatment can be
safely delayed for even a few minutes, the patient must give informed
consent before treatment continues.

A third category of exceptions to informed consent are public health
emergencies, such as epidemics. In such cases, patients may be quarantined
or treated against their will. The determination of such an emergency,
however, will not be up to the emergency physician, and, certainly, the
physician should explain to the patient why she is being treated against her
will, and, if necessary, enlist the appropriate public health authorities
before personally enforcing care.

CAPACITY

The requirement to obtain informed consent is grounded, as we saw, in the
presumptions that patients can best decide what is good for them and that

there is value in respecting their autonomy. Occasionally, however, we will encounter patients who do not appear to be able to make independent decisions as to their own good. That is, they appear to lack the capacity to make their own decisions.

As we shall see later, if a patient lacks decision-making capacity, in certain circumstances we ignore their wishes and make treatment decisions on other bases. Therefore, when the care of a patient has reached the point where a decision is needed, be it regarding an invasive procedure or admission to the hospital, it is important to know whether the patient has the capacity to make this decision.

In most cases, the question does not arise because there is little doubt as to whether or not the patient has capacity. The severely demented patient clearly lacks it, and we presume that the calm, well-groomed professional who consents to an appendectomy has capacity. However, there are cases when a patient's decision-making capacity is questionable, and we must therefore understand how to determine whether this capacity is present.

The President's Commission states that decision-making capacity consists of three attributes: (1) having a set of values and goals, (2) being able to communicate and to understand information, and (3) being able to rationally deliberate about one's choice. These attributes capture the two presumptions behind informed consent. First, it is impossible to choose what is best for oneself without having values and goals by which to measure potential outcomes, without understanding the relevant information, and without being able to process that information rationally such that one's decision will indeed move one toward one's goals. Second, one way to understand autonomy is simply as the possession of one's own goals and the ability work toward them.

Determining Capacity

To determine whether a patient has capacity, however, we need more than a set of abstract attributes. We need a procedure for determining whether a patient has these attributes. Ultimately, capacity can only be determined through attentive conversation with the patient. Such a conversation can be divided into three sections. First, we give the patient all relevant information, as discussed earlier. Second, we assess the patient's understanding by asking her to repeat what we have told her. To avoid sounding patronizing, we can truthfully present the repetition as means of making sure that we were clear. Finally, after the patient makes her choice, we ask her to explain it. This allows us to assess whether the patient has a set of goals and can rationally pursue them with the information provided.

This procedure allows us to check for the presence of all three elements of decision-making capacity described by the President's Commission. However, it focuses on the process by which the patient makes a decision. Does the decision itself matter? That is, does the fact that a patient agrees or disagrees with us affect our determination of whether he has capacity? And do the potential consequences of the decision matter?

Some authors argue that none of this matters. They say that while a patient's disagreeing with a physician may prompt the question whether the presumption of capacity with which we approach all patients is valid in this case, once we decide to assess capacity, the patient's ability to *make* the decision in question is all that matters. The physician's assessment of the risks involved or the appropriate course of action is not relevant to whether or not the patient has capacity.

Most commentators, however, believe that the risk involved in the decision the patient makes, based on both the potential consequences of the decision as well as whether she is accepting the physicians' recommendation, is indeed relevant in determining whether the patient has capacity. Patients who are considering a risky procedure or are refusing care (and thus taking on greater risk than otherwise) are held to a higher standard for demonstrating capacity than those who are undertaking less risk. What this means in practice is that we may require evidence of clearer understanding of risks and a more coherent rationale for the decision being made when the stakes are high. The principle underlying this "sliding-scale" approach to capacity is that we must balance our respect for autonomy against our obligation to protect from harm. In general, respect for autonomy trumps protecting the patient, but this is not absolute. The more impaired the patient's decision-making capacity, and hence his autonomy, the less value there is in respecting it. The greater the risk the patient is exposed to by his decision, the more value there is in protecting him from the consequences of his decision. Thus, both the patient's ability to make a reasonable decision and the risk to which he is exposed must be considered in deciding whether to accept a patient's decision.

It is important to distinguish between the sliding-scale approach to capacity and the context specificity of decision-making capacity. Even those who reject the sliding-scale approach agree that capacity assessments are question-specific. A patient may have the understanding and reasoning ability to make a simple decision, such as whether to have a superficial abscess drained, but not be able to comprehend and process all of the information involved in a more complex decision, such as whether to undergo surgery for a large but unruptured abdominal aortic aneurysm.

In addition to varying with the question at hand, capacity determinations can also vary day to day or hour to hour, just like mental status. A patient who has capacity to make a given decision on arrival may lose that capacity when she becomes delirious due to fever. Similarly, a patient who lacks capacity when he arrives may regain it when his mental status returns to normal.

A final point to keep in mind is that a refusal to communicate does not mean that a patient lacks capacity. Occasionally, patients with no lack of decision-making capacity who are refusing care also refuse to engage in a discussion of their decision. It can be difficult in these cases to determine whether the patient has capacity, and one may in fact therefore err on the side of determining that the patient does not have capacity. However, in the appropriate circumstances, when one is convinced that the patient is merely ornery and not irrational, the patient can be treated like one who has capacity.

CAPACITY AND REFUSAL OF CARE

Once we have determined whether a patient has the capacity to refuse the recommended care (or leave AMA altogether), we can decide on the appropriate response to this refusal.

Patients with Capacity

If a patient who refuses care has capacity, we must ultimately accept his refusal and allow him to decline care, and, if relevant, leave the hospital. However, if we confine our response to a patient's refusal of care to a determination of capacity, we have failed in our duty to care for the patient. Although we cannot force treatment or admission on a patient, we can work hard to make treatment acceptable.

The first step is to understand why the patient is refusing and to try to deal with those concerns. Some of these concerns may be relatively explicit and straightforward. There may be a family member or pet the patient feels he needs to care for. In that case, helping with making alternate plans for such care may allow the patient to agree to treatment. More significantly, one may discover that the patient has significantly different values than were assumed in formulating the treatment plan. For example, a patient may value quality of life over longer life. Therefore, an initial plan to admit the patient for toxic chemotherapy may be simply inappropriate, and discharge, possibly to hospice, could be the most appropriate plan and not just an accommodation to the patient's refusal to be admitted.

In other cases, the underlying reason for refusal may not be easily uncovered and may only be discovered through conversation beyond the usual capacity assessment. Such issues may include failure to adequately consider the long-term consequences of a choice, inordinate fear of pain, and failure to consider low-probability but high-cost outcomes. Other similar issues include denial, a need to maintain control, and fear of being stigmatized. Each of these can be addressed if the physician takes the time to uncover them, and the likelihood of the patient receiving proper care can thus be increased.

Sometimes, however, the plan being presented by the physician is simply not acceptable to the patient. In this case, negotiation and compromise may be called for. Any reasonable alternative to the initial optimal plan should be considered. Perhaps the patient who refuses admission will agree to further testing in the ED, even if such tests are ordinarily done only on inpatients. If so, the test should be ordered if at all possible. If it is positive, it may convince the patient to be admitted. If it is negative, it may be easier to discharge the patient comfortably. Another possibility is that a patient who refuses interventions would be willing to be admitted for observation. In many cases, this would still be better for the patient than leaving the hospital, so again, admission for "plan B" is preferable to letting the patient leave AMA. Finally, when all else fails, calling on family, friends, clergy, or a private physician to talk to the patient about his decision may be helpful.

It is vital that these discussions and negotiations be carried out in a respectful and nonthreatening manner. It should at all times be clear to the patient that you accept her right to refuse care and that you are only trying to work out the best plan of care that is acceptable to her. If at any point the patient is unwilling to continue this discussion, that decision, too, must be respected.

In truth, negotiations and discussions at the point of refusal, while better than simply allowing the patient to leave AMA, are themselves suboptimal. Refusal of care is often due to a lack of trust. Patients rarely know their ED physicians and thus have little basis on which to trust them. Fortunately, most of the time, this is not an issue, but when it is, it can manifest itself in refusal of care. Therefore, such episodes can be minimized by building the trust of the patient early in the encounter.

There are many strategies for maximizing a patient's trust. Perhaps the most vital is communicating clearly, in a way the patient can understand. This means without using medical jargon, and using a translator if necessary. It is difficult to decide to trust someone you do not understand.

The second primary way of earning trust is to display empathy and concern for the patient. Take the time to sit and give the patient your full attention when evaluating him. This may be difficult in the ED, but it is usually possible and can be very valuable. Displaying concern for the patient's comfort, even to the extent of bringing him water or a blanket, can also demonstrate your good intentions toward the patient.

Only once all of these steps have failed have we reached the point where we can accept a patient's refusal of care without failing in our duty to care.

Patients without Capacity

When a patient who is refusing care (or even who is agreeing to care) is found to lack the capacity to make the decision in question, an alternative decision-maker must be designated. Who this is is determined by local law; however, the structure is generally the same. Obviously, if the patient has been incapacitated for some time and has a legal guardian, that guardian will make medical decisions for the patient. In general, however, the first step is to determine if the patient has a *health care proxy*, also known as a *medical power of attorney*. Such a document allows a person to appoint an agent to make medical decisions should the person not be able to make them for himself. Since the currently incapacitated patient has previously made his wishes known about what to do should he lose capacity, we continue to "listen" to the patient by turning to his agent when necessary. Every state in the United States has a mechanism for appointing such an agent.

If no agent has been designated by the patient, we turn to those who presumably know the patient best and have his interests at heart – family and possibly close friends – to find a surrogate decision-maker for the patient. The closest relative or friend from among those who can be found will be authorized to make decisions. In New York state, for example, the statute provides the following ordering of potential surrogates: spouse or domestic partner, adult child, parent, (adult) sibling, close friend. The surrogate's primary role, when possible, is to make decisions for the patient based on the patient's known preferences, desires, and beliefs. If the surrogate does not know what the patient would have wanted under the circumstances, decisions should be made based on the surrogate's assessment of the patient's best interests.

Although it is important to identify an incapacitated patient's health care agent or surrogate, in most states, a person can also make specific legally binding *advance directives* (ADs) also known as a *living will*. These documents allow a person put in writing what she wants done in a particular medical situation. (For example, no artificial nutrition or no intubation.) When such a document exists, it generally takes precedence over any surrogate. That is, agents and surrogates cannot make decisions that contradict the AD, although, again, such matters are determined by local law. However, since ADs rarely apply exactly to a given case and never cover all questions, the availability of an AD does not eliminate the need for an alternate decision-maker. The AD needs to be interpreted, and other decisions need to be made.

ADs are also the first recourse when a patient without capacity has no agent or surrogate. If the patient has previously documented his wishes about a particular treatment, even if he no longer has the capacity to decide about the treatment, we follow the desires expressed in the AD.

When neither agent, surrogate, nor AD is available, it generally falls to physicians to make treatment decisions, although, as with all procedures for making medical decisions for patients without capacity, the details are determined by local law. In New York, again, the treating physician can make routine decisions based on the physician's determination of the patient's best interest. For more significant decisions, such as nonemergent surgery, the treating physician must consult with others, and another physician must concur with the treatment plan. Decisions to remove life-sustaining treatment are even more restricted.

Even though we will not act on a refusal of care by a patient without capacity, we should still try every means possible to encourage a refusing patient to agree to the treatment in question. The strategies here will be essentially similar to those discussed earlier for a patient with capacity. There are several reasons to try to obtain the patient's agreement, even if we might ultimately override their refusal. First, even patients without capacity deserve respect as people, and this respect requires that we not force them to do anything against their will unless absolutely necessary. Second, treating patients against their will, even when it is the right thing to do, can be traumatic for providers. Third, the surrogate may be more comfortable consenting to care if the patient agrees. Finally, a decision to override a patient's refusal may be moot if the patient will continue to refuse and be noncomplaint, as when postsurgical care requires particularly good wound hygiene or long-term medication compliance.

THE PROCESS

Documentation

If a patient is ultimately allowed to refuse care, it is important that the procedure that led to this be clearly documented. That is, the risks and alternatives that were discussed with the patient, the fact that the patient understood these points, the patient's reason for refusal, and the fact that the physician believes the patient to have capacity to make the decision in question must all be clearly recorded in the chart for all refusals of care. It is also helpful to document the fact that the patient had the opportunity to ask questions as well as the specific treatment the patient refused. A routine form stating that the patient is taking responsibility for the refusal of care (which usually only exists for the specific case of AMA) does not suffice, although, of course, all forms required by the hospital should be completed.

It is also important to remember that refusal of care of does not end our responsibility for the patient. In all matters other than the care they are refusing, we must treat them as we would anyone else. In particular, this means that a patient leaving AMA should receive a full set of discharge instructions and not simply be given an AMA form to sign and be allowed to leave, although the discharge form should indicated that the patient left AMA.

As noted earlier, basic AMA forms signed by the patient are not sufficient documentation. They are also not absolutely necessary. Although providing a small further measure of documentation of the patient's wishes and understanding, especially if the AMA form itself incorporates a summary of the conversation that determined the patient's understanding and capacity, no one can be forced to sign such a form. Therefore, if a patient refuses to sign, this must simply be documented. The AMA discharge is still "legitimate."

What Does Signing a Patient Out AMA Accomplish?

Documenting that a patient has left AMA (or refused any care) does not provide absolute protection against litigation. The patient or his representative could still claim, for example, that the provider did not disclose all of the relevant information or that the patient's capacity was not properly assessed. Nonetheless, a well-documented refusal of care/AMA note can provide substantial protection against a malpractice suit should the patient have a bad outcome. It can do this by explicitly documenting that the patient did receive all relevant information, as well as by showing that the patient assumed risk upon himself.

The Role of Psychiatry and Mental Illness in Capacity Determinations

It is important to note that the presence of mental illness is not in itself relevant to capacity determinations. The method laid out earlier for determining a patient's capacity is adequate even for a patient suffering from severe mental illness. Even psychoses do not necessarily interfere with all decision-making. Only when disordered thought patterns enter into the patient's decision-making does mental illness interfere with capacity. Such disordered decision-making will become clear during a careful capacity assessment.

Nor is lack of capacity a psychiatric ailment requiring specialist consultation. Any physician can assess capacity, and psychiatric consultation is not necessary. Indeed, the physician caring primarily for the patient is probably best placed to determine capacity. It is true, however, that psychiatrists are experienced at sorting out patients' underlying thoughts and motives, and thus, when there is any doubt about whether a patient's decision-making process is rational, regardless of whether the patient has underlying mental illness, a psychiatry consult may be helpful in making a final capacity determination.

Financial Impact of Leaving AMA

There is a widespread belief among physicians that patients who leave AMA will not have their ED bill paid by insurance. It is not clear where this belief originated, and it is impossible to give a blanket answer to this question because insurance companies may vary in their practices. However, multiple studies and surveys have found no evidence that leaving AMA has any effect on insurance reimbursement.

Suicide Attempts

One particularly difficult case of deciding whether to agree to a patient's refusal of treatment arises when a patient who has attempted suicide, but now appears to be rational, refuses treatment for his suicide attempt, without which he will die. Although such a patient may appear to have capacity to refuse care, the general consensus is that a suicide attempt by an otherwise healthy patient is evidence that the patient lacks capacity at that moment to make decisions about his care. A more difficult case arises when the patient has what may appear to be a rational reason for attempting suicide, in particular, terminal illness. In such a case, the refusal of care may be seen as an extension of the rational suicide attempt, and it is possible that such a refusal should be honored if all other relevant conditions are satisfied. However, there is no consensus on this matter.

Minors

Decision-making for minors is a complicated topic with many nuances. Although in general parents have the right to make health care decisions for their minor children, this right is not absolute. For details, please see Chapter 9 in this volume, "Care of Minors."

ETHICS TAKEOUT TIPS

- Every contact with a patient requires consent. When the intervention is more extensive or more risky than routine treatment, the consent must be informed and explicit and should be documented.
- The primary exception to the requirement to get informed consent for significant procedures is a true emergency in which there is no time to obtain consent.
- Any patient with decision-making capacity may refuse treatment, including admission to the hospital.
- If a patient does not have decision-making capacity, treatment decisions are made by a health care agent or close relative. ADs should also be consulted, if available.
- Only when a patient without capacity has no surrogate decision-maker or relevant AD can physicians use their best judgment in treating the patient.
- Psychiatrists are not necessary for a capacity determination, although in some cases they may be helpful.
- Before accepting a refusal of care by a patient with capacity, or treating a patient without capacity against his will, every effort must

be made to reassure the patient about the proposed treatment or arrive at an alternative plan that is acceptable to the patient.

- It is not generally true that patients who sign out AMA will be denied payment for the visit by their insurance company.

FOR FURTHER READING

Albert, H. D., & Kornfeld, D. S. (1973). The threat to sign out against medical advice. *Annals of Internal Medicine, 79,* 888–891.

Alfandre, D. J. (2009). "I'm going home": Discharges against medical advice. *Mayo Clinic Proceedings, 84,* 255–260.

Alfandre, D., & Schumann, J. H. (2013). What is wrong with discharges against medical advice (and how to fix them). *Journal of the American Medical Association, 310,* 2393–2394.

Brock, D. W., & Wartman, S. A. (1990). When competent patients make irrational choices. *New England Journal of Medicine, 322,* 1595–1599.

Callaghan, S., & Ryan, C. J. (2011). Refusing medical treatment after attempted suicide: Rethinking capacity and coercive treatment in light of the Kerrie Wooltorton case. *Journal of Law and Medicine, 18,* 811–819.

Devitt, P. J., Devitt, A. C., & Dewan, M. (2000). Does identifying a discharge as "against medical advice" confer legal protection? *Journal of Family Practice, 49,* 224–227.

Ding, R., Jung, J., Kirsch, T. D., Levy, F., & McCarthy, M. L. (2007). Uncompleted emergency department care: Patients who leave against medical advice. *Academic Emergency Medicine, 14,* 870–876.

Drane, J. F. (1984). Competency to give an informed consent. *Journal of the American Medical Association, 252,* 925–927.

Dresser, R. (2010). Suicide attempts and treatment refusals. *Hastings Center Report, 40,* 10–11.

Hwang, S. W., Li, J., Gupta, R., Chien, V., & Martin, R. E. (2003). What happens to patients who leave hospital against medical advice? *Canadian Medical Association Journal, 68,* 7–20.

Moskop, J. C. (1999). Informed consent in the emergency department. *Emergency Medicine Clinics of North America, 17,* 327–340.

Roth, L. H., Meisel, A., & Lidz, C. A. (1977). Tests of competency to consent to treatment. *American Journal of Psychiatry, 134,* 279–284.

Schaefer, G. R., Matus, H., Schumann, J. H., Sauter, K., Vekhter, B., Meltzer, D. O., & Arora, V. M. (2012). Financial responsibility of hospitalized patients who left against medical advice: Medical urban legend? *Journal of General Internal Medicine, 27,* 825–830.

Simon, J. R. (2007). Refusal of care: The physician-patient relationship and decision-making capacity. *Annals of Emergency Medicine, 50,* 456–461.

Wicclair, M. R. (1991). Patient decision-making capacity and risk. *Bioethics, 5,* 91–104.

9

Care of Minors

SARAH C. CAVALLARO, MD, AND JILL M. BAREN, MD, MBE,
FACEP, FAAP

INTRODUCTION

In general emergency departments (EDs) in the United States, pediatric patients make up an average of 20 percent of all patient visits. Emergency practitioners (EPs) may feel less comfortable with the pediatric patient due to less frequent exposure; however, given the growing number of pediatric ED visits, it is imperative to become both familiar and comfortable with this population. A unique set of ethical considerations becomes important with this population. When caring for adolescents, the EP must balance the voice of the patient along with that of the caretaker. With younger children, the EP must interface with the caretaker who is often speaking for the patient. Finally, the EP must become familiar with state laws surrounding the care of minors. This chapter highlights the major ethical principles that are operational in the emergency setting when caring for minors.

THE DIFFERENCES AMONG CHILDREN, ADOLESCENTS, AND ADULTS

From a holistic perspective, in order to provide excellent emergency care to a child, an EP must consider both the psychological presentation and state of the child. Children of the same chronological age may be at various stages of their physical, intellectual, and psychosocial development. The developmental stage and the child's relationship with his or her caretaker determine how involved the child can or should be with medical decision-making. It is important for the EP to recognize the child's stage of development to know how to appropriately involve the caretaker. The initial tone set by the EP when working with the family will likely establish the nature of the entire ED visit.

A particular challenge in the emergency setting is obtaining an accurate psychosocial history from an adolescent. Adolescents may be participating in risky behaviors that impact their overall health and emergency care needs. Complicating the task, caretakers will have varying insight into the patient's behavior. When interviewed without caretakers, adolescents may still be reluctant to share such information with the EP for fear of judgment or punishment. There have been many tools published that can aid an EP in taking an accurate adolescent history. Two widely accepted interview tools are the SHADSSS and HEADSS. These interview tools are acronyms for topics that should be covered in the interview in order of least to most sensitive topics. The HEADSS technique has the practitioner start with questions about *h*ome, *e*ducation, and *a*ctivities, and then move on to *d*rugs, *s*exual health, and *s*uicide. SHADSSS covers similar topics and guides the practitioner to raise questions about *s*chool, *h*ome, and *a*ctivities followed by *d*epression, *s*ubstance abuse, *s*exuality, and *s*afety. These interview tools can be narrowed to meet the needs and time constraints of the EP with a focus on substance abuse, depression, sexuality, and safety depending on the emergency complaint.

An emerging challenge to the care of an adolescent patient is social media. Children as young as thirteen years, as outlined in the Children's Online Privacy Protection Act, can sign up for online social media sites such as Facebook. Social media can have positive influences on an adolescent's life, such as contact with friends and access to health information. Unfortunately, social media can also be a portal for "cyber bullying" or other forms of harassment that take place online and shielded from the view of caretakers and teachers. Cell phones have facilitated the practice of "sexting," which is "sending, receiving, or forwarding sexually explicit messages, photographs or images." Participation in social media and sexting is rampant, with 22 percent of teenagers logging onto their favorite social media site more than ten times a day, and 20 percent revealing that they have sent or posted nude or seminude photographs of themselves. These portals may lead to depression, safety concerns, and risky sexual behavior that may be of concern during an emergency care encounter.

CONSENT

Modern medicine favors a culture in which a patient consults a physician and chooses the care that is most aligned with the patient's beliefs from a variety of options presented by the practitioner. This is the fundamental basis of informed consent, which dictates that a physician must explain various care options (including no care) in plain language to a consenting party who understands the options and is free to make a choice of care from among those options.

Informed consent poses a potential problem for EPs dealing with pediatric patients. A minor, defined as an individual under the age of 18 (or the age of 19 in Alabama, Nebraska, or Wyoming), may not have the emotional or cognitive maturity to fully understand and make an informed decision about his or her health care. Guardian consent by proxy is the accepted form of informed consent when treating a minor, with the expectation that the guardian is acting in the best interest of the child. If the EP feels that the guardian is not making medical decisions based on the best interest standard, the EP should consider seeking assistance from another party, such as an ethics consultant, committee, hospital administrator, or legal counsel. This is often not practical in an emergency situation but should be attempted when needed. In typical emergency circumstances, every attempt should be made to obtain parental consent for emergency care; however, if it is impossible to obtain consent in a timely fashion, life- or limb-saving care should not be delayed and, in such circumstances, consent is implied.

Older children and adolescents may not be fully autonomous in decision-making but can often participate in conversations surrounding their care together with the EP and guardian. EPs should seek *assent* from such patients. Soliciting older patients' thoughts on their care may help the EP determine patient awareness of the situation, set reasonable expectations for upcoming care, evaluate the willingness of the patient to participate in his or her care, and help the patient mature into an autonomous decision-maker. At times, a patient's refusal to assent may be binding, especially when that care has no direct benefit for that patient, such as in the context of research.

State laws provide certain exceptions to the rule for guardian consent. In some specific situations, minors are able to provide their own informed consent as if they were a competent adult. Emancipated minors are one such exception, and these include minors who are living on their own and financially independent, pregnant, a parent, in the military, or declared an emancipated minor by a court of law. Some states also grant decision-making capacity to mature minors. Mature minors are unemancipated minors seeking care for specific conditions such as sexually transmitted infection, contraception, mental health, or drug or alcohol abuse. The specifics on both emancipated and mature minors vary from state to state, and it is recommended that the EP become familiar with state guidelines in his or her area(s) of practice.

CONFIDENTIALITY AND PRIVACY

Privacy and confidentiality are fundamental to any patient–provider relationship. In 1968, the American Medical Association drafted a policy statement in strong support of confidentiality around sensitive areas of health care in adolescents, such as reproductive care. In 1988, the American Academy of Pediatrics, the American College of Obstetrics and Gynecology, and the Academy of Family Physicians created similar policy statements. Initially published in 1994 and reaffirmed in 2008, the American College of Emergency Physicians states that "confidentiality is an important but not absolute principal" and that "there are circumstances in which no societal consensus exist" with regards to minors.

To provide quality care, the EP must have as much information as possible. Research has shown that older children and adolescents are more likely to seek medical care and divulge more complete and accurate histories if they believe that their information will be kept private, including from their guardian. These issues can be particularly difficult in the pediatric patient when care and payment often include guardians.

A recommended approach to this clinical scenario is a conversation with both the patient and the guardian(s) at the onset of the visit, highlighting the EP's priority of patient confidentiality and the local legislation on mature minor laws. In order to maintain the patient's trust, it is prudent to explain the times when confidentiality, by law, must be breached. These times vary by state but generally include suspected abuse, concern for threat to self or others, and a life-threatening emergency.

Unintended breaches in confidentiality can also occur during the post-visit period. The EP should develop a plan to contact the adolescent independently of the guardian should the provider need to discuss information with the patient after the visit has concluded. If the ED visit is being covered by a guardian's insurance, an itemized bill may be sent to the policy holder. This bill may include things such as pregnancy tests. The patient should be made aware of this at the onset of the visit; hopefully, this will not dissuade the patient from pursuing care. Current research is aimed at determining a payment system that would allow for guardian insurance coverage but maintain confidentiality for adolescent patients.

Patients may desire confidentiality from their parents. Based on the emotional and cognitive maturity of the patient, it may be in the patient's best interest to include the guardian in the patient's care. Should this situation arise, confidentiality should initially be maintained so as not to delay patient care. Throughout the ED visit, the EP should then work with the adolescent to strongly encourage open communication with the parent or guardian. At times, it may be helpful for the EP to lead the family discussion (should the patient agree to disclose information) since the EP may be the most comfortable discussing sensitive topics such as pregnancy or drug abuse.

END-OF-LIFE CARE

Issues around end-of-life care are one of the greatest challenges for any EP. Often, an EP has just met a family for the first time and has had little to no ability to create a relationship prior to having an end-of-life care discussion. Such a discussion with the family of a pediatric patient can be even more difficult depending on provider experience or provider emotion surrounding pediatric death. The American Academy of Pediatrics recognized the need for experts in end-of-life care and, in 2006, created the board certified specialty of *pediatric palliative care.*

Pediatric palliative care is similar to adult palliative care, in which a multidisciplinary team of physicians, nurses, social workers, psychologists, spiritual leaders, bereavement specialists, child life specialists, and others work to improve the quality of life and decrease suffering for the patient and family. Unlike some adult end-of-life care models, the pediatric palliative care model does not exclude those patients who continue to receive life-sustaining treatment should that be in the best interest of the patient. In fact, the Patient Protection and Affordable Care Act states that pediatric patients can receive both hospice and/or palliative care services along with life-sustaining therapy. Therefore, the palliative care team is an extra layer of medical, social, and financial support in the hospital, outpatient office, or patient home for the patient, the family, and the providers.

Family support is a critical part of pediatric end-of-life care. The death of a child may be particularly traumatic for a family. The EP must have a face-to-face conversation with caregivers when a death happens in the ED; it is helpful to involve primary care doctors or specialists who have an established relationship with the family if possible. Siblings should also be considered in the bereavement process because they are at risk of feeling neglected while caregivers react to grave loss. Bereavement specialists, psychologists, social workers, spiritual leaders, and other members of the palliative care team can aid the EP in this process because it will extend well beyond the ED visit.

To help families with bereavement, the American Academy of Pediatrics believes that families should be given the option to be present during cardiopulmonary resuscitation (CPR). When interviewed after the death of their child, parents who witnessed CPR felt more satisfied with their child's care. These parents were more likely to believe that nothing else could be done to help prolong their child's life and that they were a comfort in the last moments of their child's life. These parents report that witnessing CPR helped their grieving process.

Social workers are an invaluable resource to the EP. They can facilitate crucial aspects of care in the settings of child abuse, psychiatric disease, and complex coordination of outpatient care. They can also address schooling needs, assist in obtaining medications, and help in dealing with financial difficulty, bereavement, and much more. Each ED will have different access to social work support. It is recommended that the EP become familiar with his or her own resources and the social worker's comfort with the issues faced by pediatric emergency patients. An EP may even need to consider the transfer of a child to another ED or hospital if psychosocial needs cannot be met at a particular institution and if it is in the best interest of the patient.

End-of-life care may be even more difficult with an unanticipated death. This difficulty extends out of the ED to our first responders. In 2003, the National Association of EMS Physicians and the Committee on Trauma of the American College of Surgeons offered guidelines on terminating resuscitation in the field for adults with out-of-hospital cardiac arrest from blunt trauma. Pediatric patients were excluded from these guidelines. In 2014, the American Academy of Pediatrics published a policy statement on traumatic out-of-hospital cardiac arrest. Although this statement calls for further research to be done in order to develop a guideline for such patients, the current standard is to resuscitate and transport these patients to the ED, aside from cases clearly incompatible with life such as decapitation, rigor, or greater than 30 minutes of cardiac arrest. This recommendation is based on limited data that show the outcomes of pediatric patients are still poor but better than adult outcomes. The recommendation also allows grieving families to have access to the counseling and bereavement resources based in the hospital.

ETHICS TAKEOUT TIPS

- Determine the child's stage of development early to adequately balance the participation of the patient and the parent in medical decision-making. Setting the tone of the ED visit early will make it proceed more smoothly.

- It can be difficult to obtain an accurate history from adolescent patients. Structured interview tools such as SHADSSS or HEADSS are effective techniques.
- Social media, when used inappropriately, can be dangerous to a child's health, and this is not always recognized by parents.
- A minor is defined as a person under the age of 18 in most states or under the age of 19 in Alabama, Nebraska, and Wyoming. Guardian consent by proxy is the accepted form of informed consent when treating a minor.
- Emergent life-saving care should not be delayed if the EP is unable to find a guardian for consent; in these cases, consent is implied
- An EP should seek assent from older children. Refusal to assent to care is binding if care does not provide a direct benefit to the patient.
- Emancipated minors are minors who are living on their own with financial independence, pregnant, a parent, in the military, or declared an emancipated minor by a court of law. Many states give emancipated minors the ability to consent to medical care without a parent.
- Mature minors are unemancipated minors seeking care for specific conditions such as sexually transmitted infections, contraception, mental health, or drug or alcohol abuse. Some states give mature minors the ability to consent to medical care regarding these specific conditions only.
- At the onset of an interview, the EP should explain to both the parent and patient the importance of confidentiality and privacy. The EP should also note when confidentiality must be breached. In cases where confidentiality can be maintained, the EP should work with the patient to disclose information to a trusted adult who can support the patient through his or her medical care.
- The pediatric palliative care team can help facilitate care within the ED in the context of end of life and can support families with bereavement care long after the ED visit has concluded.
- Pre-hospital providers should transport blunt cardiac arrest patients to the ED aside from cases clearly incompatible with life such as decapitation, rigor, or greater than 30 minutes of cardiac arrest. This allows families access to end-of-life resources and counseling available in the hospital.
- Parents should be presented with the option to be present for CPR of their child.

- An excellent resource for providers is the Guttmacher Institute website: www.guttmacher.org/. This site provides both information and state-based policies, resources, and statistics on many of the topics discussed throughout this chapter.

FOR FURTHER READING

AMA Council on Scientific Affairs. (1993). Confidential health services for adolescents. *Journal of the American Medical Association, 269,* 1420–1424.

American College of Emergency Physicians. (1994). Patient confidentiality. *Annals of Emergency Medicine, 24,* 1209. *Reaffirmed in October 2008 by the ACEP Board of Directors.* www.acep.org/Clinical-Practice-Management/Patient-Confidentiality/

American College of Surgeons Committee on Trauma, American Academy of Pediatrics, Committee on Pediatric Emergency Medicine Committee, National Association of EMS Physicians and American College of Emergency Physicians, Pediatric Emergency Medicine. (2014). Withholding or termination of resuscitation in pediatric out-of-hospital traumatic cardiopulmonary arrest. *Pediatrics,* 133, e1104–e1116.

American Academy of Pediatrics, Committee on Bioethics. (1995). Informed consent, parental permission, and assent in pediatric practice. *Pediatrics,* 95(2), 314–317.

American Academy of Pediatrics, Committee on Media and Communication. (2011). The impact of social media on children, adolescents, and families. *Pediatrics,* 127(4), 800–804.

American Academy of Pediatrics, The Committee on Psychosocial Aspects of Child and Family Health. (2012). Supporting the family after the death of a child. *Pediatrics,* 130, 1164–1169.

American Academy of Pediatrics, Section of Hospice and Palliative Medicine and Committee on Hospital Care. (2013). Pediatric palliative care and hospice care commitments, guidelines, and recommendations. *Pediatrics,* 132, 966.

American College of Emergency Physicians. (1994). Patient confidentiality. *Annals of Emergency Medicine, 24,* 1209. *Reaffirmed in October 2008 by the ACEP Board of Directors.* www.acep.org/Clinical-Practice-Management/Patient-Confidentiality/

Clark, L. R., & Ginsburg, K. R. (1995). How to talk to your teenage patients. *Contemporary Adolescent Gynecology, 1,* 23–27.

Cohen, E., Mackenzie, R. G., & Yates, G. L. (1991). HEADSS – A psychosocial risk assessment instrument: Implications for designing effective intervention programs for runaway youth. *Journal of Adolescent Health, 12,* 539–544.

English, A. (1990). Treating adolescents: Legal and ethical considerations. *Medical Clinics of North America, 74,* 1097–1112.

Jacobstein, C. R., & Baren, J. M. (1999). Emergency department treatment of minors. *Emergency Medical Clinics of North America, 17*(2), 341–352.

Merrill, C. T. (Thomson Healthcare), Owens, P. L. (AHRQ), & Stocks, C. (AHRQ). (2008). *Pediatric emergency department visits in community hospitals from selected states, 2005.* HCUP Statistical Brief #52. Rockville, MD: Agency for Healthcare Research and Quality. www.hcup-us.ahrq.gov/reports/statbriefs/sb52.pdf

Rainey, D. Y., Brandon, D. P., & Krowchuk, D. P. (2000). Confidential billing accounts for adolescents in private practice. *Journal of Adolescent Health*, 26(6), 389–391.

Tinsley, C., Hill, J. B., Shah, J., Zimmerman, G., Wilson, M., Freier, K., & Abd-Allah, S. (2008). Experience of families during cardiopulmonary resuscitation in a pediatric intensive care unit. *Pediatrics*, 122(4), e799–e804.

10

The Difficult Patient

JAY M. BRENNER, MD, FACEP, AND JAVAD T. HASHMI, MD

Emergency physicians practice under stressful work conditions. One patient may be the victim of a gunshot injury, while at the same time another may be suffering from an acute myocardial infarction. Emergency physicians are obligated ethically and legally to care for all patients who present to the emergency department (ED), even patients who may be difficult. In this busy setting, emergency physicians may have little time to dedicate to the difficult patient, and such a patient may seem to consume valuable resources that could be allocated to other patients. The difficult patient, however, should not be seen as a hassle to be avoided but instead as a rewarding opportunity to connect with someone who has been marginalized by a sometimes unforgiving health care system.

The definition of *difficult patient* remains somewhat elusive, and no universally accepted definition exists. Groves and Hanke use the term *hateful patient* to describe one "whom most physicians would dread to treat." It seems antagonistic and unnecessarily cruel to refer to a patient as "hateful."

Harrison and Vissers refer to the difficult patient as one "who through maladaptive behavior causes the physician to have a negative reaction towards the patient, resulting in an impaired patient–physician relationship." This definition inaccurately ascribes the difficulty solely to the patient.

Similarly, Anstett describes the difficult patient as one "who engages in counterproductive behavior," thereby harming the doctor–patient relationship. These definitions place great emphasis on some shortcoming or failing on the part of the patient. Such culpatory definitions could further stigmatize the difficult patient, reinforcing in the mind of the physician the patient's "hatefulness" and "maladaptive behavior."

Simon et al. uses less judgmental language and broadens the definition of the difficult patient to one "who interferes with a physician's attempts to establish a normal therapeutic relationship." He goes on to note that such interference need not be intentional or malicious on the part of the patient. Although this definition still assumes the physician's noble efforts, it is much more palatable for the sake of discussion.

It would be helpful for physicians, at least on a conceptual level, to move away from the difficult patient paradigm to that of the more neutral model of the *difficult patient–physician encounter*. In this way, it is the encounter and not the patient that is labeled as "difficult." The inclusion of the word *physician* in difficult patient–physician encounter is appropriate because it recognizes that there may be certain physician factors that can also lead to, or at least contribute to, the difficult encounter. The sole emphasis on "the maladaptive behavior" of the patient, with no consideration of physician factors, is a reflection of the outdated paternalistic model of medicine. Contemporary medicine has moved toward a patient-centric model of care, and the concerns of the patient, including the frustrations of the patient toward the "difficult physician," ought to be duly considered. This chapter will seek to address both patient and physician factors leading to the difficult patient–physician encounter. We will engage in an ethical analysis and review the ethical dilemmas that arise out of it. Finally, we will offer solutions to ameliorating the difficult patient–physician encounter (see Table 10.1).

PATIENT FACTORS, PHYSICIAN FACTORS, AND THE PATIENT–PHYSICIAN RELATIONSHIP

Case: Kelly is a forty-six-year-old woman with a known history of depression, anxiety, fibromyalgia, and chronic abdominal pain. She presents to the ED for an acute exacerbation of abdominal pain associated with nausea but no vomiting. She has nonbloody diarrhea, feels lightheaded, and starts to complain of some shortness of breath as well. This is Kelly's fourth visit to the ED in the past month, and she has had two computed tomography (CT) scans in the same time period, which did not reveal an etiology of her pain. Kelly says Tylenol does not help her pain, and she is allergic to ibuprofen. She is rude to the nursing staff and yells at the doctor when he enters the room, "I've been waiting here for five hours and nobody has done anything about my pain!"

TABLE 10.1. *The BATHE technique*

	BATHE Technique	Verbalization
B	**Background:** Assess the **b**ackground of the situation	"Tell me what has been happening."
A	**Affect:** Assess the patient's **a**ffect	"How does that make you feel?"
T	**Troubling:** Determine the problem that is most **t**roubling for the patient	"Which of these symptoms are you most concerned with?"
H	**Handling:** Evaluate how the patient is **h**andling the problem	"How have you been managing this problem?"
E	**Empathy:** Convey **e**mpathy	"You seem to be going through a lot. I understand how that can be frightening."

Emergency physicians can use these verbalizations of the BATHE technique, initially described by McCulloch et al., to address "difficult" patients' underlying psychological and emotional needs. They should be tailored carefully to specific situations so that they are infused with authenticity.

Hahn and colleagues showed that approximately 15 percent of patients in the primary care clinic could be considered difficult. Even though these difficult patients account for a relatively small fraction of the patients an emergency physician will examine in any given shift, they often require more time and attention than other patients. Furthermore, due to an inherent recall bias, physicians may perceive that they expend much more of their time and attention in the service of these patients than they may do in reality. These patients disrupt the normal flow, efficiency, and harmony of the ED, which frustrates the emergency physician. It is believed that difficult patients not only impede their own care but also that of the other patients in the department.

Physicians and nursing staff may consistently regard certain patients as "difficult." Hahn and colleagues found a strong correlation between difficult patients and mental illness. Difficult patients are almost twice as likely to have a mental illness as compared to other patients. Physicians found fewer than a tenth of patients without mental illness to be difficult, whereas a full quarter of those with mental illness were deemed to be so. Common psychiatric disorders associated with the difficult patient include generalized anxiety, panic disorder, dysthymia, major depressive disorder, probable alcohol abuse or dependence, and multisomatoform disorder. It is reasonable to assume that psychiatric illness may remain underdiagnosed in the difficult patient population.

Aside from underlying psychopathological disorders, 90 percent of difficult patients were found to have abrasive personality types or personality disorders. The psychiatric literature has documented such personality disorders, including paranoid, schizoid, schizotypal, antisocial, borderline, histrionic, narcissistic, avoidant, dependent, and obsessive-compulsive personality disorder.

In addition to mental illnesses and personality disorders, a third factor has been identified in the difficult patient: they often present with multiple physical complaints. Emergency physicians may pejoratively label such patients as having a "pan-positive review of systems." The vagueness of their symptoms can often be frustrating to the physician and thwart the physician's attempts to zero in on the diagnosis. For example, a patient who presents with sudden-onset right lower quadrant abdominal pain secondary to acute appendicitis is rarely viewed as being difficult. The patient has pain in one location resulting from an organic pathology, which can objectively be identified with CT imaging. With a clear diagnosis, the treatment is also straightforward: the emergency physician consults the surgery team, who whisk the patient away to the operating room. For the emergency physician, such a patient is perspicuous to diagnose and manage. Meanwhile, a patient like Kelly, with her vague, chronic, and diffuse abdominal pain, is less satisfying. The diagnostic workup is unclear and often does not reveal a diagnosis; the patient is often deemed manipulative, factitious, and/or drug-seeking.

Multiple physical complaints can result in extensive diagnostic testing, including CT imaging and other invasive tests. Often, these diagnostic workups are unremarkable, confirming in the mind of the emergency physician that "nothing is wrong with the patient" and "it is all in the patient's head." This reinforces a negative view of the patient and further hampers the patient–physician relationship. Conversely, some difficult patients receive minimal or no workups if they have presented similarly multiple times in the past. Physicians can become frustrated with trying to maintain this delicate Goldilocks balance of ordering not too much, not too little, but just the right amount of diagnostic testing. For example, Kelly presents with an acute exacerbation of chronic abdominal pain and has undergone multiple CT scans of her abdomen in the past, but now she comes in with excruciating pain. Should the physician repeat the CT imaging in order not to miss a diagnosis? Or abstain from it in order to save the patient from excess radiation exposure?

Multisomatoform disorder has been identified as an association with the difficult patient, which, by definition, consists of multiple physical complaints. The emergency physician is primarily trained in the diagnosis and treatment of acute and subacute diseases and may have less comfort or capability with more chronic, unremitting disorders. Psychiatric disorders by their very nature often require weeks to months to years of treatment and cannot be cured in the average span of an emergency visit. Therefore, emergency physicians believe that they have little to offer these patients, whereas these patients reciprocate this negativity by expressing dissatisfaction toward the emergency physician. The attitude of the physician toward the difficult patient can be mitigated if the physician bears in mind the association between the difficult patient and psychopathology, which is often outside the immediate control of the patient. In other words, the physician ought to remember that the difficult patient is likely not consciously or maliciously intending to be difficult, but rather certain underlying factors contribute to such a disposition.

> *Case: Dr. Marsh is a thirty-three-year-old emergency physician who recently completed his residency at a Level 1 trauma center. Now, he works as a solo doctor in an outlying community hospital. Dr. Marsh is going through a divorce and is suffering from symptoms of depression. This is his fourth night shift in a row, and his ED is now overcapacity, with patients filling the hallways and the waiting room. Dr. Marsh evaluates Kelly, our example patient, a forty-six-year-old woman with multiple complaints. She is upset and yells at him about the wait, saying, "I've been waiting here for five hours and nobody has done anything about my pain!" Dr. Marsh looks at his watch. He says, "No, ma'am. It's actually only been four hours."*

Krebs et al. surveyed the characteristics of physicians who report more frustration with patients. Physicians vary considerably in the percentage of patients they perceive as difficult. Those who report higher frustration with patients tend to share certain characteristics. Age seems to be one such factor, with physicians under the age of forty reporting higher levels of frustration with patients. The number of work hours was also found to be a contributing factor, especially for those working more than fifty-five hours per week. In light of the accelerated pace of the ED and the abnormal diurnal rhythms of shift workers, this number of hours may in fact be much lower for emergency physicians. Additionally, physicians who reported higher frustration with patients tended to have more symptoms of anxiety, depression, and stress.

Viewing these three factors together – age of the physician, number of work hours, and stress levels – a clear picture emerges: a young, less-experienced doctor working long hours in a stressful environment will more likely be frustrated by patients. Working long hours in stressful conditions means that physicians have less tolerance for the patient who may require extra time and effort, especially if it is perceived that the patient's symptoms are due to a psychosomatic complaint. Seasoned physicians have had time to perfect their craft and might be less likely to feel overwhelmed, as compared to younger doctors. Furthermore, younger emergency physicians are more likely to work longer and less desirable hours than their senior colleagues for a number of reasons. The constant rotating of shifts, to which the younger emergency physician is often subjected, may lead to social isolation and clinical depression. When dealing with patients who have been labeled difficult, physicians may benefit from pausing to reflect and to ask themselves if there are outside factors leading to their frustration, which is then being transferred to and superimposed on the patient.

> *Case: The triage nurse asks Kelly accusingly, "Why are you back again?" The staff understands that she is a "frequent flyer" and decides to let her wait for two hours in the waiting room because "we need to take care of our sick patients first." Once she is placed in a hallway in the ED, Kelly overhears the primary nurse telling the triage nurse that "she's here all the time." When she asks the primary nurse for pain medication, she is told that the doctor must evaluate her first. The emergency physician doesn't see her for another two hours, and, by this time, Kelly's pain is unbearable and her patience has run out. She yells, "I've been waiting here for five hours and nobody has done anything about my pain!"*

In countering the pervasive paternalistic model of the patient–physician relationship, it is not sufficient to merely elaborate the physician factors contributing to the difficult encounter. Instead, what is needed is a complete paradigm shift away from the older approach to a more patient-centric model. Here, the concerns of the patient take precedence, even when it involves a patient's grievances toward staff. As Fiester reasons, "[t]he conventional explanation for these [patient–physician] conflicts lays the blame squarely at the feet of the patient, typically via mental disorders or maladaptive personality traits... If there are grounds to reconceive the 'difficult' patient as someone reacting to the perception of ill treatment ... then there is an ethical obligation to address this perception of harm." In this view, the "maladaptive" behavior is seen as a response to the perceived injustice. As Fiester puts it, "[p]ersons who feel indignation, resentment, or offense are susceptible to manifesting their moral grievance in counterproductive ways." For example, Kelly's frustration toward the physician is a reaction to the "indignation, resentment, or offense" she may have felt due to the judgmental statements made by the hospital staff.

If a wrong is done to the patient, then there is an ethical duty to investigate the harm and remove it if possible. This approach to the difficult patient–physician encounter shifts the focus from frustration to action. Physicians receive little formal training in dealing with difficult patients. Furthermore, the treating physician is not an impartial arbiter but a vested party and is, therefore, impossible to extract completely from bias. In the case of Kelly, Dr. Marsh is likely already biased against the patient in favor of his nursing staff. Did Dr. Marsh delay evaluating the patient because he himself agreed with the assessment of the nursing staff? It is difficult to consider Dr. Marsh an impartial arbiter in this situation. If it is accepted that there are both patient and physician factors at play in the difficult patient–physician encounter, then it may indeed be problematic to have the treating physician as the arbiter. Fiester argues for the role of the clinical ethicist, which should be consulted to act as an impartial arbiter in such scenarios. This would mean an expansion of the role of the clinical ethics service to include the difficult patient–physician encounter, but Fiester points out that the difficult patient–physician encounter is usually a part of many ethics consultations anyway. It can be argued that the difficult patient–physician encounter, especially if the patient feels wronged in some way, is by definition an ethical issue that in turn necessitates an ethics consultation. Including an ethicist in such conflicts may not always be practical in the ED, but the concept of a third party is an important step in recognizing the two sides of the difficult patient–physician equation.

ETHICAL ANALYSIS

Emergency physicians have an ethical duty to care for patients, a duty that extends to difficult patients. The Emergency Medical Treatment and Labor Act (EMTALA) is U.S. law. Emergency physicians are legally bound to provide medical care for all patients, regardless of how pleasant or difficult they may be. Physicians found in violation of EMTALA can expect disciplinary as well as legal action against them.

EMTALA establishes a legal mandate, but emergency physicians should also adhere to the ethical codes established by the American Medical Association and the American College of Emergency Physicians. They both mention that even difficult patients must be treated with compassion and respect. Furthermore, the physician must refrain from denying treatment to a patient because of a judgment based on discrimination. This implies that the physician may not refuse to treat based merely on her dislike of the patient.

The duty to care for the patient is balanced with the physician's right to avoid harm. While it is often understood that the physician must avoid harming the patient, it is also true that the physician has the right to avoid harm from the patient. The physician should not need to suffer physical or emotional abuse from the patient. Reconciling the duty to care with the right to avoid harm means that the emergency physician has a duty to care for all, even the patient considered to be difficult, unless the patient is directly threatening the physician either verbally or physically. Therefore, the factors commonly linked to the difficult patient, such as mental illnesses or personality disorders, are not sufficient grounds to terminate the patient–physician relationship.

The four principles of medical ethics, as enumerated by Beauchamp and Childress, must be considered in dealing with the difficult patient. The patient has the right to autonomy, which means that she not only has the right to make her own medical decisions, but also that she has the right to her own self-identity. The patient has a right to be difficult and may actually benefit herself by being an advocate for herself, even if the physician considers this effort self-defeating. The twin principles of beneficence and nonmaleficence compel a physician to do what is best for the difficult patient and to abstain from harming her. The ethical principles of autonomy, beneficence, and nonmaleficence must be balanced with justice, understood as the fair distribution of limited health resources among all patients in the ED. However, the emergency physician must adhere to justice based not on how pleasant or difficult a patient is but rather based on the dictates of the medical need – just as the judge rules not on the disposition of the defendant but based on the dictates of the law.

> *Case: On physical exam, Kelly is found to have tenderness at McBurney's point, with rebound and guarding. A previous entry in the patient's medical chart reads, "Consider drug-seeking behavior." The patient is difficult, being hostile to staff, and demanding pain medication in a loud voice. The nurse turns to Dr. Marsh, the emergency physician, and asks him, "Do you really want me to line and lab her up?"*

Iserson's Rapid Ethical Decision-Making Model, a three-step tool, can help emergency physicians navigate this common ethical dilemma. First, the physician asks herself if there is a precedent case from which a rule can be applied to the new case. In this case, Dr. Marsh is faced with a difficult patient who presents with an acute exacerbation of chronic abdominal pain. Should the nurse obtain an IV catheter to administer pain medication and to facilitate CT imaging with IV contrast? The CT scanner will not only expose the patient to radiation, but it is also a limited resource that must be shared with other patients. Furthermore, the CT imaging will result in a delay in disposition of the patient, meaning that the patient's bed will not be ready for a new patient in the waiting room. In this case, Dr. Marsh can ask himself, "In the previous patient I had taken care of who had a similar history and physical exam – with right lower quadrant tenderness, rebound, and guarding – did I administer pain medication and obtain a CT scan?" When asked in this way, the clinical decision may become obvious: the patient is at risk for acute appendicitis, a condition that indicates pain medication and CT imaging. The emergency physician should seek to apply clinical decision-making tools to aid decision-making in caring for difficult patients because these tools often consider signs and symptoms as opposed to patient personality.

If, however, there is no precedent case or rule that can reasonably be applied to the situation, Iserson's approach dictates that the physician ask herself whether or not the clinical decision can be delayed. In the case of the difficult patient, this is often appropriate because the patient–physician relationship may sometimes improve with time. In our example case, if the patient's physical examination were a bit less worrisome, then Dr. Marsh could potentially order pain medication and carry out serial abdominal examinations. Kelly may become more pleasant once she is given pain medication, and her physical exam may become more reliable as well. However, delay in decision-making can only be done so long as no harm is expected to come to the patient as a result of it. In our example, there is enough concern for acute appendicitis that decision-making cannot reasonably be delayed.

The third step of Iserson's method requires the physician to ask herself three questions: (1) the Impartiality Test asks whether or not the physician would accept the clinical decision if she were in the place of the patient, (2) the Universalizability Test asks whether the physician's colleagues would make the same clinical decision in the given scenario, and (3) the Interpersonal Justifiability Test asks whether or not the clinical decision is defensible to others, namely, the physician's colleagues, supervisors, and the general public. All three of these questions would give Dr. Marsh clear guidance as to how to proceed: he knows that he would want his right lower quadrant pain taken seriously if he were the patient (Impartiality Test), that another provider would be expected to follow an acute appendicitis protocol if taking care of a similar patient (Universalizability Test), and that he would not have a well-substantiated defense if brought before a court for a missed appendicitis based on that particular patient presentation (Interpersonal Justifiability Test).

ETHICAL DILEMMAS

Groves describes four specific types of difficult patients: dependent clinger, entitled demander, manipulative help-rejecter, and self-destructive denier. Although such names are accusatory and may be unfair to patients, these descriptors are helpful in that the emergency physician may identify patients as such.

> Case: Rebecca is a forty-two-year-old woman with a history of chronic lower extremity edema, for which she presents to the ED at least weekly. She usually requests compression stockings, ibuprofen, and a meal. She is very grateful to the emergency physician, Dr. Marsh, but she has gained displeasure from the ED staff due to her repeated visits, almost always for minor complaints. She seeks to establish long-term care with Dr. Marsh, even asking if she can add him to her social media account.

Rebecca is, in Groves's classification scheme of difficult patients, a "dependent clinger." Dependent clingers differ from other difficult patients in that they are often very friendly toward physician staff. Unlike other difficult patients who may not listen to physician advice, dependent clingers request physician advice and guidance to an excessive degree. For example, Rebecca seeks repeated physician guidance for chronic pain in her lower extremities instead of simply trying over-the-counter ibuprofen at home. Her dependence is frustrating to the busy ED staff, which becomes exasperated when they see her return again and again for the same complaint, especially when the ED is busy. The extra handholding desired by these patients tests the patience of the emergency physician. Additionally, the patient seeks to establish a long-term relationship with the emergency physician, which not only is inconsistent with the role of the emergency physician but may also encroach on the physician's privacy. For example, Rebecca needs physician guidance so much in her day-to-day life that she wishes to add Dr. Marsh to her social media account. Groves argues that dependent clingers ought to be handled by establishing boundaries early on. For example, Rebecca should be reminded that the ED is intended for acute or subacute medical problems and that she should schedule an appointment with her own primary care doctor for her chronic lower extremity edema. Additionally, Dr. Marsh can let her know that it would not be appropriate for Rebecca to add him to her social media account. Instead, he would be happy to treat her in the ED in the case of an emergency.

It should be noted that the terminology of "the dependent clinger" is unnecessarily demeaning toward the patient, and the concept itself is questionable. Rebecca may, in fact, have a low IQ and may *need* some extra "handholding" in life. A social worker consultation may be needed to help the patient obtain regular follow-up appointments with a primary care provider. This will establish the long-term care the patient requires instead of simply blaming the patient for seeking it in the wrong place. In lieu of characterizing this patient as a "dependent clinger," such a patient can be thought of as the "needy patient." It is the duty of a physician to provide help, and therefore the emergency physician should feel satisfied in providing it. An ED functions as more than just a facility to treat individual patients; it is an institution that acts as a safety net for the entire community, especially the weak and vulnerable. Therefore, any physician pursuing a career in emergency medicine ought to be prepared to help the patient who requires extra help, even when that help may involve more than traditional medical workup and treatment.

Case: Megan is a pleasant thirty-seven-year-old woman who presents to the ED with lower back pain. The patient has sciatica, but the H&P does not indicate acute spinal cord compression. Dr. Marsh does not think emergent radiological imaging would be warranted at this time. Megan's husband John is in the room. He demands "strong pain medication" and magnetic resonance imaging (MRI) of the spine. John exclaims, "I've worked in health care before, and I know a lot more than many doctors!" He mentions that several previous doctors have "bungled" his own medical care, and he doesn't want the same for his wife. Finally, he threatens, "I should let you know that I know the CEO of the hospital and I will make sure you get fired if you do not do as I say."

In this example case, the patient herself is very easygoing, but her husband is being difficult. The difficult patient–physician relationship sometimes arises not from the patient or the physician but rather from the patient's family or other advocates. This is especially so in the case of pediatric patients, where overbearing parents can be classically difficult. Groves refers to this type of difficult patient as the "entitled demander."

The patient's husband, John, is the CFO of a large company and therefore feels "entitled" to "VIP treatment" in the ED. He is also threatening because he feels that this will enable him to get his way. Groves writes of these patients: "[T]hey use intimidation, devaluation, and guilt-induction . . . [S]uch patients often exude a repulsive sense of innate deservedness as if they were far superior to the physician." It is not surprising that the physician would in turn dislike such a patient.

Not only does the entitled demander demean the physician on a personal level, but also his demands and threats often encroach on the physician's sphere of autonomy and expertise. Although patient autonomy is rightfully valued and protected, it should not be understood to give patients the power to unilaterally dictate their management. Rather, the physician offers the patient choices, and the patient is able to pick from among those choices through informed consent; alternatively, the patient can seek a second opinion from another physician. However, the patient's autonomy does not extend to dictating management, such as demanding an MRI when there is no indication for one. The emergency physician should not simply acquiesce to the demand of an emergent MRI, because the MRI is a limited resource and must be saved for those patients who have emergent conditions warranting its use, such as those suspected of having acute spinal cord compression.

If it can be said that some patients feel "entitled," so, too, can it be said that some physicians may also feel "entitled." In fact, just as the CFO may feel superior to the physician, so, too, can physicians feel superior to their patients due to their respected status in society. Was Dr. Marsh's ego bruised by John the CFO's threat? As has been discussed earlier, difficult patient–physician encounters consist of both patient and physician factors. Physicians are certainly not immune to feeling "entitled." It would be unethical for Dr. Marsh to let his personal feelings hamper his care of the patient.

Groves also points out that the hostility exhibited by entitled demanders may be "born of terror of abandonment." Such patients may feel that making threats is the only way that they will be adequately cared for. It is also a coping mechanism: the entitled demander acts in this manner as a way of exerting control over her medical condition. Groves argues, "'[e]ntitlement' serves for some persons the functions that faith and hope serve in better adjusted [persons]." Physicians are in the service of helping those in need. If demanding patients express their need in a different way, they are still in need of help from the physician, and the physician is ethically bound to help. Once the patient's hostile attitude is understood to be a defense mechanism, it seems inappropriate to refer to them as "entitled demanders." Instead, a less judgmental term would be "the demanding patient."

Dealing with such demanding patients can indeed be very difficult and should involve de-escalation, bargaining, and boundary establishment. In the case of John, Dr. Marsh can de-escalate the situation by saying, "I understand your frustration. I'm very sorry that your previous encounters with physicians have not been positive. I value the fact that you want to protect your wife from a similar fate." By starting the conversation with a validation of the patient's grievances, the emergency physician can often defuse the situation or at least lower the patient's defenses. The next two steps involve bargaining and boundary establishment. John demanded "strong pain medication" and an MRI. Although the emergent MRI may be difficult to obtain, the first request is easy to fulfill. Dr. Marsh can say, "I will notify the nurse immediately to administer morphine, which is a powerful pain killer." The use of the word "immediately" conveys the urgency of treating the patient's pain, which is ethical because good pain control is to be offered to all patients, not only "VIPs." Establishing boundaries often occurs in tandem with bargaining: in this case, Dr. Marsh can explain that an emergent MRI cannot be ordered for the patient's condition, but that he could call the patient's primary care provider to recommend an outpatient MRI.

ETHICS TAKEOUT TIPS

- The emergency physician should acknowledge the psychiatric conditions contributing to the difficult patient.
- The emergency physician should recognize the physician factors leading to the difficult patient–physician encounter.
- The terminology and conceptual framework of "the difficult patient" ought to be changed to "the difficult patient–physician encounter."
- The emergency physician should use ethical principles to guide the management of difficult patient encounters.

FOR FURTHER READING

Anstett, R. (1980). The difficult patient and the physician-patient relationship. *Journal of Family Practice*, 11, 281–288.

Baruch, J. (2007). *Fourteen stories: Doctors, patients, and other strangers.* Kent, OH: Kent State University Press.

Beauchamp, T. L., & Childress, J. F. (2001). *Principles of biomedical ethics.* New York: Oxford University Press.

Council on Ethical and Judicial Affairs. (2014). *AMA code of medical ethics.* www.ama-assn.org/ama/pub/physicianresources/medical-ethics/code-medi cal-ethics.page

Fiester, A. (2012). The "difficult" patient reconceived: An expanded moral mandate for clinical ethics. *American Journal of Bioethics, 12*(5), 2–7.

Groves, J. E. (1978). Taking care of the hateful patient. *New England Journal of Medicine, 298*(16), 883–887.

Hahn, S. R., Kroenke, K., Spitzer, R. L., Brody, D., Williams, J. B., Linzer, M., deGruy, F. V., 3rd. (1996). The difficult patient: Prevalence, psychopathology, and functional impairment. *Journal of General Internal Medicine, 11*, 1–8.

Hanke, N. (1984). The problem patient. In W. R. Dubin, N. Hanke, & H. W. Nickens (Eds.), *Psychiatric emergencies: Clinics in emergency medicine* (Vol. 4, pp. 153–168). New York: Churchill Livingstone.

Harrison, D. W., & R. J. Vissers. (1997). Approach to the difficult patient in the emergency department. In P. Rosen, R. Barkin, D. F. Danzl, et al. (Eds.), *Emergency medicine: Concepts and clinical practice* (4th ed., pp. 2841–2852). St. Louis: Mosby-Year Book.

Krebs, E. E., Garrett, J. M., & Konrad, T. R. (2006). The difficult doctor? Characteristics of physicians who report frustration with patients: An analysis of survey data. *BMC Health Services Research, 6*, 128–135.

Mayer, M. L. (2008). On being a 'difficult' patient. *Health Affairs, 27*(5), 1416–1421.

McCulloch, J., Ramesar, S., & Peterson, H. (1998). Psychotherapy in primary care: The BATHE technique. *American Family Physician, 57*(9), 2131–2134.

Simon, J. R., Dwyer, J., & Goldfrank, L. R. (1999). The difficult patient. *Emergency Medicine Clinics of North America, 17*(2), 353–370.

11

Law Enforcement in the Emergency Department

EILEEN F. BAKER, MD, FACEP

INTRODUCTION

Emergency physicians often come in contact with law enforcement agents during their daily practice. Victims or perpetrators of crime may be brought to the emergency department (ED) accompanied by the police. Motor vehicle collisions also prompt investigation by officers of the law. Certainly, emergency physicians wish to maintain a mutually respectful relationship with law enforcement agents. Nevertheless, it is essential that emergency staff remember that their first duty is to the care of their patients. Ethical issues that may surface include patient privacy concerns, duty to warn of a potential threat of harm, and intoxication and drug ingestion. Emergency physicians may be called upon to collect evidence in the ED. Issues may surface regarding the treatment of undocumented immigrants or criminal suspects. Also, law enforcement and security personnel may be requested to provide for the safety of the ED staff.

This chapter addresses the ethical issues practitioners may encounter in the clinical practice of emergency medicine. Where applicable, emergency physicians are encouraged to familiarize themselves with federal, state, and local laws that pertain to these subjects. The American College of Emergency Physicians (ACEP) Code of Ethics can be found in Appendix A and outlines the ethical duties of the emergency physician.

PRESENCE OF LAW ENFORCEMENT AND SECURITY PERSONNEL IN EDS

The degree to which security and law enforcement personnel can be found in EDs varies quite widely. Large, urban centers may employ armed security forces or have police substations located on the hospital grounds.

Some may be stationed in the ED itself. In rural areas, however, no security guards may be available at all. Metal detectors staffed by security personnel may also be utilized in some urban centers. In addition, security guards may be armed with lethal weapons, incapacitating weapons (stun guns, electrified batons, or tasers), or not at all.

Although armed security staff members are intended to provide increased protection against violence by patients and hospital visitors, the presence of weapons in the ED may actually increase the potential for harm. In one study of hospital-based shootings in the United States from 2000 to 2011, 23 percent of injuries in the ED resulted from weapons obtained by perpetrators who disarmed law enforcement personnel.

Nevertheless, security and outside law enforcement personnel play an essential role in assisting the medical staff to care for violent patients who threaten hospital workers, other patients, or themselves. They may be called upon to disarm patients or secure weapons brought into the ED. In addition, the simple presence of security or police in the department (a show of force) may be sufficient to diffuse a potentially violent situation. Some facilities employ a "panic button" that when pressed activates recording devices and notifies local authorities of an escalating or dangerous situation in the ED.

CONFIDENTIALITY

The physician's first duty is to the health of the patient. An essential component of the physician–patient relationship is the element of confidentiality. The Health Insurance Portability and Accountability Act (HIPAA) regulates the use and disclosure of protected health information. Certain "covered entities," such as health care clearinghouses, employer sponsored health plans, health insurers, and medical service providers, may disclose protected health information to law enforcement officials for law enforcement purposes as required by law. This includes court orders, court-ordered warrants, subpoenas, and administrative requests, or to identify or locate a suspect, fugitive, material witness, or missing person.

Physicians may be pressured by police to disclose information such as toxicology screen results, blood ethanol levels, or other medical information. Medical conditions such as diabetic emergencies, seizure disorders, or other neurologic or psychiatric diagnoses may be relevant to a police investigation. Physicians should only make the medical record available when proper releases have been signed. This may require a subpoena in some cases. Furthermore, physicians should obtain ethanol levels at their discretion, when such information is relevant to patient care, rather than in the interest of investigators alone. During the course of some investigations, such as traffic accidents, police may require an ethanol level be drawn. In some states, physicians need not order this test because law enforcement agencies have protocols in place so that laboratory personnel may draw blood samples on their behalf when the law compels that the sample be provided.

RELEASE OF INFORMATION

There are times when the release of patient information is appropriate or even mandatory. Famously, *Tarasoff v. Regents of the University of California* involved the failure of a psychologist and supervising psychiatrist to warn a woman, identified to them by their patient, of his threat to harm her. She was later murdered by the patient. The judge ruled that "Protective privilege ends where public peril begins." In all states but Nevada, North Dakota, North Carolina, and Maine, medical personnel have the duty to warn potential victims of those who pose an imminent threat to them. In some institutions, consulting service providers orchestrate a plan for disposition from the ED.

General threats and homicidal ideation without reference toward any one individual present a challenge to health care personnel. Because no particular individual is singled out, the duty to warn cannot be implemented. Both practitioners and law enforcement agents have expressed concern and frustration with the law as written. It may allow persons suffering from mental illness not only to be released (when they deny intent to harm any one individual), but potentially to have access to weapons. Laws such as Florida's Baker Act hold the strong position that those suffering from mental, emotional, and behavioral disorders should not be treated as criminals.

POTENTIAL IMPAIRMENT

Virtually all states have laws mandating that neurologically impaired drivers be identified. Delaware, New Jersey, and Nevada have mandatory reporting laws for epilepsy. California and Utah mandate reporting of dementia and other cognitive impairments. Requirements to report unfit drivers in Canada vary by province. Physicians in both Canada and the United States may face legal action by victims of motor vehicle collisions involving impaired drivers if the court finds that the physicians could have foreseen the danger of their patients' continuing to drive.

Similarly, it should be the policy of physicians to warn patients of potential impairment after receiving or when prescribed medications that may alter perception, coordination, or mental alertness. Caution also should be exercised after procedural sedation. The American College of Emergency Medicine's "Clinical Policy for Procedural Sedation and Analgesia in the Emergency Department" recommends postprocedure monitoring and ensuring that patients return to preprocedure baseline before discharge. Alternatively, the patient may be discharged under the care of a responsible third party after meeting discharge criteria. The College recommends advising the patient that the medications they received could cause "confusion, sleepiness or clumsiness." Adults are advised not to engage in "any activity that requires alertness or coordination" for the next twenty-four hours, including driving, operating heavy machinery, using power tools, cooking, climbing, or riding a bicycle. Swimming, baths, and hot tub use should be avoided. The policy also advises patients not to make important decisions such as signing contracts or making expensive purchases or important commitments for the ensuing twenty-four hours.

It may be appropriate to discharge an intoxicated but alert patient home. At issue is who accompanies the patient and the type of supervision than can be expected at home (a sober adult). A distinction exists between alcohol intoxication and impairment. Intoxication refers to the clinical state of intoxication due to ingestion, whereas impairment involves the diminished ability to do various tasks. Patients may be impaired, yet not obviously intoxicated. Failure of the physician to advise patients not to drive or operate machinery after obtaining a serum alcohol level creates the potential for medico legal liability. For this reason, some recommend explicit and well-documented instructions be provided to alcohol-induced impaired patients, just as one would for head-injured patients.

Generally speaking, there is no legal requirement to report drug or alcohol use/abuse in ED patients. Mandatory reporting of substance use in pregnancy, as was adopted in Florida in 1987, resulted in discrepancies such that black women were ten times more likely to be reported than whites. This racial difference persisted even with a comparison of public versus private health care. The results demonstrate the preconception that substance abuse, especially in pregnancy, is a problem affecting minority groups, urban populations, and lower socioeconomic groups, which biases physicians in identifying substance exposure.

MINORS AND THE LAW

At times, minors may become involved with infractions of the law. Although it is clear that some infractions must be reported, such as acts of violence involving a weapon, others may not be so clear. In general, activities such as underage consumption of alcohol may be handled by the minor's guardian. Underage drinking by adults over the age of eighteen, but under the legal drinking age is not uncommon. Research demonstrates that more than 80 percent of college students drink alcohol, and almost 50 percent report binge drinking in the past two weeks. Some universities have developed programs to assist students who engage in underage consumption who may be at risk for developing a drinking problem. Mandatory alcohol evaluation for students identified as problem drinkers may be the best solution to address this issue. In one study, lower rates of binge drinking were found at colleges in areas with greater numbers of laws regarding underage drinking.

In situations in which child abuse or neglect is suspected, appropriate reporting to child protection agencies is warranted.

TREATMENT OF CRIMINALS, SUSPECTS, AND PRISONERS

As always, the physician's duty is to the patient, even when that patient is in police custody. As discussed earlier, patient confidentiality is of utmost importance. Furthermore, the physician should demonstrate respect for the patient as a person, despite the patient's legal status.

Concomitantly, it is the physician's duty to maintain a safe environment for ED staff, as well as for visitors and patients. Prisoners may require hand or ankle cuffs or other restraints to ensure the safety of others. At times, violent patients may need to be subdued. Subjects who do not respond to verbal calming and de-escalation techniques require pharmacologic treatment for agitation. Use of sedative agents may help facilitate adequate physical control. Pharmacological intervention in the violent or unruly patient, such as the use of benzodiazepines, dissociative agents (such as ketamine), and butyrophenones (such as haloperidol) may be necessary. Bear in mind, however, that such interventions should never be used as a means of punishment or for staff convenience.

The physician may be called upon to treat patients in whom tasers, stun guns, or other electrical control devices have been utilized by law enforcement or security personnel. The physician must ensure that the patient is not harmed by such interventions. Patients in a state of excited delirium or psychosis present a significant challenge to the ED staff. Treatment for agitation, hyperthermia, acidosis, rhabdomyolysis, and hyperkalemia must be initiated where appropriate. Again, it is the physician's duty to maintain a safe environment for all those in the ED.

At times, law enforcement personnel may accompany a suspect to the ED but release the individual on his or her own recognizance, with a summons to appear in court to face charges. In such a case, the onus is on the patient (or his or her insurance company) to pay for the ED visit, rather than on the law enforcement agency. This practice is ethically questionable because the patient may be unable to afford to pay for his or her care. In cases where the patient is not impaired by drugs, alcohol, or a medical condition, he or she may refuse care under such circumstances. However, if there is cause for the physician to be concerned that the patient is unable to provide informed consent, appropriate care should be provided in light of this fact.

NONINTERFERENCE WITH MEDICAL CARE

Frequently, emergency staff will come in contact with victims and perpetrators of crime. Care must be taken by the physician and staff to preserve evidence whenever possible. In the case of death, the patient's hands should be bagged to preserve evidence that may be found on the skin or under the fingernails. Patients may also be swabbed at the bedside for ballistics evidence. Clothing should be preserved, with care taken to avoid cutting through entrance/exit wounds. Similarly, procedures such as chest tubes or thoracotomies should be performed without transecting wounds whenever possible. Protocols for documentation of photographic or recorded evidence should be followed, and these include proper patient identification and site and measurement of injuries. In addition, staff must be prepared to authenticate the evidence they collect and ensure that the chain of custody is intact when handing it over to law enforcement authorities. It is essential, however, that evidence collection does not interfere with life-saving interventions.

The sexual assault examination may be conducted by a physician, but frequently a specially trained nurse performs the Sexual Assault Nurse Exam (SANE). In this case, the physician's role may be more limited. Rather than provide documentation of the SANE, the physician may be asked to prescribe medications, such as antibiotics for possible sexually transmitted infection exposure or emergency contraception. In addition, the physician may address any injuries that may have occurred. When conducting the sexual assault exam, standardized kits often are employed. The physician and staff should follow the instructions to the letter and ensure that proper chain of custody is followed.

Medical personnel are mandated reporters for suspected child abuse/neglect, elder abuse (in some states), interpartner violence (in some states), and assault with a deadly weapon (e.g. knives and guns). There may be no mandate to report injury due to punching or kicking in some states where abuse, interpartner violence, or assault are not suspected. However, if the victim of a crime wishes to report it, the ED staff should assist the victim in whatever way they can.

Drug and alcohol abuse are not reportable unless the patient poses a danger to self or others. A drug overdose may qualify in some instances. As discussed in earlier, minors under the influence of drugs and alcohol may be a reportable offence.

At times during the course of treatment the ED staff may discover that the patient is in possession of controlled substances or weapons. Institutions such as hospitals and psychiatric facilities may implement regulations regarding possession and confiscation of these items to ensure the safety of patients and staff members. Fourth Amendment protection against unreasonable search does not apply to searches conducted by private individuals, so this protection does not apply to searches conducted by staff of a private facility. Weapons and controlled substances should be secured either by hospital security or the police. Physicians, nurses, and other nonsecurity personnel should not take it upon themselves to disarm a patient who might escalate to violence.

In the absence of an arrest or search warrant, law enforcement personnel may not retain confiscated items. In the ED, such items may be returned to the individual upon discharge, with appropriate caveats. Hospital policy may allow for continued holding of weapons and controlled substances during a patient's hospitalization. Most facilities do not want their staff to destroy controlled substances themselves under the worry that the substances may not actually be destroyed. Law enforcement will usually accept custody of illegal substances but not legal intoxicants such as alcohol. Hospital staff may choose to dispose of intoxicating beverages rather than accept the liability of returning such substances to the patient on discharge. Some have recommended that law enforcement, when taking possession of controlled substances, not be given any identifying information about the patient. However, there is case law that allows for discovery of illicit substances in public areas or in plain sight, which can result in criminal charges against the patient. Such cases hinge on the expectation of privacy that patients may or may not enjoy in treatment areas of the ED.

Patients who are released after psychiatric hold and for whom there are safety concerns should not have weapons returned to them. Reasons for not returning a patient's personal effects should be documented in the clinical record. However, such items may be returned to the patient's relative, guardian, advocate, or representative who assumes responsibility for the safe keeping of potentially harmful items.

An estimated 11.2 million undocumented immigrants reside in the United States. Illegal immigration (uncodumented persons) status is not reportable, and hospitals legally cannot discriminate between illegal immigrants and citizens. Furthermore, only the federal government and its agents are in a position to enforce immigration law. Patients brought in by border patrol agents following a failed attempt at illegal entry to the United States should be treated as is medically appropriate. Patients who do not require hospitalization may be released to boarder patrol agents, if such agents have retained custody of the patient in the ED. It is not the physician's responsibility to report or detain undocumented persons. The ACEP opposes federal and state initiatives that require physicians and health care facilities to refuse care to undocumented persons or to report suspected undocumented persons to immigration authorities.

Under the federal Emergency Medical Treatment and Active Labor Act (EMTALA), hospitals are required to provide (1) a medical screening examination to determine the type of care needed and (2), based on the evaluation, treatment to stabilize patients with an emergency condition. Studies have shown that undocumented immigrants are less likely to seek medical attention due to fear of their immigration status being discovered. As a result, such patients do not avail themselves of preventive services and may delay seeking care until their condition has worsened. Chronic medical conditions such as cancer therapies and renal dialysis cannot be provided under the EMTALA provision. This means that although a patient's condition may be stabilized in the ED, the undocumented person has few financial resources for long-term treatment and intervention in the United States. Many immigrants also face language barriers and may be wary of providing identifying information to health care workers.

Under the Affordable Care Act of 2010, U.S. citizens must purchase health insurance or pay a penalty. However, the individual mandate and additional care provided by the resulting increased pool of insured patients is not applicable to undocumented persons. Legal immigrants who have lived in the United States for less than five years also cannot qualify for Medicaid. Although undocumented persons cannot be covered by Medicaid, the state-federal health insurance program for the poor reimburses hospitals for delivering emergency treatment to illegal immigrants. Federal Disproportionate Share Hospital (DSH) funds are tied to the percentage of the hospital's emergency patients not qualifying for Medicaid, the number of uninsured patients it serves, and the number of illegal immigrants cared for in the ED. The Medicare Modernization Act of 2003, Section 1011, included $250 million per year between 2005 and 2008 to help pay for emergency care for undocumented patients. Unfortunately, as more hospitals ask to be repaid from a limited pool of money, each receives less reimbursement. Furthermore, under the Affordable Care Act, 75 percent of DSH funds have been cut. Some fear that hospitals in financial trouble will cut uncompensated nonemergency medical services or even refuse to treat undocumented persons and opt to pay a potential fine instead.

Some medical ethicists argue that denying care to undocumented persons constitutes a violation of autonomy because the decision to accept or refuse care is taken out of the patient's hands. Physicians, they argue, have the professional obligation to treat those in need (the bioethical principle of beneficence). Conversely, others argue that providing care to undocumented persons takes resources away from citizens and people who have entered the United States legally, thus violating the principle of justice. Viewing moral codes from the perspective of the physician–patient relationship ignores the greater interests of society. Those who defend limiting expenditures on undocumented patients point out that the interests of other members of the community are violated by the resulting lack of resources.

The ACEP Code of Ethics states:

> Emergency Medical Treatment and Active Labor Act (EMTALA), has established access to quality emergency care as an individual right that should be available to all who seek it. Recognizing that emergency care makes a substantial contribution to personal well-being, emergency physicians endorse this right and support the universal access to emergency care. Denial of emergency care or delay in providing emergency services on the basis of race, religion, sexual orientation, real or perceived gender identity, ethnic background, social status, type of illness or injury, or ability to pay is unethical. Emergency physicians should act

as advocates for the health needs of indigent patients, assisting them in finding appropriate care. Insurers, including managed care organizations, must support insured patients' access to emergency medical care for what a prudent layperson would reasonably perceive as an emergency medical condition. Society, through its political process, must adequately fund emergency care for all who need it.

Ultimately, resource allocation decisions are made more appropriately at the policy level than at the level of an individual physician–patient encounter. Although the patient's best interests are the emergency physician's primary concern, medically nonbeneficial testing or treatment is not morally required. Hence, the emergency physician should allocate resources prudently while honoring his or her ethical duty to the patient.

ETHICS TAKEOUT TIPS

- The physician's first duty is to the patient. Physicians should adhere to HIPAA regulations in disclosing a patient's medical information.
- The physician's duty to treat entails respect for the patient as a person, even when in police custody or detained due to immigration status.
- Physicians must ensure the safety of patients and staff. Violent patients may be subdued using physical and/or chemical means where appropriate. Such interventions should not be a form of retribution.
- Weapons and contraband should be secured by trained hospital staff and/or law enforcement agents. Return of weapons is permissible if the patient does not pose a threat. Drugs and contraband are the purview of law enforcement.
- Most states mandate a duty of physicians to warn individuals who are threatened by a patient in their care. This does not extend to nonspecific threats of violence.
- Neurologically impaired drivers, those receiving procedural sedation, and intoxicated patients should be warned not to drive or operate machinery.
- Intoxication and drug ingestion generally are not reportable. Some patients may be sent home with a responsible adult where appropriate.
- Practitioners should attempt to preserve evidence of a crime whenever possible and follow documentation guidelines. Preservation of the chain of evidence is essential.

- Specially trained staff (Sexual Assault Nurse Examiners) may conduct the examination after sexual assault.
- Child abuse, elder abuse, and interpartner violence should be reported as per state law.
- Immigration status is not reportable. Resource allocation decisions are best made at the policy level than at the level of an individual patient–physician encounter.

FOR FURTHER READING

American College of Emergency Physicians. (1998). Clinical policy for procedural sedation and analgesia in the emergency department, *Annals of Emergency Medicine*, 31, 663–677.

Berger, J. T., Rosner, F., Kark, P., & Bennett, A. J. (2000). Reporting by physicians of impaired drivers and potentially impaired drivers. *Journal of General Internal Medicine*, 15(9), 667–672.

Berlinger, N., & Raghavan, R. (2013). The ethics of advocacy for undocumented patients. *Hastings Center Report*, 43(1), 14–17.

Chasnoff, I. J., Landress, H. J., & Barrett, M. E. (1990). The prevalence of illicit-drug or alcohol use during pregnancy and discrepancies in mandatory reporting in Pinellas County, Florida. *New England Journal of Medicine*, 322(17), 1202–1206.

Kelen, G. D., Catlett, C. L., Kubit, J. G., & Hsieh Y. H. (2012). Hospital-based shootings in the United States: 2000 to 2011. *Annals of Emergency Medicine*, 60(6), 790–798.

National Conference of State Legislatures. (2013). *Mental health professionals' duty to warn.* //www.ncsl.org/research/health/mental-health-professionals-duty-to-warn.aspx

National Institute on Alcohol Abuse and Alcoholism. (2013). *College drinking.* http://pubs.niaaa.nih.gov/publications/CollegeFactSheet/CollegeFactSheet.pdf

Petit, J. R. (2005). Management of the acutely violent patient. *Psychiatric Clinics of North America*, 28, 701–711.

Rocca, P., Villari, V., & Bogetto, F. (2006). Managing the aggressive and violent patient in the psychiatric emergency. *Progress in Neuro-Psychopharmacology and Biological Psychiatry*, 30, 586–598.

Simel, D. L., & Feussner, J. R. (1989). Does determining serum alcohol concentrations in emergency department patients influence physicians' civil suit liability? *Archives of Internal Medicine*, 149, 1016–1018.

Simel, D. L., & Feussner, J. (1990). Driving-impaired patients leaving the emergency department: The problem of inadequate instructions. *Annals of Internal Medicine*, 112, 365–370.

Sultan, B. (2014). The domestic and international ethical debate on rationing care of illegal immigrants. *Voices in Bioethics*, April 1.

Tarasoff v. Regents of the University of California, 17 Cal.3d 425, 131 Cal. Rptr 14, 551 P2d 334 (1976).

U.S. Department of Health and Human Services. (n.d.). *Summary of the HIPPA privacy rule.* www.hhs.gov/ocr/privacy/hipaa/understanding/summary/index. html

Wechsler, H., Lee, J. E., Nelson, T. F., & Kuo, M. (2002). Underage college students' drinking behavior, access to alcohol, and the influence of deterrence policies: Findings from the Harvard School of Public Health College alcohol study. *Journal of American College Health, 50*(5), 223–236.

12

Research Ethics

LAUREN M. SAUER, MSC, RICHARD E. ROTHMAN, MD, PHD,
AND GABOR D. KELEN, MD

RESEARCH ETHICS IN EMERGENCY MEDICINE

The nature of emergency medical practice presents distinct ethical challenges both for clinical care and research. Because emergency medicine remains a relatively young specialty, it does not yet have a long historical tradition to address all the unique ethical precepts inherent to human subjects investigations conducted in this setting. Understanding basic broad principles of the ethics of research relevant to studies conducted in acute care settings, as well as the growing body of experiences of investigators in our field, however, serves as a useful framework for emergency medicine investigators.

WHY IS ETHICAL RESEARCH IMPORTANT?

The need for an ethical framework to guide research is based on a fundamental principle that human dignity and autonomy should be respected. In the past, novice researchers primarily learned the basic ethical principles of research from seasoned mentors, absorbing their practices and habits without the benefit of standardized processes or pathways. History warns us, however, that without a structured code the conduct of research is susceptible to harm of subjects, either human or animal. In fact, it is the callousness toward subjects throughout history, some in very modern times, that has shaped the current framework for ethical conduct of research.

Historical Context

One of the greatest advances in human research over the past hundred years was the international dissemination of the Nuremburg Code, established in 1947, in response to the horrific offenses of the Nazis under the guise of "research." This code advanced several fundamental ethical research principles, most importantly, the need for voluntary consent of human subjects. The World Medical Association's *Declaration of Helsinki*, first issued in 1964 and most recently revised in 2013, remains as one of the most relevant documents for the governance of the conduct of research. The document reinforced the basic principles of biomedical research articulated in the Nuremburg Code, articulating several key provisions including:

1. The goal of research or societal priority can never take precedence over the rights and interests of individual research subjects.
2. Participation (or declining to participate) in research must not put patients/subjects at a disadvantage with respect to medical care.
3. Research requires the consideration and guidance of an independent committee.[1]

Further regulation resulted from several watershed studies conducted between 1960 and 1980 that forever changed the manner in which clinical research is overseen and conducted. These events include the Tuskegee Syphilis Study, the Willowbrook Study, and the Jewish Chronic Disease Hospital Case. Each brought to light the need to codify ethical conventions in research (see Table 12.1). The Tuskegee Syphilis Study in particular was at least partially responsible for the enactment of the National Research Act of 1974 by the 93rd Congress of the United States. This act created the National Commission for the Protection of Human Subjects of Biomedical and Behavioral Research, charged with developing human subjects-related public policy, and was ultimately responsible for the landmark Belmont Report.

The Belmont Report, published in 1979, provides a broad ethical framework for experimentation on human subjects. The framework stressed three ethical principles: respect for persons, beneficence, and justice. These principles, along with requirement for personal and professional responsibility, still guide ethical research today. Sound personal and professional decision-making is the foundation for the conduct of ethical research; it guides appropriate research methodology, protects the safety and welfare of research subjects, and safeguards the validity of reported outcomes. Additionally, it ensures the continued trust of the public in research and researchers, which is critical to continued improvements in medical care.

---

[1] The modern Institutional Review Board (IRB).

TABLE 12.1. *Unethical human subjects studies examples*

Tuskegee Syphilis Experiment
A study conducted by the U.S. Public Health Service between 1932 and 1972 researching
   the natural progression of untreated syphilis in rural, impoverished African
   American men from Macon, Alabama. The study subjects were promised free health
   care, meals, and insurance and kept uninformed about both their condition and
   alternatives to care for their syphilis.

Willowbrook Hepatitis Studies
Multiple studies conducted on mentally disabled children with hepatitis between 1955
   and 1970 at a state-run institution for disabled children in Staten Island, New York.
   Children at Willowbrook were deliberately exposed to hepatitis, were exposed
   naturally to hepatitis, and were not fully informed of the risks of participation in the
   studies.

Jewish Chronic Disease Hospital Case
A series of studies conducted on chronically and mostly mentally ill patients at the
   Jewish Chronic Disease Hospital in 1963 attempting to understand how the spread of
   cancer was impacted by a weakened immune system. Participants were exposed to
   live cancer cells without consent in order to understand how otherwise-healthy
   bodies fight off malignant cancer cells.

ETHICAL PRINCIPLES GUIDING RESEARCH

Respect for persons is the concept stating that all people deserve the right to
fully exercise their autonomy and that persons with diminished capacity
for autonomy are entitled to protection.

Through the concept of autonomy, study participants are guaranteed rights when they agree to participate in a research study. Through
the process of informed consent, potential subjects are given the information necessary to make a determination regarding their own willful
participation. It is important to note that informed consent is not
simply a document or form that needs to be signed or acknowledged,
but is instead a critical process that continues from initial interaction
with a potential subject through to the completion of participation in
the study. Consent may be changed or withdrawn at any time, without
consequence, and is a mandatory essential component of ethical
research.

Beneficence speaks to the risk–benefit analysis of the study or
research, or balancing of the risk to the participant with the benefit
to the participant or society. This balance is not consistently easy to

determine. However, the investigator is obliged to make every effort to detail the foreseeable risks and benefits for the participant. Such knowledge allows the potential subject to weigh the risks with the benefit to self and, where applicable, to society. Beneficence also addresses the responsibility of the investigator to make every effort to design the study in favor of the benefits while diminishing risks to participants as much as possible.

Justice, the third principle voiced in the Belmont Report, speaks to the just distribution of benefits, burdens, and harms of the research. Fundamentally, given the risks, research should engage the population for whom the benefit is envisioned. Additionally, this precept is understood to indicate that study subjects should be drawn from an appropriate representation of the population intended to ultimately benefit. Important characteristics in this regard may include ethnicity, race, gender/sex, socioeconomic status, age, comorbidities, or other potential subject attributes relevant to the area of study.

INSTITUTIONAL REVIEW BOARDS

Tasked with monitoring research activities for appropriate application of the three essential principles, institutional review boards (IRBs) are independent groups whose primary function is to guide protection of the welfare of human subjects. The National Research Act of 1974, noted earlier, required the establishment of IRBs at the local level and mandated review of all federally funded research involving human subjects. The *Common Rule*, the short name for the Federal Policy for the Protection of Human Subjects, was adopted by a number of federal agencies in 1991. Through Title 45 of the Code of Federal Regulations Part 46, the U.S. Food and Drug Administration (FDA) established IRB procedures to carry out the federal mandate. The FDA and the Department of Health and Human Services (DHHS), through the office for Human Research Protection, have empowered IRBs with responsibility for oversight of any research conducted on humans. Local IRB committees are accordingly tasked with reviewing initial protocols, guiding informed consent process, and weighing the benefits of the study against the risks. IRB committees are also responsible for reviewing adverse events (even if judged insignificant), with the onus to report on the investigator, and for making decisions about the continuation of the study and/or modification of the study protocol or procedures as the risks and benefits are better perceived during the actual conduct of the study.

INFORMED CONSENT

In most instances of human subjects research, informed consent will be obtained from all participants. According to CFR 45, "no investigator may involve a human being as a subject in research covered by this policy unless the investigator has obtained the legally effective informed consent of the subject or the subject's legally authorized representative." There are several components of appropriate, valid, and comprehensive informed consent (see Box 12.1). Potential research participants must be as informed to extent possible of (1) the foreseeable risks, even if of low likelihood; (2) benefits; (3) nature of the research; and (4) alternatives to enrollment in the research protocol. Additional requirements include language that permits subjects to withdraw from the study at any point without bearing on their medical care and an explanation of protocols and procedures should participants suffer an adverse event and who to contact if they have any questions under any circumstances.

BOX 12.1. *Valid informed consent components*

- Explanation that the study involves research
- Description of the nature, purpose, expected duration, and experimental components
- Expected or foreseeable risks and discomforts
- Benefits to individual, others, or general population
- Description of alternatives to participation
- Assurance that personal information will be held in confidence
- Compensation/reimbursement of costs information
- Information on handling of adverse events or harm due to or during participation
- Information on who to contact with questions or concerns related to any aspect of the study
- Statement that participation is voluntary and without consequence for nonparticipation or withdrawal from the study at any time
- Documentation of participant's (or surrogate) consent
- No exculpatory language waiving participant's legal rights

Summary of information from 21 CFR 50.25

ALTERNATES TO STANDARD CONSENT

There are specific instances in which standard, written, informed consent may not be required or is unobtainable and yet the research can still be undertaken. In general, this includes two scenarios: (1) when obtaining written consent is not appropriate or impractical and (2) for certain emergency research, in which case standard consent is not feasible because of a life-threatening medical condition requiring an urgent intervention. The first assertion applies to situations where there is no more than minimal risk to the participant *and* where obtaining written consent is either not practical (or would detract from the study due to introduction of potential biases). Oral consent may, in certain instances, better protect the interests of the participants. For example, in some studies, obtaining written consent may introduce identifiers to the study that would otherwise not have been collected. In low-literacy study populations, written consent may undermine the relationship of trust between the researcher and the study participant, whereas oral consent may actually strengthen it. Oral consent must still contain all the required components of the consent process (Box 12.1); however, the actual consent is verbal and the participant is often given an unsigned document with the same key study details as written consent would entail.

The second assertion, emergency research, is directly germane to the field of emergency research and allied fields of disaster health. Emergency research enrolment protocols address subjects whose condition precludes traditional informed consent in real-time prior to initiating a research protocol. There are numerous instances in which it has been determined that there is critical value in studying the potential efficacy of life-saving or other clinical interventions, but study subjects may not be able to consent due to the nature of their condition. Still, however well-intentioned or of potential importance, the ethical question raised is whether such research should be conducted at all because it violates a key ethical precept of ensuring individual autonomy. The distinguishing feature of emergency research without consent is that autonomy is not being removed from the participant by the nature of the research or researcher, but rather autonomy was removed prior to their potential enrollment. Several excellent examples of this type of research have been well-described in our field.

Implied consent is a long-standing practice in the health care setting for patients who are incapacitated, in need of a life-saving intervention, and cannot provide consent. Although it seems as though this would be a straightforward extension to the conduct of emergency research, it is not.

"Implied consent" is a nonresearch concept allowing medical treatment and management by qualified individuals in situations where obtaining written or oral consent is not possible. In contradistinction, the concept of emergency research without consent is restricted to research protocols only and is independent of any implied need of treatment.

The following two alternatives (waiver of informed consent and deferred consent) to the standard informed consent process may be considered in emergency research or other settings in which informed consent is not obtainable.

Waiver of Informed Consent

A waiver of informed consent may be issued for specific cases of emergency or resuscitation research under strict guidelines from the FDA and DHHS. In 1996, the FDA Final Rule for Waiver of Informed Consent was issued to provide regulations for proceeding with emergency research with a waiver of informed consent.'

There are multiple specific and narrow criteria required for conducting research with a waiver of informed consent (Box 12.2). It is important to note that the federal guidelines regarding emergency research do not supersede any state laws on the subject. IRBs are tasked with the responsibility of knowing and interpreting state laws on the subject of emergency research prior to granting waivers.

BOX 12.2. *Criteria for waiver of informed consent*

1. Participants must be in a life-threatening situation requiring immediate intervention.
2. Clinical equipoise must exist (i.e. the research must be operating with a null hypothesis).
3. Collection of data on the intervention must be necessary to determine safety and efficacy.
4. Consent is not feasible, either from the patient or appropriate legal surrogate.
5. There is no way to pre-identify potential participants.
6. Participation in the research may directly benefit the participant.
7. The research could not practicably be carried out without the waiver (i.e. study with consent is not practical).

In addition to the listed steps, there are several practical steps that local IRBs may require researchers to address prior to permitting a waiver of informed consent.

Community Consultation, Consent, and Public Disclosure

Often, the local IRB may deem it appropriate for the investigator to discuss research aims directly with the community on which the researcher intends to focus the investigation in order to gain a better understanding of concerns, assess potential barriers, and solicit their input. There are several different ways to approach community consultation. It should be noted, however, that community consultation is not synonymous with consent itself.

Community consultation is directed at the local level, which may influence the approach appropriate for a given project. The nature of the study may help further refine the population of interest. Community engagement forums includes town hall or public forum meetings, call-in talk shows (radio and television), focus groups within the community supported by community leadership, random digit dialing to solicit feedback from a representative sample of individuals, or booths at local health fairs. Social media may provide an excellent means of assuring representative community engagement. If the specific targeted group is not accessible in the local community, the investigator may consider alternate surrogate or representative communities where the study population of interested is appropriately represented.

Findings from the community should be determined prior to engagement. Indeed, community consultation is assumed to be a dialogue (i.e. a two-way communication) and advisory to the IRB, and it should be structured as such. It is not intended to be an explanation of importance or of why the study must take place.

Community consent occurs after community consultation and, critically, does not waive the necessity for informed, individual consent. Although not a mandatory step in obtaining waiver of consent for emergency research, community consent often is used as a means for community leadership to permit researcher access to the community by consenting on their behalf. However, in most instances, another method of or alternative to informed consent will be sought.

In addition to community consultation, the FDA recommends that community consultation should include public disclosure of the research program for all approved emergency research. Public disclosure is essentially informing the general public that the research is or will be taking place without standard informed consent. The disclosure must summarize the research, including researcher contact information, a study timeline, location, study population, risks and benefits, alternatives, a discussion of the reasoning for exception to informed consent, and opt-out pathways if appropriate. Following completion of the study, public disclosure includes informing the community of the termination of the study and the results of the research, both positive and negative.

Deferred Consent

Deferred consent is an approved alternative means of obtaining consent after enrollment for those studies in which prospective informed consent is not possible. The process of deferred consent, also known as *retrospective consent*, involves obtaining consent from the participants after they are lucid or from a legal representative who can be identified after the subject has been enrolled and received a treatment or intervention. For longitudinal studies, if possible, the subject should be consented prior to continuation of the intervention or treatment. For minimal-risk studies, such as request for use of excess sample, deferred consent may be an alternative option to obtaining consent when written informed consent was not an option at the time the participant was present in the emergency department (ED). Ultimate agreement to participate may prove challenging in deferred consent studies but has still been shown to be an effective strategy.

Independent Data Monitoring

Because of the vulnerable populations involved in emergency research and the seriousness of the research itself, all emergency research studies using a waiver of informed consent must have an independent data monitoring committee. It is the responsibility of this committee to oversee study implementation and advise both the study sponsor (if applicable) and the investigator regarding the conduct of the investigation.

SPECIAL AND VULNERABLE POPULATIONS

One of the most challenging aspects of conducting research in the emergency medicine setting is that the ED population is arguably inherently vulnerable. Vulnerability is neither defined by nor dependent solely on medical condition or severity of illness, but ultimately is related to a clinician's finding of questionable or diminished autonomy. Patients seeking ED care may be in pain, in crisis, suffering from altered sensorium, or otherwise lack decision-making capacity at the time or their ED visit, which may create or enhance vulnerability. Failure of the investigator to properly consider that the target population of the research may include vulnerable members will essentially render obtained consent invalid. Most IRBs and research grant agencies compel investigators to address whether vulnerable populations are included in the study and, if so, define the approach for assessing capacity and obtaining consent.

Table 12.2 details populations generally accepted as vulnerable for the purposes of research. Note that despite this assertion, the ED as a setting is not included in the definition or examples of vulnerable populations. However, virtually all ED patients are likely to fall under one of the rubrics, thus requiring the ED investigators consideration in the design and conduct of the study

ETHICAL CONDUCT IN EMERGENCY MEDICINE RESEARCH

Research misconduct is defined as fabrication, falsification, or plagiarism in proposing, performing, or reviewing research or in reporting research results according to 42 CFR Part 93. It does not include inadvertent error, differences of opinion, interpretations, or judgments of data. Public trust in medicine is based on the integrity of the underlying research. Even unintentional error may lead to erosion in public trust of medical practice or public health measures.

One of the most impactful recent occurrences of research misconduct involved Andrew Wakefield who, in order to perpetrate an elaborate fraud, willfully falsified data implying a link between the mumps, measles, rubella (MMR) vaccine and autism. This small study of only twelve children, published in *The Lancet* in 1998, was widely reported in the lay media. Although since retracted, the public damage continues through to today.

Relationship between Investigator and Subjects

A particular situation that the emergency medicine investigator should be aware of relates to the duality of roles that is present when the investigator is also the treating physician. However unintended, the physician-investigator dyad potentiates undue influence. Modern IRBs are highly vigilant for this situation and will assist in determining the appropriateness of

TABLE 12.2. *Vulnerable populations*

Population Type	
Examples	Special Considerations
Cognitive/Communicative	
Children, infants, mentally ill or cognitive impairment, intoxicated, gravely ill, non-English speakers	May lack capacity to consent; may require designee; may not fully understand consent language
Institutional or Deferential	
Students, prisoners, patients, elderly, children	May be unduly influenced by caretaker, provider, custodian, or guardian; may agree to participate to avoid returning to custody
Medical	
Patients in severe pain, terminally ill, pregnant	May lack ability to weigh risks and benefits; may have short-term cognitive impairment due to medical condition
Economic	
Impoverished or low-income, individuals without access to health care or underinsured	May be influenced by excessive inducement, may not appropriately weight benefits against risks
Social	
Minorities, disease populations, domestic abuse victims	Participation may result in social stigmatization or other undue consequences

physician as investigator. There are ways to mitigate the potential for undue influence, such as having an impartial assistant (e.g. a study coordinator) obtain consent from the subject/patient possibly removed from the treatment area.

Safety and Welfare of Subjects

The safety and welfare of the study subject(s) must be the highest priority for the researcher. Researchers should make every effort to identify potential risks and adverse events that may impact their study population. Adverse events may occur in any study, even when all ethical and regulatory guidelines are followed. Investigators are obliged to have protocols in place a priori to address how adverse events will be categorized and handled should they occur. Participants must be informed of the process for dealing with injury or adverse events as part of the informed consent process. Adverse events are an expected component of clinical research and do *not* constitute research misconduct; however, misconduct has occurred if the researcher hides, ignores, or avoids reporting these events to the IRB, even if the researcher judged the adverse event as minor, temporary, or believed he or she was acting in the best interest of the participants.

Another important aspect of human subjects protections is that, with few exceptions, study subjects cannot be deceived about the purpose of the research in which they are participating. Deception includes absence of full disclosure to a potential study participant. Deception in research undermines trust between the public and researchers and jeopardizes the integrity of the informed consent process. Should a study, by the nature of the research, require deception, alternative approaches to address the question must be sought, and only if no other methodology is feasible can deception even be considered as a valid approach. Importantly, all studies using deception must reveal the true nature of the study once concluded.

Data Interpretation

One area that can often lead to ethical misconduct is data analysis and interpretation. Whereas intentional fraud such as fabricating, deleting, or falsifying data is a rather clear-cut ethical violation, there are less clear violations as well. For example, selective representation or inclusion of data that can result in a predetermined or desired outcome is inappropriate and can significantly impact future research and outcomes. Thus, investigator vigilance to appropriate data usage and interpretation is critical.

Authorship

Once a study has concluded, the next step is to disseminate results of the research through publication of a manuscript. In the absence of advanced planning, potential ethical dilemmas may arise regarding authorship. The International Committee of Medical Journal Editors offers a set of accepted guidelines for appropriate crediting. Although these recommendations are not all-inclusive and not always followed, they are guidelines for standardization of authorship in the medical literature.

Two issues are traditionally the most contentious: the inclusion and exclusion of authors and the appropriate order of authorship. In the modern era, credited authors should have contributed intellectually to the study or the actual drafting of the manuscript. Extensive involvement in the conduct of the study, as may occur with assistants, students, and others in and of itself, does not by itself qualify for authorship, and it is considered unethical to include such individuals in the authorship roster. More easily understood is the failure to include participants among the authorship group who have provided true intellectual input into the study. This may occur when students or residents are part of the research team. Order of authorship can be quite controversial, especially in a mentor–mentee relationship. Typically, the first author position goes to the person responsible for the majority of writing of the major draft(s), regardless of seniority. However, the senior investigator does have the ability to mentor or oversee the writing of the manuscript and retain the first author position, as long as the order of the authorship is made clear prior to writing. Recently, many journals have permitted dual first authorship, which can mitigate potential conflicts.

Conflict of Interest and Research Sponsorship

In theory, ethical research should be performed without any secondary or competing interest and without any predetermined outcome expectation. In practice, this can be challenging, especially in the clinical environment. Researcher dollars are increasingly sparse, and funded investigators may feel pressured to report research results that are favorable to sponsors. Even if not intentional, researchers can interpret study results in a sponsor-preferred manner; thus, various blinding techniques should be used in all aspects of the study to ensure that the process is objective and free from biases from beginning to end. Furthermore, potential conflicts of interest should be disclosed when reporting results.

EVOLVING AREAS OF EMERGENCY MEDICINE RESEARCH

Although the foundational ethical principles in any area of emergency medicine research are the same, evolving subspecialties and disciplines carry their own unique ethical dilemmas. This section examines a few emerging areas of emergency medicine research that may have distinctive ethical issues. The issues listed here are not comprehensive but may give insight into the challenging path to conducting ethical research in these evolving disciplines.

Disaster Medicine

Much like ED populations, disaster populations are inherently vulnerable, and their study must take this into consideration. In addition to the vulnerability of the population, the environment in which disaster research is undertaken may be chaotic, stressful, and dangerous. Historically, breakdown in ethical conduct in disaster setting has been more frequently related to investigator(s) carelessness or lack of awareness, rather than to willful misconduct. The environment in which disaster research is conducted may actually foster the disregard for following standard ethical precepts. Given that disasters usually occur with no notice or occur in unpredictable locals, there is often need for rapid deployment of research resources for effective study. As such, typical IRB review and approval are not always possible. In light of this, emergency IRBs such as the Public Health Emergency Research Review Board (PHERRB) and local rapid response IRBs have been put in place to address real-time decisions associated with the need for rapidly developed human subjects protocols.

Low-resource and International Emergency Medicine

Several unique issues arise when considering emergency medicine research in low-resource and certain international settings. For example, the country or local jurisdiction may or may not have its own IRB or equivalent. Although not a research ethical issue in and of itself, in some settings, nonscientific agents of the host government serve as de facto IRBs, and their approval will need to be procured. There may be language or other cultural barriers to obtaining true informed consent. As important as the research may be for future preparedness, there may be no benefit whatsoever to the population studied. Research methods and goals may conflict with local cultural norms or be otherwise inappropriate or insensitive, and the researcher should consider how population will be impacted following the conclusion of the research. For example, a clinical intervention may require long-term follow-up care once the study is complete, and the population's medical infrastructure may not be able to support this. The Council for International Organizations of Medical Sciences provides guidelines for the conduct of research in low-resource settings. The guiding principles stated are that the research should be responsive to the needs and priorities of the population and that the outcome of the research should intend to benefit the population or community studied. This latter tenet is in distinction to accepted research conduct in well-resourced settings, where research is considered appropriate even if it only benefits society at large.

CONCLUSION

Scientists are charged with upholding the public's trust through the appropriate and ethical conduct of research. Nowhere is this more important than in emergency medicine, a setting with opportunities for conducting clinically important research, but also one with considerable challenges. ED populations are inherently vulnerable, and obtaining true informed consent can be particularly challenging in the emergency environment. Considered attention to the ethical precepts discussed in this chapter – some unique to emergency medicine – will facilitate the adoption of appropriate methods to ensure properly conducted research and avoidance of problems that may harbor misconduct.

ETHICS TAKEOUT TIPS

- Understanding the basic broad principles of the ethics of research and how they apply to acute care settings is critical.
- Research ethics has evolved from the outcomes of several sentinel events including:
  * The Nuremburg Trials of Nazi Germany and resulting Nuremburg Code
  * The World Medical Association's *Declaration of Helsinki*
  * The Tuskegee Syphilis Study
  * The Willowbrook Study
  * The Jewish Chronic Disease Hospital Case
  * The National Research Act of 1974
- Three main principles guide appropriate human subjects research:
  * *Autonomy* speaks to the guaranteed rights of subjects when they agree to participate in a research study.
  * *Beneficence* speaks to the risk–benefit analysis of the study or research or to a balancing of the risk to the participant with the benefit to the participant or society.
  * *Justice* speaks to the just distribution of benefits, burdens, and harms of the research.
- IRBs govern the responsible and appropriate conduct of human subjects research.

- When conducting human subjects research, participants must be appropriately consented using the guidelines of CFR 45.
- When conducting research in situations where consent is not obtainable, researchers must obtain a waiver of informed consent, preapproved by their institution's IRB and following the guidelines of CFR 45.
- Special considerations must be given to vulnerable populations, of which ED patients are inherently part.
- Vulnerable populations include those:
  * Those with cognitive/communicative defects
  * Those who are institutionalized
  * Those in deferential relationships
  * Those with medical needs
  * Those with economic needs
  * Those with social needs
  * Those in dependent relationships
- Emergency medicine investigators should be aware of the duality of roles when the investigator is also the treating physician because the relationship may cause undue influence during consent.
- Researchers must be particularly careful to avoid ethical misconduct in data analysis and interpretation, must be vigilant to appropriate data usage, and must understand that interpretation is critical.
- The International Committee of Medical Journal Editors offers a set of accepted guidelines for authorship.

FOR FURTHER READING

Biros, M. H., Fish, S. S., & Lewis, R. J. (1999). Implementing the Food and Drug Administration's final rule for waiver of informed consent in certain emergency research circumstances. *Academic Emergency Medicine*, 6, 1272–1282.

Biros, M. H., Lewis, R. J., Olson, C. M., Runge, J. W., Cummins, R. O., & Frost, N. (1995). Informed consent in emergency research: Consensus statement from the Coalition Conference of Acute Resuscitation and Critical Care Researchers. *Journal of the American Medical Association*, 273(16), 1283–1287.

Emanuel, E. J., Grady, C. J., Crouch, R. A., Lie, R. K., Miller, F. G., & Wendler, D. D. (Eds.). (2008). *The Oxford textbook of clinical research ethics.* New York: Oxford University Press.

Fish, S. (1999). Research ethics in emergency medicine. *Emergency Medical Clinics of North America*, 17(2), 461–474.

Godlee, F., Smith, J., & Marcovitch, H. (2011). Wakefield's article linking MMR vaccine and autism was fraudulent. *British Medical Journal*, 342, 7452.

International Committee of Medical Journal Editors. (2014). *About the recommendations*. www.icmje.org/recommendations/browse/about-the-recommendations/

Council for International Organizations of Medical Sciences. (2002). *International ethical guidelines for biomedical research involving human subjects*. www.cioms.ch/publications/guidelines/guidelines_nov_2002_blurb.htm

Jesus, J. E., & Michael, G. E. (2009). Ethical considerations of research in disaster-stricken populations. *Prehospital and Disaster Medicine*, 24(2), 109–114.

National Research Act, H.R. 7724, Public Law 93–348, July 12, 1974, 42 U.S.C. 289: Public Health and Social Welfare, Statute 88, pp. 342–354. www.gpo.gov/fdsys/pkg/STATUTE-88/pdf/STATUTE-88-Pg342.pdf

The National Commission for the Protection of Human Subjects of Biomedical and Behavioral Research. (1979). *The Belmont Report: Ethical principles and guidelines for the protection of human subjects of research*. www.hhs.gov/ohrp/humansubjects/guidance/belmont.html

The Nuremburg Code: Regulations and ethical guidelines. www.research.buffalo.edu/rsp/irb/forms/Nuremberg_Code.pdf

U.S. Department of Health and Human Services, Food and Drug Administration. (2013). *Exceptions from informed consent requirements for emergency research* (21 CFR 50.24). Silver Spring, MD: Authors.

U.S. Department of Health and Human Services, Food and Drug Administration. (1996). Protection of human subjects: Informed consent and waiver of informed consent requirements in certain emergency circumstances: Final rule (45 CFR 46.101). Silver Spring, MD: Authors.

Ward, R., Krugman, S., Giles, J. P., Jacobs, A. M., & Bodansky, O. (1958). Infectious hepatitis – Studies of its natural history and prevention. *New England Journal of Medicine*, 258, 407–416.

World Medical Association. (n.d.). *World Medical Association Declaration of Helsinki – Ethical principles for medical research involving human subjects*. www.wma.net/en/30publications/10policies/b3/index.html

13

Conflicts of Interest

ERIKA NEWTON, MD, MPH, AND ADAM J. SINGER, MD

An Ancient Problem

A conflict of interest (COI) is a clash between two interests held
by an individual or institution wherein one interest threatens to
undermine advocacy or impartiality toward the other. COI has been
a source of concern and debate since ancient times. Plato's *Republic*
considered its political ramifications, while Hippocrates wrote of the
profit motive in medicine: "Any wisdom ... wherein works some
scientific method, is honourable if it be not tainted with base love of
gain and unseemliness."

COI in Medicine

In the United States, as in most places, physician earnings are largely
independent of the benefits that accrue to patients from effective medical care. Fee-for-service medicine, the dominant U.S. practice model,
creates a COI for physicians by enabling them to earn more by doing
more – for example, more procedures – even when more may not be
needed. The other major financial COI in medicine is created by financial largesse on the part of the drug and medical device industry. Gifts
and payments to physicians and financial support for medical research,
education, and informational resources have, together with congres-
sional lobbying, placed industry in a position of considerable influence
over patient care.

  Physicians also face an array of nonfinancial interests that may sometimes be at odds with the needs of patients. These include personal beliefs,

ideals, and predilections; professional ambition; social obligations, such as to one's family; and practical concerns.

A Duty to Avoid COI

Central to any discussion of COI in medicine is an understanding of physicians' professional obligations toward patients. These obligations are generally defined in terms of Beauchamp and Childress' "four principles" approach to medical ethics: beneficence (providing benefits and preventing or lessening harm), nonmaleficence (not causing harm), respect for autonomy (respecting and fostering informed choice), and justice (fairly distributing benefits, risks, and cost). A COI represents a threat to the fulfillment of one or more of these obligations. Physicians are therefore ethically bound to avoid COI wherever possible.

Key Steps in the Management of COI

An essential first step in managing COIs is to identify them when or before they arise. Recognizing COIs, however, may be a challenge. It is important to understand that a COI resides in a set of conditions, not in any resulting action or attitude. It comes into being as soon as an individual or institution faces two competing interests, one of which might reasonably be expected to affect decisions involving the other.

Once identified, situations involving a COI should generally be avoided, if at all possible. For example, physicians are discouraged from treating family members lest emotional ties cloud professional judgment. Mere effort of will cannot be counted on to help one resist the influence of a competing interest. Research has shown that people are unreliable judges of their own biases and tend to greatly underestimate their susceptibility to COI, even rationalizing their actions after the fact.

When a physician cannot completely avoid a COI, the best approach is transparency and disclosure. For example, a physician in a financial relationship with a drug manufacturer should make this known to any patients for whom she prescribes proprietary drugs by this manufacturer. However, disclosure alone cannot be relied on to mitigate COI. First, COIs often go undeclared, whether because they are awkward to acknowledge, because failure to disclose them is rarely detected and penalized, or because they are not recognized. Second, even with disclosure, conflicts continue to pose a risk to objectivity and judgment.

MEDICINE AND INDUSTRY

A Strong Bond, an Inherent COI

Close ties have been forged between medicine and the drug and medical device industry, as shown in Figure 13.1. Industry funds the lion's share of U.S. biomedical research, contributes heavily to medical education, and has provided countless individual physicians with compensation for services and with outright gifts. With the shrinking of research support from federal sources in the past decade, it is a commonly held view that U.S. medical research could not manage without industry support; a similar argument is made for medical education.

As durable as it has proved to be, the relationship between medicine and industry suffers from a profound conflict: the prevailing aim of industry is to maximize its profits in order to meet the expectations of its

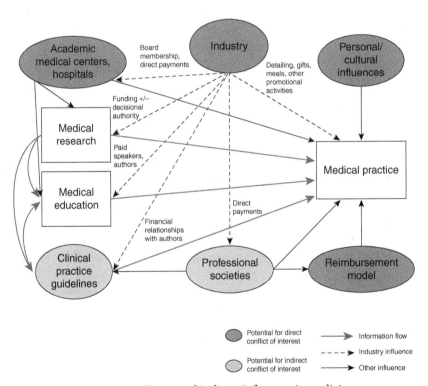

FIGURE 13.1. Direct and indirect influences in medicine.

shareholders, an aim not compatible with putting patients' interests first. This inherent COI has become a pervasive presence in U.S. health care and a source of concern to many. To be profitable and remain in business, companies must promote and sell their products. When physicians' medical decision-making is influenced to this end, patients' interests may be subverted in the process.

CHAPTER OVERVIEW

For simplicity's sake, the chapter will be divided into conflicts in medical practice, medical research, and medical education. These categories are nevertheless closely intertwined, as shown in Figure 13.1. The final section will discuss approaches to dealing with COI in medicine, along with possible future directions.

COI IN MEDICAL PRACTICE

Financial Conflicts

Gifts, Food, and Money from Industry
The drug industry invests heavily in marketing and drug promotion– as much as $27 billion in 2012, nearly 90 percent of it aimed at physicians – a staggering $27,000 per physician. The greater portion of this goes toward *detailing*, face-to-face interactions between sales representatives and physicians. Along with product information and free drug samples for patients, physicians receive gifts such as pens and notepads, reference books, meals – even tickets to sporting events. In a recent survey, 94 percent of physicians reported receiving something of monetary value from industry in the previous year, including gifts (83 percent) and reimbursement for attending an educational meeting (35 percent). In addition, drug companies pay physicians handsomely for a variety of services such as consulting, serving on speakers bureaus, and participating in clinical research.

A large body of evidence indicates that physician–industry interactions of this kind alter physician behavior. Prescribing practices, formulary choices, and assessment of medical information have all been found to favor drugs promoted in this way. Even free drug samples lead to increased prescribing of sample drugs, despite their usually higher cost and second-line status. Such effects are consistent with social science research from the mid-1900s demonstrating that the

BOX 13.1. *Self-referral*

A forty-three-year-old woman presents to the emergency department (ED) following a low-speed motor vehicle collision. She has no specific complaints, but examination reveals tenderness to the right lower ribs and subcostal region; her vital signs are normal. While awaiting chest and rib x-rays and an abdominal computed tomography (CT) scan, the resident performs a bedside ultrasound (FAST scan) because his program director feels he needs the practice. The ultrasound is supervised by the attending physician on shift. Should the department bill for the ultrasound? Why or why not? What conflict(s) of interest are involved?

receipt of a gift or free service creates in the mind of the recipient a social obligation to reciprocate, regardless of the monetary value of the gift.

A serious COI is established when physicians accept gifts from drug companies. Through their ability to influence prescribing, such gifts represent a direct threat to physicians' fulfillment of their duty to put patients' interests first. A second ethical problem is that patients, or their insurers, bear the cost of the gifts. Finally, gifts from industry may weaken society's trust in the medical profession.

Most physicians are unaware of how much their behavior is influenced by gifts from industry. Likewise, a study of medical students found that most felt they were entitled to the gifts and that even among students who did not feel entitled, most had accepted them. In contrast, patients are much more likely to perceive industry gifts as inappropriate or influential over medical practice.

Fee-for-Service Medicine

By the fee-for-service practice model long-dominant in the United States, physician earnings tend to increase in proportion to the volume of procedures and services provided. This has the unintended effect of rewarding physicians for care that patients may not need. The line between necessary and unnecessary care is often subjective, but truly unnecessary care drives up costs and increases patients' risk of harm, with little likelihood of benefit. *Self-referral* is the referral of a patient for tests or care in which the physician has a financial interest (see Box 13.1).

Emergency physicians frequently work as salaried hospital employees rather than as fee-for-service providers. They may nevertheless experience pressure to increase their billing for the good of their department or institution. A decision to perform a procedure such as a bedside ultrasound or a splint or to add documentation to the medical record may augment revenue for the hospital and department – and boost a physician's incentive pay. Insofar as such incentives (and disincentives) risk influencing medical decision-making independent of patients' needs, they represent a COI.

Of note, financial COI plagued the converse incentive system under managed care in the 1980s, with similarly problematic results: physicians and health centers were rewarded for restraint in the use of health services and, inadvertently, for withholding even necessary patient care services at times. Public fears about this COI were a large part of the backlash that resulted.

Nonfinancial Conflicts

Not all COI in medical practice is financial. *Defensive medicine*, medical care aimed specifically at avoiding a malpractice claim, is common among emergency physicians, often resulting in more testing than is medically indicated. Likewise, pressure to reduce turnaround times may contribute to an emergency physician's preference for imaging over observation, for example, in a patient with abdominal pain. COI among consultants may also affect the care of ED patients: on-call physicians wishing to limit their workload, particularly after hours, may downplay the need for their involvement in a case; emergency physicians may in turn be reluctant to insist, not wishing to antagonize a colleague.

Teaching hospitals and their trainees face an educational mandate that may not align seamlessly with the needs of patients. A resident seeking more experience with a specific procedure and not mindful of the COI involved is at risk of placing this goal ahead of a patient's need for the procedure. *Postmortem procedures* on newly deceased patients constitute a unique dilemma wherein the duty of medical educators to teach procedural skills to trainees runs up against the ethical and legal obligations to seek – and risk being denied – permission from patients' surviving family members.

Finally, a variety of sources of COI at the level of the individual, too numerous to list, may have a significant influence on medical decision-making. Beliefs, predilections, and unconscious biases have been shown to act on a large scale in health care. For example, research continues to find

BOX 13.2. *Research sponsorship*

A team of clinical investigators at a university is offered a $1.5 million industry grant to lead a large-scale clinical trial comparing a new drug to placebo; 5,000 patients are to be enrolled. The contract stipulates that publication of the study is subject to sponsor approval upon study completion. Should the investigators sign the contract? Why or why not? What conflict(s) of interest are involved?

systematic differences in the provision of pain medication by patient ethnic group. Religion, to name just one other example, may affect how a physician or a health care facility provides family planning and abortion services.

COI IN MEDICAL RESEARCH

Conflicts for Investigators

Clinical investigators face a variety of interests (see Box 13.2). To begin with, they are legally and ethically bound to protect human research subjects from harm to the extent possible, to obtain informed consent, and *to ensure that the potential benefits of a research study justify even small risks of harm.* ED patients serving as research subjects are a vulnerable study population, with typically higher acuity presentations and no ongoing relationship between patient and researcher to establish trust. When ED patients are unable to give consent because of the urgency of their clinical status, a waiver of consent or emergency exception must be sought.

At the same time, investigators have obligations to science, society, their employers, and their sponsors. Commercial sponsorship of medical research is often accompanied by enormous financial stakes. To the extent that this threatens the scientific independence of investigators, it represents an important COI. Companies are highly motivated to present their products in a favorable light, and a strong association has been demonstrated between industry sponsorship of a study and pro-industry findings.

Pressure to Publish

Academic researchers are under considerable pressure to publish, both for academic advancement and to maintain funding. This pressure may result in a number of undesirable effects on the medical literature. These include the undertaking of trivial studies that can be completed rapidly but contribute little; *duplicate publication*, the reporting of a study more than once or in installments; *guest authorship*, the use of prominent-name researchers as "authors" despite marginal involvement in a study; and even outright fraud.

Pressure to Achieve Positive Results

Positive studies – studies with statistically significant results, implying, for example, that a drug works – are overrepresented in the medical literature. In fact, positive studies are nearly twice as likely to be published as negative ones, according to a Cochrane review. This *publication bias* appears in large part to reflect the greater number of positive manuscripts submitted for review.

Publication bias is motivated by several factors. Positive studies receive more citations. Investigators may assume positive studies are also more likely to be accepted. Most important, for academic investigators with industry sponsors, positive results may be more likely to secure renewed funding, as the perceived performance of a company's product can mean up to billions of dollars in sales.

Such real and perceived advantages of positive studies represent a COI for investigators and sponsors alike, with a number of undesirable consequences. The first is the failure to publish studies with negative results. Jones et al. found that of 585 large randomized controlled trials registered in the ClinicalTrials.gov database, more than one-fourth – involving nearly a million planned or actual participants – were never published, and industry-sponsored trials were nearly twice as likely as other trials to go unpublished.

Similar in concept, *selective reporting* or *outcome-reporting bias* is the reporting of only a portion of the findings in a study – a deviation from a study's original design. One study found that in nearly half of registered clinical trials, the previously selected primary outcome had been changed to favor a statistically significant result. Industry-sponsored studies have been found up to four times as likely to report favorable results.

Design bias is the framing of the research question and selection of the methodology so as to yield favorable results. Common sources of design bias are (1) *inappropriate comparators* (comparison of a drug with placebo, no therapy, or a reduced dose of another agent); (2) the use of endpoints lacking clinical importance; (3) *subgroup analysis*, with publication of only the most favorable results; (4) and the reporting of relative rather than absolute risk reduction.

The systematic skewing of the literature toward positive studies by such means invalidates conclusions about a body of research, biases systematic review articles and meta-analyses, and poses considerable safety risks to patients. The drug manufacturer GlaxoSmithKline was fined an unprecedented $3 billion for, among other charges, suppression of safety and efficacy data for the drugs Paxil (paroxetine) and Avandia (rosiglitazone) – data that indicated that the former was no more effective than placebo in young patients with major depression and might increase suicidal behavior in these patients and that the latter increased the risk of heart attack in diabetics.

When clinical research is not conducted in good faith, investigators fail in their obligations toward subjects as well. Failure to publish negative studies violates subjects' rights by exposing them to risks unbalanced by the potential to benefit others and cheats future subjects and investigators if studies are needlessly repeated. With respect to design bias, clinical trials configured to achieve desired outcomes run afoul of the principle of clinical *equipoise*, or a starting point of uncertainty as to which treatment arm is superior. Although controversial in its details, this principle reflects an important ethical consideration in clinical trials: the need to protect human subjects from interventions known to be inferior to available alternatives.

Conflicts for Medical Journals

As its gatekeepers, journal editors and peer reviewers have a considerable impact on the medical literature. A journal submission may meet with a biased reception if an editor or reviewer sees the author as a competitor or has a personal financial interest at stake. One study found that manuscripts were twice as likely to be accepted when authors had excluded particular reviewers.

Editors also face financial COI on behalf of journals themselves by way of their publishers. *Reprint sales* represent a major source of income for many medical journals – 41 percent of the Lancet's total income at one point – and command profit margins as high as 70 percent. Industry-funded studies are associated both with more reprint orders and more citations or *impact factor*. Incentives such as these for favoring industry-funded studies are at odds with journals' fiduciary obligation to accept manuscripts strictly on their merits.

BOX 13.3. *Speakers bureaus*

A resident attends a departmental grand rounds led by a nationally recognized trauma specialist and lecturer. The speaker begins by acknowledging participation in speakers bureaus for several drug companies. She then highlights the benefits of a new class of pro-coagulant drugs but does not single out a specific agent. After the talk, the resident completes an evaluation form and is asked whether the lecture contained commercial bias. The resident is unsure how to answer because the lecturer was up-front about her financial interests – which involve competing manufacturers of drugs of the class discussed – and did not promote a specific drug. Is the question answerable? Why or why not? What conflict(s) of interest are involved?

COI IN MEDICAL EDUCATION

Medical education comes in many forms: classroom instruction, bedside teaching, expert lectures, written materials, observation of physician role models, and hands-on clinical experience. All but the last of these are vulnerable to the influence of secondary interests.

Financial interests exist on the part of industry and frequently also academic medical centers (AMCs), physician educators, and physician role models. The extensive involvement of industry in medical education has until recently been widely accepted. Policies at the national and institutional level concerning physician–industry interactions are becoming more restrictive over time.

COI at AMCs

AMCs, where most medical training takes place, may have financial ties to industry at a number of levels. In a recent study, sixteen of seventeen U.S. drug companies had board members – paid a mean of more than $300,000 – serving in leadership positions at AMCs, many of them top-ranking institutions. AMCs have received monetary awards from industry of up to several million dollars annually. Sixty percent of medical school chairs in 2006 reported personal ties to industry. Many clinical departments accept industry funds for residency and fellowship training. In addition to research funding, clinical investigators at AMCs often have other paid industry connections (e.g. serving as speakers or consultants), and most AMCs hold equity in drug companies sponsoring their research. Gifts and other perquisites from industry to academic physicians have also long been the norm at AMCs, although they are now increasingly discouraged.

Fee-for-service patient care is another source of financial COI at AMCs, as elsewhere in medicine. Faculty mentors may teach trainees by example that increasing one's billing is a goal worth pursuing in its own right.

COI among Educators and Speakers

Industry-sponsored lectures, whether at grand rounds, resident teaching conferences, or continuing medical education (CME) events, typically involve a loss of independence for speakers and should be considered promotional. *Speakers bureaus* consist of speakers – usually well-regarded academic physicians, or *key opinion leaders* (KOLs) – paid generously by drug companies to provide lectures to physicians and trainees encouraging the use of specific agents; companies retain control over lecture content (see Box 13.3). In addition to creating a sizeable COI for physician speakers, the payments are passed on to patients in the form of higher drug prices.

COI among Authors

Industry ties are common among authors of written informational materials. Even medical textbooks have been sponsored by industry.[1] Intentional misattribution of authorship – guest authorship (described earlier) and *ghost authorship*, the failure to list individuals who have made substantial contributions to a manuscript – is widespread among industry-sponsored medical research articles and review articles.

Systematic Review Articles and Meta-analyses
Systematic review articles and meta-analyses are typically authored by content-area experts. Concerns have been raised that such authors' pre-existing beliefs may bias the questions addressed, the data included, and the resulting conclusions, whereas experts in systematic review methodology would be less likely to introduce bias. Evidence of financial COI and associated pro-industry bias has also been identified in these articles.

Clinical Practice Guidelines
COI among clinical practice guideline panelists may bias guidelines, particularly when strong evidence is lacking and guidelines draw on panelist

consensus. *Panel stacking* refers to the slanting of panels toward a particular view through biased member selection. More concerning, financial relationships between guideline panels and drug companies have become the norm. A majority of panelists voting on the American Heart Association (AHA) 2000 stroke guidelines recommending fibrinolytic use had ties to Genentech, maker of the fibrinolytic agent rTPA (alteplase), and the company had contributed a total of $11 million to the AHA in the preceding years. Conflicts have likewise been found for guidelines endorsing high-dose steroids for acute spinal cord injury and aggressive erythropoeitin use for anemia in chronic renal failure, among others. Financial COI among guideline authors is rarely disclosed in published guidelines.

COI and Medical Trainees

Medical trainees are the target of extensive promotional efforts by industry. A 2005 study found that third-year medical students were offered a mean of one industry-sponsored gift or activity per week, and nearly all had been asked or required to attend at least one industry-sponsored lunch. In another study, 97 percent of residents were found to be carrying at least one item bearing a drug company insignia.

Trainees may be ill-prepared to manage potential COI with industry. Education on drug promotion is inconsistent, with most medical schools devoting less than half a day to the topic. Studies continue to find that most students and residents believe only others are influenced by drug promotion and feel entitled to at least modest gifts and sponsored activities. For their part, physician educators comfortable with high levels of financial COI unwittingly teach trainees to feel the same.

The Association of American Medical Colleges (AAMC) concluded in 2008 that the relationship between academic medicine and industry had a negative impact on physician autonomy, objectivity, and altruism; a subsequent Institute of Medicine (IOM) report went further, declaring that its risks outweighed any potential benefits. Trainees entrust their early professional development to their teaching faculty and clinical role models. Patients, too, place their trust in this process. Partisan medical educators and educational resources risk conveying biased information, to the detriment of both trainees and patients. When this partisanship goes unchecked, the threat extends to medical professionalism and the primacy of patient welfare on the larger scale.

COI in CME

CME is required for most U.S. physicians as a condition of relicensure, specialty certification, and hospital privileges. It is also a multibillion dollar industry with profit margins for CME providers as high as 31 percent. The drug and device industry has assumed a sizeable role in CME funding – at peak, commercial sources contributed half of all CME funding or up to $1.2 billion per year.

Industry funding of CME typically takes the form of "unrestricted educational grants," with most contracts going to physician societies, AMCs, or "medical education and/or communications companies" (MECCs). MECCs are private, for-profit companies that plan CME meetings, prepare educational programs, and recruit and pay academic physicians to deliver the programs. In what amounts to an unusually overt COI, the same companies serve in a marketing capacity for their industry sponsors, and some have openly acknowledged subordinating educational to marketing aims. MECCs currently comprise a small minority of all accredited CME providers but continue to account for a substantial 34 percent of physician participation in CME activities. More than a quarter of CME funding continues to come from commercial sources.

Industry funding of CME comes with financial advantages for many – physicians earn CME credit at lower out-of-pocket cost, academic physicians are well compensated for providing lectures, and CME providers make substantial profits. In return, however, industry sponsors have been in a position to influence educational program content – by selecting the speakers, choosing the lecture topics, even preparing the slides – and evidence has indeed shown that industry-sponsored CME boosts sales of sponsors' products. Changes to the Accreditation Council for Continuing Medical Education (ACCME) Standards for Commercial Support now stipulate that commercial sponsors not suggest or select speakers or topics. However, the opportunity remains for the biasing of speakers and material toward sponsors' interests.

APPROACHES TO COI IN MEDICINE

A variety of approaches have been taken to mitigate the effects of COIs on medical practice, research, and education and to eliminate some conflicts outright. Position statements and guidelines issued by the IOM, AAMC, and other national groups are in broad agreement on these approaches; increasingly, AMCs have instituted COI policies in accordance with them.

Disclosure

Efforts to manage COI in medicine, whether in practice, research, or education, have until recently been focused on disclosure and transparency. Patients want disclosure from their physicians, and a new federal law mandates it on their behalf: the so-called Sunshine Act requires the reporting by industry of all payments to U.S. physicians and teaching hospitals exceeding $10, and patients and others may view these at OpenPaymentsData.CMS.gov.

The 2009 IOM report on COI calls disclosure a "critical but limited first step." Several problems limit the utility of disclosure. First, it can have paradoxical consequences. Listeners tend to underestimate bias following disclosure of a conflict, perhaps believing that disclosure signals honesty, whereas speakers become more likely to exhibit bias, perhaps feeling absolved of the need for impartiality. Second, audiences, readers, and patients may lack sufficient knowledge to assess information for bias, even when aware it may be present. Third, judgment appears to be influenced by the first information encountered, even information one is trying to ignore; this is known as *anchoring bias*.

Rules on disclosure frequently lack standardization, clarity, and comprehensiveness and tend to rely on self-report, generally without verification or enforcement. Recusal policies are uncommon. For example, in 2011 the IOM came out with standards for the development of clinical practice guidelines, but fewer than half of subsequent guidelines were found to adhere to at least half of these standards. Medical journals, too, tend to leave COI reporting to authors' discretion. A study of ninety-five articles by researchers paid at least $1million by industry sponsors found that fewer than half had disclosed the relationship. Honorary and ghost authorship also persists despite a requirement by many journals to report author contributions.

Disclosure should not be a substitute for more effective solutions. As *New Yorker* writer James Surowieki wrote, "Transparency is well and good, but accuracy and objectivity are even better."

AMC Policies Restricting Physician-Industry Interactions

The American Medical Student Association (AMSA) issues an annual scorecard assessing how effectively medical school COI policies address interactions among students, faculty, and industry. Criteria for assessment have become more stringent, in keeping with recommendations of the IOM, AAMC, and a task force of AMC leaders recently convened by the

TABLE 13.1. *Domains of potential conflict of interest at academic medical centers, assessed by the 2014 AMSA Scorecard*

1. Gifts
2. Meals
3. Industry-funded promotional speaking relationships (not ACCME-accredited)
4. Industry-support of ACCME-accredited continuing medical education
5. Attendance of industry-sponsored promotional events
6. Industry-supported scholarships and awards
7. Ghostwriting and honorary authorship
8. Consulting and advising relationships
9. Access of pharmaceutical sales representatives
10. Access of medical device representatives
11. Conflict of interest disclosure
12. Conflict of interest curriculum
13. Extension of conflict of interest policies to community affiliates
14. Enforcement and sanctions of policies

Pew Charitable Trusts. Of the 161 U.S. medical schools surveyed in 2014, 17 percent received A's (best practices in at least half of fourteen domains), 50 percent B's (good practices in all domains), and 16 percent C's (poor practices in more than one domain); for the remainder, insufficient information was available (see Table 13.1 for domains).

Noteworthy results of the 2014 survey include the following:

- About half of all U.S. medical schools have banned industry-funded gifts of any value; more than half have banned industry-funded meals except in association with CME programs; and about half effectively ban faculty from serving on promotional speaker's bureaus for industry – the latter up from 27 percent in 2013 and 2 percent in 2008.
- Few schools prohibit detailing or have policies limiting marketing activity by industry representatives (although the number of those that do has doubled yearly since 2012), and almost none prohibit industry funding for trainee travel to conferences, although many prohibit such funding if earmarked for individual students.
- Nearly all schools continue to permit industry funding of CME that allows companies to target specific topics, courses, or departments.

McCormick et al. identified a lasting effect on the beliefs and behaviors of physicians exposed as residents to a policy of no contact with pharmaceutical representatives. By establishing clear guidelines and limitations on industry interactions with physicians and trainees, AMCs have the potential to reduce COI on a large scale.

COI Education for Trainees

AMSA, AAMC, the Council of Emergency Medicine Residency Directors (CORD), and others have advocated formal education for medical trainees about COI, the critical evaluation of information, and the prevention of marketing activities from inappropriately influencing treatment decisions. About one in five medical schools currently provides COI education at the desired level, according to AMSA.

Academic Detailing and Computerized Decision Support

A key step toward reducing the inappropriate influence of secondary interests on medical decision-making is ensuring physician access to unbiased information sources. Educational outreach or *academic detailing* – personal visits by a trained person to educate physicians about evidence-based practices – is one approach that has shown some success. Another is decision support in the form of "pop-up" computer alerts, which have been found capable of preventing the rise in prescriptions typically seen for heavily marketed medications.[2]

COI Policies for Research

Institutions whose investigators conduct research funded by the National Institutes of Health (NIH) must comply with federal regulation aimed at promoting objectivity in clinical research. Revised in 2011, this regulation requires institutions to maintain and enforce a policy on financial COI in research; ensure disclosure of such COI by investigators; establish guidelines for assessing disclosures; establish a plan for managing COI, for enforcing disclosure, and for applying sanctions where appropriate; and report back to the Public Health Service.

Clinical Trials Registries

Clinical trials registries are official platforms and catalogs for registering clinical trials. By allowing access to data that may never be published, they offer a more complete view of the evidence in a given area than would otherwise be available. This also makes possible the retrospective identification and quantification of publication bias and selective report-ing. The World Health Organization (WHO), the 2008 revised Declaration of Helsinki, and the International Committee of Medical Journal Editors (ICMJE) all consider registration of interventional trials obligatory. ClinicalTrials.gov, run by the U.S. National Library of Medicine (NLM), is the largest and most widely used trial registry today. All clinical trials conducted in the United States are required to be registered in the registry.

Despite exhortations at the international, national, and journal levels, compliance with registration requirements has been found to be poor.[3] Moreover, failure to publish remains a problem even among registered trials, particularly those funded by industry, and the results of unpublished trials are often unavailable on ClinicalTrials.gov.

COI Policies for Medical Journals

The ICMJE developed and maintains a set of best practice and ethical standards for medical journals and the publication of scholarly work. These standards, which target financial COI, aim to ensure "accurate, clear, unbiased" articles and are intended for authors, peer-reviewers, editors, and others involved in the publication process. A 2005 survey found that a minority of journals had disclosure policies for peer reviewers and editors, very few published such disclosures, and few required recusal for COI.

Noncommercial CME

Arnold Relman, former editor-in-chief of the *New England Journal of Medicine,* defined high-quality CME as "critical, unbiased, and based only on the highest level of evidence." The IOM and others have called for development of a mechanism for funding CME that is free from commercial influence. In a 2011 survey, physicians acknowledged commer-cial bias in industry-sponsored CME but said they would be unwilling to accept higher registration fees in exchange for elimination of commercial support. Noncommercial CME has in fact been found financially viable, however, in one case raising tuition fees by only $100–125 and receiving high ratings by participants.

Alternative Practice Models

The Affordable Care Act includes a variety of reforms intended to encou-rage adoption of alternatives to fee-for-service medicine. In *global budget programs*, health care provider organizations are given an overall budget to care for patients, with rewards for improved outcomes and lower health care spending. *Bundled payments* are fixed amounts paid to health care providers for all the services a patient is expected to need during a period of time. In *shared savings arrangements*, groups of health care providers work together as *accountable care organizations*, sharing responsibility for coordinating lower cost, higher quality care for a group of patients.

Many physicians, particularly employees of AMCs or health maintenance organizations, are paid on a salary basis, rather than by patient volume or by the service. Increasingly, too, physician payment may be based in part on evaluation of the provider's performance for a given population, in a *pay-for-performance* (P4P) arrangement.

CONCLUSION

COI is a widespread problem in medicine. Its principal sources are financial ties with industry and the fee-for-service practice model. COI in medicine is a serious concern because of its potential to adversely affect patient care, whether through direct influence on physicians' decision-making or through the biasing of their information sources and educators.

Important steps have been taken toward eliminating or mitigating some forms of COI in medicine. These steps include institution-level restrictions on gifts and money from industry, stricter federal regulations on COI in research, mandated registration of clinical trials, an increase in noncommercial funding of CME, and practice models offering alternatives to the fee-for-service incentive structure.

Change on many additional fronts will be required, however, to achieve true independence on the part of practitioners, researchers, educators, and other contributors to the field (peer reviewers, editors, guideline authors, etc.). For example, disclosure of COIs would need to be both mandated and enforced, with penalties for failure to disclose and greater use of recusal. Separation would need to be maintained between clinical investigators and those standing to benefit financially from the findings of a research study. Registration of clinical trials would need to be more closely monitored, with enforcement of penalties for noncompliance. For clinical guideline panels, an emphasis on methodological rather than content-area expertise has been recommended, along with an impartial panel selection process and recusal for financial conflicts.

Ultimately, meaningful reduction in COI will come down to a shift of norms within the medical profession. Physicians must consider for themselves, both as individuals and at the level of institutions and professional associations, what they expect from their profession. Influential professional organizations may effect change through a gradual process of increasingly strict corrective guidelines. At the same time, young physicians who have been educated on the issues may opt to take a stand against threats to integrity, independence, and purpose in the profession. They, too, may make a difference by advocating in large numbers for the adoption of such guidelines and for other necessary changes.

ETHICS TAKEOUT TIPS

- Physicians have a duty to avoid COI where patient care might be affected.
- Fee-for-service medicine and physician–industry interactions create COI by, respectively, (1) rewarding physicians for patient care independent of its value to patients and (2) establishing ties known to influence drug prescribing independent of medical appropriateness.
- Clinical investigators face financial and other COI that may distort the research literature through design bias, selective reporting, and failure to publish negative studies.
- Financial relationships with industry are widespread in medical education among speakers, clinical and academic role models and educators, and authors of informational resources such as clinical practice guidelines.
- Important steps in the management of COI in medicine include

  * Disclosure, with verification, enforcement, and greater use of recusal
  * Academic medical center policies limiting physician–industry interactions
  * COI education for trainees
  * Strict COI policies for clinical investigators
  * Clinical trials registries
  * Development of noncommercial CME
  * Professional society guidelines that actively aim to reduce COI

FOR FURTHER READING

American Medical Student Association. (2014). *AMSA Scorecard 2014*. www.amsascorecard.org/
Association of American Medical Colleges. (2008). *Protecting patients, preserving integrity, advancing health: Accelerating implementation of COI policies in*

human subjects research. AAMC-AAU Advisory Committee on Financial Conflicts in Human Subjects Research. www.aamc.org/jointcoireport

Asher, S. L., Schears, R. M., & Miller, C. D. (2011). Conflicts of interest in human subjects research: Special considerations for academic emergency physicians. *Academy of Emergency Medicine,* 18(3), 292–296.

Bekelman, J. E., Li, Y., & Gross, C. P. (2003). Scope and impact of financial conflicts of interest in biomedical research: A systematic review. *Journal of the American Medical Association,* 289(4), 454–465.

Cain, D. M., & Detsky, A. S. (2008). Everyone's a little bit biased (even physicians). *Journal of the American Medical Association,* 299(24), 2893–2895.

Campbell, E. G., Gruen, R. L., Mountford, J., Miller, L. G., Cleary, P. D., & Blumenthal, D. (2007). A national survey of physician-industry relationships. *New England Journal of Medicine,* 356(17), 1742–1750.

Campbell, E. G., Weissman, J. S., Ehringhaus, S., et al. (2007). Institutional academic industry relationships. *Journal of the American Medical Association,* 298(15), 1779–1786.

Fortuna, R. J., Zhang, F., Ross-Degnan, D., Campion, F. X., Finkelstein, J. A., Kotch, J. B., ... Simon, S. R. (2009). Reducing the prescribing of heavily marketed medications: A randomized controlled trial. *Journal of General Internal Medicine,* 24(8), 897–903.

Institute of Medicine. (2009). *Conflict of interest in medical research, education, and practice.* Washington, DC: The National Academies Press.

Jones, C. W., & Platts-Mills, T. F. (2012). Quality of registration for clinical trials published in emergency medicine journals. *Annals of Emergency Medicine,* 60(4), 458–464.

Lexchin, J., Bero, L. A., Djulbegovic, B., & Clark, O. (2003). Pharmaceutical industry sponsorship and research outcome and quality: Systematic review. *British Medical Journal,* 326(7400), 1167–1170.

Loewenstein, G., Cain, D. M., & Sunita, S. (2011). The limits of transparency: Pitfalls and potential of disclosing conflicts of interest. *American Economic Review,* 101(3), 423–428.

Lundh, A., Barbateskovic, M., Hrobjartsson, A., & Gotzsche, P. C. (2010). Conflicts of interest at medical journals: The influence of industry-supported randomised trials on journal impact factors and revenue – cohort study. *PLoS Medicine,* 7(10), e1000354.

Petersen, M. (2003, May 30). Court papers suggest scale of drug's use: Lawsuit says doctors were paid endorsers. *New York Times.* www.nytimes.com/2003/05/30/business/court-papers-suggest-scale-of-drug-s-use.html

Pew Charitable Trusts. (2013). *Persuading the prescribers: Pharmaceutical industry marketing and its influence on physicians and patients.* www.pewtrusts.org/en/research-and-analysis/fact-sheets/2013/11/11/persuading-the-prescribers-pharmaceutical-industry-marketing-and-its-influence-on-physicians-and-patients

Stamatakis, E., Weiler, R., & Ioannidis, J. P. (2013). Undue industry influences that distort healthcare research, strategy, expenditure and practice: A review. *European Journal of Clinical Investigation,* 43(5), 469–475.

Wazana, A. (2000). Physicians and the pharmaceutical industry: Is a gift ever just a gift? *Journal of the American Medical Association,* 283(3), 373–380.

14

Medical Errors and Patient Safety

JOHN C. MOSKOP, PHD

INTRODUCTION: TWO CASES

Case 1: Dr. Abel is an attending emergency physician on duty in the emergency department (ED) of a large urban teaching hospital. It is a midsummer Saturday afternoon, and the ED is crowded, with patients in every ED bed and several more on gurneys in ED hallways. Dr. Abel is currently supervising Dr. Baker, a first-year resident, as she performs an endotracheal intubation on Mr. Chase, a COPD patient who presented to the ED with severe shortness of breath. Dr. Baker is having some difficulty completing this procedure, and Dr. Abel advises her about how to proceed. He is aware that this is an essential skill for Dr. Baker to master, and he does not want to take over the procedure because that will prevent her from gaining this experience and will undermine her confidence. Dr. Abel also recognizes, however, that delay in completing this procedure poses some risk to Mr. Chase, and it is also increasing the waiting time of the many other patients in the ED. How should he handle this situation?

* * *

Case 2: Dr. Doyle is the emergency physician on duty this morning in the ED of a small community hospital. Mr. Ellis, a physician assistant working with her in the ED, asks for her help. He tells her that Mr. Ford presented to the ED late last night with symptoms of recurrent headache, cough, and nasal congestion, and Dr. Grey, the emergency physician on duty overnight, prescribed an antibiotic for a presumed sinus infection. Mr. Ellis reports that Mr. Ford has just returned to the ED, and his symptoms, including shortness of breath, nausea, and sweating, are much worse after beginning the antibiotic. When Dr. Doyle reviews Mr. Ford's medical record, she discovers that he had previously reported an allergy to this class of antibiotics, and she realizes that this is the likely cause of his worsened condition. How should she handle this situation?

199

These two cases illustrate different issues of medical error and patient safety that occur in the setting of the hospital ED. Errors raise important questions about the scope and limits of professional responsibilities to keep patients safe and to inform them about their medical condition and its treatment. After examination of these questions, this chapter will conclude with reflections on the two cases.

A Brief History

Until the turn of the twenty-first century, medical errors were largely a hidden subject, rarely discussed outside of the professional medical literature. That situation changed abruptly in 2000, when the prestigious U.S. Institute of Medicine (IOM) published a report entitled *To Err Is Human: Building a Safer Health System* (Kohn et al., 2000). This IOM report estimated that as many as 98,000 deaths each year in U.S. hospitals were due to medical errors. National news media highlighted this estimate, pointing out that the annual incidence of fatal medical errors was equivalent to the deaths that would occur if there were a crash of a jumbo jet every day of the year, and so the topic of medical error found its way onto the national agenda.

In *To Err Is Human*, and in several subsequent reports, the IOM offered a variety of strategies for preventing medical errors and for creating a new "culture of safety" in the U.S. health care system. Other professional and regulatory organizations addressed the problem of medical error in a variety of ways. In 2003, for example, the American Medical Association (AMA) adopted an ethics opinion entitled "Ethical Responsibility to Study and Prevent Error and Harm." This opinion asserts that "physicians must strive to ensure patient safety and should play a central role in identifying, reducing, and preventing health care errors" (American Medical Association, 2003). It calls on physicians to participate in establishing error reporting mechanisms, investigating error reports, identifying impaired or incompetent colleagues, and disclosing errors to patients.

Between 2004 and 2008, the Institute for Healthcare Improvement, a nonprofit association of U.S. hospitals, organized two major hospital error prevention programs. The 100,000 Lives Campaign (2004–2006) promoted six interventions to prevent 100,000 avoidable hospital deaths, and the 5 Million Lives Campaign (2006–2008) proposed twelve additional interventions to prevent 5 million patient injuries. Many U.S. hospitals during this period established their own institutional patient safety programs to develop and implement local safety initiatives.

In addition to their concern for the welfare of their patients, hospitals have implemented patient safety initiatives in response to new patient safety standards and regulations. The Joint Commission, the primary U.S. accreditation agency for hospitals and other health facilities, has adopted multiple safety standards in recent years, including standards requiring leadership attention to safety issues, staff safety education, incident reporting systems, and disclosure of medical errors. A growing number of insurance reimbursement rules also impose financial penalties for failure to protect patient safety. In 2008, for example, Medicare implemented new rules that deny reimbursement for the treatment of eight "preventable complications," including transfusions with the wrong blood type, retained objects after surgery, and central line infections.

Concepts and Types of Medical Error

To address ethical issues of medical error and patient safety, one must have a basic understanding of central concepts and conceptual distinctions in this area. This section will offer definitions of medical error and related concepts, make two important conceptual distinctions, identify major types of error, and consider features of the ED setting that may contribute to errors.

Definitions

What, exactly, is a medical error? Multiple definitions of error have been proposed, and there is no clear consensus on a single definition. Consider, for example, the following three definitions:

1. "The failure of a planned action to be completed as intended or the use of a wrong plan to achieve an aim" (Kohn et al., 2000)
2. "An unintended act or omission, or a flawed system or plan, that harms or has the potential to harm a patient" (American Medical Association, 2003)
3. "An act or omission with potentially negative consequences for the patient that would have been judged wrong by skilled and knowledgeable peers at the time it occurred" (Wu et al., 1997)

As the first definition from the IOM report suggests, errors can occur both in the choice of a treatment plan and in the execution of that plan. The AMA definition adds that both acts and omissions can be errors and links error with harm or potential harm. The Wu et al. definition includes an additional requirement that the action or omission in question would have been judged wrong by peers at the time it occurred, not just in retrospect.

Commentators have described multiple different types of medical error and other concepts related to error. See Table 14.1 for definitions of some of the most widely used concepts in the literature on medical error and patient safety.

Conceptual Distinctions
Error and harm. Two of the definitions in Table 14.1 of medical error refer to harm or the potential for harm as part of the meaning of error. Our concern about medical errors is primarily a result of their potential to cause harm to patients, but it is also important to note that there is no necessary connection between medical errors and harm to patients. On the one hand, some clear errors do not cause any harm; for example, a patient may receive a medication intended not for him but for another

TABLE 14.1. *Common patient safety and medical error concepts*

Active error	An error that occurs at the level of the frontline operator and whose effects are felt almost immediately
Adverse event	An injury resulting from a medical intervention
Latent error	An error in design, organization, training, or maintenance that leads to operator errors and whose effects typically lie dormant in the system for lengthy periods of time
Near miss	An event or situation that could have resulted in an accident, injury, or illness, but did not, either by chance or through timely intervention
Patient safety	Freedom from accidental injury; ensuring patient safety involves the establishment of operational systems and processes that minimize the likelihood of errors and maximize the likelihood of intercepting them when they occur
Systems error	An error that is not the result of an individual's actions but the predictable outcome of a series of actions and factors that comprise a diagnostic or treatment process
Unpreventable adverse event	An adverse event resulting from a complication that cannot be prevented given the current state of knowledge. (In contrast, an adverse event or near miss that is preventable given the current state of medical knowledge is a medical error.)

Definitions from Kohn et al. (2000) and Quality Interagency Coordination Task Force (2000).

patient but suffer no ill effects from that medication. On the other hand, some patient harms are not the result of a medical error; for example, a patient may receive the "correct" medication for her condition (i.e. the medication that most skilled physicians would recommend for that condition) but still suffer an unforeseeable but severe complication from that medication.

Reporting and disclosure of errors. Both of these terms refer to communication of information, and they may appear to be synonyms. The literature on patient safety, however, makes a clear distinction between them. It uses the term "reporting" to refer to the communication of information about medical errors or other adverse events to institutional, professional, or public authorities, including institutional safety officers, professional licensure boards, and public health insurance officials. In contrast, the term "disclosure" is used to refer to communication of information about errors or adverse events to patients or to patients' surrogate decision-makers.

Types and Incidence of Medical Errors
What are the major types or categories of medical error? Medical errors can be categorized in multiple different ways. In a 1991 study of serious injuries to 1,133 hospitalized patients caused by medical treatment, for example, physician reviewers classified errors contributing to these injuries into the following five broad categories:

1. Errors in the performance of procedures, including technical errors and inadequate monitoring
2. Errors of prevention, including failure to take indicated preventive measures
3. Errors of diagnosis, including misdiagnosis and delay in diagnosis
4. Errors in drug treatment, including use of an inappropriate drug or dose
5. System errors, including inadequate staffing or training and defective equipment (Leape et al., 1991)

The incidence and distribution of these different types of error is likely to vary in different treatment settings. A 2003 study of errors in a busy academic medical center ED, for example, identified eighteen errors per one hundred ED patients (Fordyce et al., 2003). Croskerry and Sinclair (2001) argue that the ED is an error-prone practice setting. High patient volume, high acuity of illness, and the lack of continuity of care are all common features of the ED setting. These features may increase the risk of error because physicians must often act quickly and with limited information about the patient's condition and past medical history. Frequent ED patient "handoffs" from one physician or nurse to another may also result in errors due to incomplete, inaccurate, or poorly organized transfer of information or to failure to re-evaluate the patient or the treatment plan.

ETHICAL ISSUES IN PATIENT SAFETY

Error Reporting, Investigation, and Prevention

Moral Foundations

Physician duties to report, investigate, and prevent medical errors are grounded in fundamental bioethical principles of beneficence and non-maleficence. These principles enjoin physicians to act for the benefit of their patients and to refrain from actions likely to do more harm than good. Medical errors violate these principles: they do not promote the goal of benefitting patients, and they expose patients to potential or actual harm. Physicians therefore have very powerful reasons to avoid making errors in the care of their patients. When they do make an error, physicians have similarly strong reasons to report and investigate the error. Reporting and investigation of the error are essential to identifying the causes of the error. Knowing how and why the error occurred is, in turn, essential to formulating and implementing changes in treatment procedures or systems to prevent future errors of the same type. Error reporting, investigation, and practice modification thus enable physicians to provide beneficial care and avoid harm to future patients.

There is, however, a seemingly paradoxical tension between the commitment, on the one hand, to avoid errors and, on the other hand, to report and investigate them. Physicians taught to strive relentlessly for error-free practice may reach an implicit conclusion that they must achieve infallibility in clinical judgment and technical execution. They may, therefore, view failure to reach this unrealistic goal as inexcusable. Rather than accept and report an error that they view as an inexcusable failure, they may seek to deny or conceal the error or to shift responsibility for the error to another provider or to the patient.

Competing Interests

As noted earlier, physicians have a strong moral interest in promoting the welfare of their patients, and this interest provides a powerful reason to keep patients safe by preventing medical errors. Indeed, the Physician Charter on Medical Professionalism, a statement endorsed by multiple medical professional associations, asserts that patient welfare must be the physician's primary concern (ABIM Foundation et al., 2002). Individual patient welfare is not the only interest that guides physician behavior, however. Rather, there are a variety of other interests that influence physicians' decisions and actions, and attention to these interests can motivate physicians to limit or compromise their efforts to maximize an individual patient's welfare. These interests may, for example, result in exposing patients to increased risk of harm or in decisions not to report an apparent medical error. Leung et al. (2012) report on a number of interests identified by surgeon informants as influences on their intraoperative decision-making that may contribute to medical errors or other adverse patient outcomes. I group these competing interests into three categories: other-patient-based interests, third-party-based interests, and personal interests.

Other-patient-based interests. In addition to patient welfare, the Physician Charter endorses two other fundamental principles: patient autonomy and social justice. Respect for these latter principles may require physicians to take actions that compromise a patient's welfare. Surgeons in the Leung et al. study, for example, described situations in which patients' expressed wishes to avoid surgery influenced their decision to forgo beneficial interventions and other situations in which the pressure of patients waiting for surgery caused them to hurry to complete a procedure. Pressures of time or scarce human or material resources may thus limit the ability of physicians to meet all the needs of their patients. Even if physician decisions in these situations lead to adverse patient outcomes, they may not constitute medical errors but rather decisions that are justified by principles of patient autonomy or social justice.

Third-party-based interests. Patients have strong interests in their medical care, to be sure, but so do a number of others, including patients' family members and members of the health care team, including trainees. The interests of these third parties can and do influence medical treatment decisions in at least some circumstances. A patient's children, for example, may decide that they cannot pay the substantial sum needed to provide a very expensive new chemotherapy that offers a modest survival benefit for a parent with advanced cancer. As a result, the patient may die sooner, not as a result of medical error, but of the unavailability of resources for treatment. In a different situation, a neurology resident who is admitting an unstable patient to the hospital at 3:00 a.m. may have some slight uncertainty about an initial treatment plan, but decide not to interrupt the sleep of his supervising attending physician to seek assistance. In Case 1 at the opening of the chapter, the attending emergency physician allows a first-year resident to intubate a patient, likely posing some increased risk to the patient due to the resident's relative inexperience. In each of these three situations, physicians' treatment decisions are influenced by the interests of third-party stakeholders (family members and other health care providers) in addition to patient interests.

Personal interests. A variety of personal interests of physicians may also compete with attention to the interests of patients. Surgeons in the Leung et al. study, for example, acknowledged that concern for their own personal self-esteem and professional reputation may incline them not to admit uncertainty or seek assistance in a difficult case. They also observed that their desire to keep their jobs may prevent them from questioning the decisions of a department chair or senior colleague. Finally, these surgeons recognized that financial considerations in a fee-for-service system may influence them to operate in marginal cases or to proceed to surgery sooner than necessary. Another personal interest that influences physician decisions is responsibility to family members: a physician might, for example, cut short an appointment with a patient in order to respond to a request from a spouse for assistance with their child's sudden illness.

In response to the increasing pressure of market forces in medicine, the Physician Charter and other codes of professional ethics assert that physicians must place the interests of patients above personal interests. This assertion requires careful interpretation, however. Does it require that physicians always act in the best interests of their patients, so as, for example, to achieve a marginal increase in patient safety even when that requires a great sacrifice of their own personal interests? Such an absolute priority for patient interests over personal interests seems unrealistic and indefensible; we do permit physicians to make choices based on financial and family considerations, and those choices do have consequences, both positive and negative, for their patients. Making defensible choices, therefore, often requires comparative assessment of the moral significance of several competing interests.

These competing interests may arise in the reporting, investigation, and prevention of medical errors in a variety of ways. An ED nurse, for example, may observe a treatment that she believes is not appropriate for the patient's condition. She may contemplate reporting this incident, but fear that if she does so, the treating physician will retaliate against her for this action. If the hospital does not protect its staff from retaliation for reporting such incidents, it may be unreasonable to require that the nurse submit such a report. In another situation, an emergency physician may judge that an ED patient she is evaluating has a condition severe enough to require intensive care. When she requests immediate admission of the patient to the hospital's ICU, however, she is told that no bed is currently available, and the patient will have to remain in the ED for several more hours. The emergency physician expresses great concern for the safety of the patient, but sees no obvious way to prevent delay in securing the definitive treatment that this patient urgently needs.

Error Disclosure to Patients and Surrogates

Moral Foundations

The previous section examined moral reasons for reporting, investigating, and preventing medical errors. Despite the best intentions and best efforts of health care institutions and professionals to prevent medical errors, however, both individual and system performance will remain imperfect, and so some medical errors will continue to occur. When a medical error is identified, what, if any, information about that error should be disclosed to the patient or to a representative of the patient, if the patient lacks the ability to understand this information? Is error disclosure a professional responsibility whenever an error is made or only in some cases of error? What is the moral rationale for error disclosure?

The primary moral rationale for disclosing medical errors, I argue, is the professional duty to be truthful. Truthfulness is widely recognized as a central professional responsibility of physicians and other health care professionals. The Principles of Medical Ethics of the AMA, for example, assert that "A physician shall ... be honest in all professional interactions." Similarly, the American College of Emergency Physician's Principles of Ethics for Emergency Physicians, described as "fundamental moral responsibilities of emergency physicians," affirms that "Emergency physicians shall communicate truthfully with patients." There are several persuasive moral reasons for a professional duty of truthfulness. Truthful communication shows respect for patients as moral agents who are entitled to information about their health and medical treatment. Deception of another person, in contrast, is typically a sign of disrespect for that person. Truthful communication with patients provides them with information that they require in order to make informed treatment decisions. The practice of truthfulness also fosters a therapeutic relationship of trust and cooperation that promotes beneficial patient outcomes.

It is also important to recognize that the professional duty to be truthful is not absolute or unlimited, however. That duty is limited to information about the patient's medical condition and treatment. Physicians thus have no duty to disclose personal information about themselves, and they have a positive duty *not* to disclose confidential patient information to anyone who is not entitled to that information (Moskop et al., 2005). Neither does the duty of truthfulness require disclosure to the patient of all medical information about that patient. Physicians are not required, for example, to disclose medical information that is highly technical or is insignificant. So-called *total disclosure* is neither practical nor desirable for patients or physicians.

In view of these clear limits of the professional duty to communicate truthfully, how should physicians determine how much and what kind of information to disclose to their patients? The U.S. law of informed consent offers a standard, called the "reasonable person standard," to determine how much information patients should receive in order to provide their informed consent to treatment. According to that standard, the physician should disclose what a reasonable person in the patient's position would want to know in order to make a treatment decision. This legal standard applies specifically to disclosures for the purpose of obtaining a patient's informed consent to treatment, but it can be extended as a moral guideline to the broader context of physician–patient communication in general.

What would adoption of a reasonable person standard imply regarding disclosure of medical errors? Multiple studies provide evidence that patients do want to know about errors that occur in their medical care. In two survey studies, for example, 99 percent of health plan members and parents reported that they wanted to be informed about *all* errors in their or their children's care (Hobgood et al., 2005; Mazor et al., 2004). In two studies of patients who sued their physicians, a commonly expressed reason for taking this action was the patients' desire to find out what had happened to them (Beckman et al., 1994; Hickson et al., 1992).

Which medical errors should be disclosed to patients or their representatives? In a focus group study, patients unanimously reported a desire to know about any error that caused harm to them (Gallagher et al., 2003). Reasonable people would presumably want to know about harmful medical errors because these errors have serious health consequences and are likely to require decisions about continuing medical care, even though it may be difficult for physicians to acknowledge that their error has harmed the patient. What about "minor errors," that is, errors that did not cause any harm to patients? The lack of significant consequences may make it less important to disclose minor errors, but these errors may be easier for physicians to disclose, and most patients report that they want to know about both minor and more serious errors in their care.

I conclude that the professional responsibility of truthfulness provides compelling moral grounds for affirming a specific duty of physicians to disclose medical errors to patients or their representatives. This is a widely shared conclusion in published studies of the ethics of error disclosure. Surveys of physician behavior, however, suggest that many physicians are nevertheless reluctant to disclose medical errors. It appears, therefore, that there remain significant barriers to error disclosure.

Barriers to Disclosure
This section considers barriers to physician disclosure of medical errors in four categories – system barriers, patient barriers, physician barriers, and liability barriers.

System barriers. During the long period in which medical errors were a largely hidden problem, U.S. health care systems did not generally support or encourage the reporting or disclosure of medical errors. When errors did occur, system responses were often counterproductive; for example, risk management staff might attempt to minimize or cover up the error in order to protect the institution, or physicians might convene a morbidity and mortality conference designed to identify and blame the clinician guilty of committing the error. These responses discouraged physicians from freely disclosing the commission of errors to their patients.

As noted earlier, greater attention to medical errors in recent years has required health care systems and institutions to implement procedures to report, investigate, and prevent errors, and systems have also developed explicit guidelines and procedures for the disclosure of errors to patients or their representatives. These error disclosure procedures must address complex questions about when errors should be disclosed, who should disclose them, and whether responsibility for errors should be ascribed to individual providers or to the larger system of care.

The hospital ED setting poses several distinctive system-based barriers to error disclosure. Frequent transitions of care from one ED provider to another may increase the risk of error, and they also raise questions about who should assume responsibility for disclosing an error that occurred earlier in a patient's ED stay. Emergency physicians may not be able to disclose an error when it is discovered because the patient has already left the ED via admission as an inpatient or discharge from the institution. Emergency physicians may also be reluctant to disclose errors to patients because they usually lack a previous relationship with their patients and so cannot rely on established bonds of trust to enable patients to receive this information with acceptance rather than anger.

Patient barriers. Additional barriers to error disclosure are a result of patient characteristics. These characteristics may be found more frequently in ED patients than in patients treated in other settings. The physician may not be able to disclose a medical error discovered after the patient has left the ED because the patient has not provided contact information, as is likely in patients who are homeless, migrant workers, or fugitives. Other patients cannot receive information about a medical error because they are disoriented, unconscious, have another impairment of mental capacity, or have died. If the patient cannot receive this information, the physician should disclose the error to the patient's authorized representative or to the next of kin of a deceased patient, if that person can be identified and contacted.

Physician barriers. No one wants to make errors, and no one (except perhaps sadists and sociopaths!) wants to injure other people. This desire is likely intensified in medical practice because physicians are taught that nonmaleficence – avoiding harm to patients – is a basic professional obligation. When physicians make serious medical errors, they are prone to experience feelings of failure, inadequacy, shame, guilt, and fear of exposure. To protect themselves from these negative feelings, physicians may try to deny the error and may decide not to report or disclose it. Even if a physician recognizes the need to disclose an error, he or she may feel ill-equipped to do so. In a study of attending physicians and residents working in an academic ED, only 12 percent reported any formal instruction in disclosing errors to patients (Hobgood et al., 2004). Physicians who are arrogant, slothful, avaristic, or aloof may avoid disclosure of errors in order to avoid undesired consequences for themselves. Finally, physicians may decide not to disclose an error because they fear that disclosure will cause the patient to be anxious, to lose trust in them, or to terminate the therapeutic relationship.

Liability barriers. Both individual physicians and institutional health care providers are concerned about this final kind of barrier to error disclosure. Their concern is that disclosure of errors may increase the risk of malpractice liability. A physician may, for example, reason as follows:

1. Unless a medical error is obvious, or I decide to disclose the error, most patients will never know that I made an error in their treatment and that it was my error, and not just their disease or injury, that caused them harm.
2. My disclosure of errors thus reveals to patients that harms they have experienced are the result of my medical errors.
3. With this knowledge, patients may take legal action against me to receive compensation for their injuries.
4. Therefore, choosing not to disclose my (nonobvious) medical errors will reduce my risk of malpractice liability.

Furthermore, disclosure of error may be admissible as evidence that one is at fault for an iatrogenic injury. For these reasons, defense attorneys, at least until recently, have counseled physicians not to disclose errors, especially if there is any uncertainty about the cause of an adverse event. Protecting oneself from malpractice liability is certainly an understandable, if not an especially admirable, reason for nondisclosure of medical errors.

Some legal commentators, however, have challenged the claim that disclosure of errors increases one's liability risk. These authors point out that patients have many reasons for initiating lawsuits, including financial compensation for injuries, to be sure, but also a desire to learn what happened to them, a feeling of abandonment by their physician, a perception of physician indifference to their suffering, and a desire to prevent future errors. Many of these patient interests can be satisfied if physicians disclose errors promptly and apologize sincerely, provide continuing treatment, and describe initiatives implemented to prevent future errors of the same kind. When an error has harmed a patient, it will also be appropriate to offer fair compensation for injuries the patient has suffered.

Empirical data on the relationship of error disclosure and malpractice liability remain limited. Proponents of disclosure often cite reports from the University of Michigan Health System (Boothman et al., 2009). Following implementation of an aggressive error disclosure and patient compensation policy in 2001, this health system reports greater patient satisfaction, fewer lawsuits, and lower overall costs. Other scholars, however, argue that full disclosure of harmful errors will increase legal claims and their associated costs (Studdert et al., 2002). The effect of a practice of error disclosure on malpractice claims remains uncertain, but even if disclosure does not reduce liability risks, there remain powerful moral and psychological reasons to adopt this practice.

Strategies for Disclosure

This section reviews strategies to promote medical error disclosure at the public policy, health system, and individual practice levels.

Public policy strategies. Perhaps the most sweeping policy proposal to increase medical error disclosure is replacement of the current medical malpractice system with a no-fault compensation system for medical injuries or with an enterprise liability system in which health systems, not individual practitioners, assume liability for injuries due to medical errors. Under either system, physicians could disclose errors without fear of individual liability. Such a fundamental policy change would be welcomed by most physicians but strongly opposed by plaintiffs' attorneys, and so its implementation in the United States is unlikely in the foreseeable future.

A more modest change in policy in recent years is the enactment of so-called *apology statutes*. Thirty-six states have passed laws making physician disclosures and apologies for adverse outcomes inadmissible in lawsuits. These statutes are designed to remove one barrier to physician disclosure of errors: namely, the concern that admission that a physician has made a medical error can be used as evidence against him or her in a malpractice lawsuit. This protection may not be as robust as it appears at first glance, however. Several commentators caution that many of these statutes protect only "partial apologies," that is, apologies that express sympathy for a patient's suffering, but not admissions of error or responsibility for a patient's iatrogenic injury (Cohen, 1999; Dresser, 2008). Patients, however, may desire more than sympathy; they may want clear disclosure that an error occurred in their care and an apology for that error.

System strategies. Individual health systems can also adopt measures to encourage error disclosure in their facilities. Error disclosure is less onerous when there are fewer errors to disclose, so the institutional error identification, investigation, and prevention programs described earlier may make a significant contribution to error disclosure.

Health systems may also implement explicit error disclosure policies and procedures. Systems have a clear incentive to undertake this task because the Joint Commission has adopted a performance standard that requires hospitals to disclose information about unanticipated outcomes of treatment that result in significant harm to patients. These procedures typically address questions of who should participate in error disclosure to patients and when and how disclosure should occur.

Health systems can also provide opportunities for error disclosure training for staff and resident physicians. Clearly, there are better and worse methods for disclosing sensitive information about medical errors to patients and their representatives. Truog et al. (2011) have recently published a comprehensive guide for the teaching and practice of medical error disclosure.

Practice strategies. What can individual physicians do to improve their practice regarding disclosure of medical errors? In an *Annals of Emergency Medicine* review of this topic, emergency physicians Joel Geiderman, Cherri Hobgood, and Gregory Luke Larkin joined me in making the practice recommendations listed in Table 14.2 (Moskop et al., 2006).

We believe that this combination of practices, implemented in a health system that supports and encourages error disclosure, provides a consistent and effective approach to error disclosure that can help physicians overcome the many barriers to carrying out this professional responsibility.

THE CASES REVISITED

Case 1 describes a kind of situation that occurs with some frequency in the busy EDs of academic medical centers. In this situation, Dr. Abel must attend simultaneously to several different and competing interests, and the decisions he makes are likely to have both positive and negative consequences for multiple stakeholders. He has responsibilities to provide appropriate emergency medical treatment for Mr. Chase, the patient with COPD; to supervise and teach Dr. Baker, the resident working with him; and to play a major role in providing timely and effective medical care for the multiple other patients present and waiting in the ED. No course of action can eliminate the risk of medical error in this situation, but some actions may reduce that risk more than others. Given her relative inexperience, for example, Dr. Baker may be more likely to make a procedural error in intubating Mr. Chase than Dr. Abel. If Dr. Abel and his attending physician colleagues always deny Dr. Baker the opportunity to perform this procedure due to that higher risk of error, however, Dr. Baker will never gain the experience she needs, and she will be more likely to perform this procedure incorrectly in a future independent practice situation. If Dr. Abel chooses to spend a long period of time preparing and coaching Dr. Baker through the procedure, that may reduce the risk of a procedural error, but it may increase the risk of overlooking a life-threatening condition in a hurried assessment of one of the many other waiting ED patients.

As this case suggests, preventing medical errors is one of many important professional responsibilities of physicians. There is no single or simple algorithm for making practice decisions in the face of these multiple competing professional responsibilities. Dr. Abel must, therefore, make a considered judgment about how to manage and prioritize competing goals based on an assessment of which goals are the most important and urgent in the specific circumstance. He may, for example, decide to guide Dr. Baker's intubation efforts more directly, so that the procedure is completed quickly and effectively: Mr. Chase receives the ventilator support he requires, and Drs. Abel and Baker can proceed to care for other ED patients.

In Case 2, Dr. Doyle discovers an apparent medication error made during a patient's previous visit to the ED. Mr. Ford has now returned to the ED with a serious allergic reaction to that medication. Dr. Doyle must decide how to address this situation. Obvious courses of action are to evaluate the patient, to confirm the patient's allergy history if time allows, and to begin appropriate therapy for the patient's allergic reaction. Dr. Doyle must also decide whether to disclose the medication error and, if so, when and how to make that disclosure. Does the professional responsibility to disclose one's own medical errors also apply to errors made by other health care professionals, as in this case? This remains a controversial question. A letter written in response to the Moskop et al. (2006) article on error disclosure, for example, asserts that emergency physicians should not disclose errors committed by other physicians (O'Shaughnessy, 2007). The author argues that these judgments can be mistaken and that they can expose other professionals to unwarranted liability exposure.

Dr. Doyle may, however, conclude that the medical error in this case is readily apparent and that Mr. Ford deserves an explanation of the probable reason for the serious condition that has prompted his return to the ED. If so, several other questions present themselves. Should Dr. Doyle herself make this disclosure to Mr. Ford, or should she communicate with her colleague Dr. Grey, who prescribed the medication, and ask him to assume this responsibility? Should disclosure be delayed until Mr. Ford's medical condition has responded to treatment, or should it be part of the explanation provided to Mr. Ford about his condition and recommended treatment? Should other hospital staff, as, for example, a risk management officer, participate in the disclosure process?

This situation illustrates the value of clear institutional guidelines for the process of error disclosure. If such guidelines are clear, well understood, and effective, Dr. Doyle, Dr. Grey, and their colleagues in the ED and throughout the hospital can confidently and sensitively carry out their responsibilities to disclose medical errors.

ETHICS TAKEOUT TIPS

- When medical errors occur, make disclosure a routine, habitual activity.
- To develop proficiency and comfort in this practice, disclose both minor and major errors.
- Avoid delay in disclosing errors. ("Information delayed is information denied.")
- When the cause of an adverse event is not clear, disclose what is known and provide further information when it becomes available.
- Speak simply, clearly, and directly; avoid euphemisms that may be misunderstood.
- When trainees or other ED staff make errors, assist them in the error disclosure process.

FOR FURTHER READING

ABIM Foundation, ACP-ASIM Foundation, and European Foundation of Internal Medicine. (2002). Medical professionalism in the new millennium: A physician charter. *Annals of Internal Medicine*, 136, 243–246.

American Medical Association. (2003). Opinion 8.121 – Ethical responsibility to study and prevent error and harm. In *AMA code of medical ethics*. www.ama-assn.org/ama/pub/physician-resources/medical-ethics/code-medical-ethics/opinion8121.page

Beckman, H. B., Markakis, K. M., Suchman, A. L., & Frankel R. M. (1994). The doctor-patient relationship and malpractice: Lessons from plaintiff depositions. *Archives of Internal Medicine*, 154, 1365–1370.

Boothman, R. C., Blackwell, A. C., Campbell, D. A., Jr., Commiskey, E., & Anderson, S. (2009). A better approach to medical malpractice claims? The University of Michigan experience. *Journal of Health and Life Sciences and Law*, 2, 125–159.

Cohen, J. R. (1999). Advising clients to apologize. *Southern California Law Review*, 11, 1009–1069.

Croskerry, P., & Sinclair, D. (2001). Emergency medicine: A practice prone to error. *Canadian Journal of Emergency Medicine*, 3, 271–276.

Dresser, R. (2008). The limits of apology laws. *Hastings Center Report*, 38(3), 6–7.

Fordyce, J., Blank, F. S., Pekow, P., Smithline, H. A., Ritter, G., Gehlbach, S., . . . Henneman, P. L. (2003). Errors in a busy emergency department. *Annals of Emergency Medicine*, 42, 324–333.

Gallagher, T. H., Waterman, A. D, Ebers, A. G., Fraser, V. J., & Levinson, W. (2003). Patients' and physicians' attitudes regarding the disclosure of medical errors. *Journal of General Internal Medicine*, 289, 1001–1007.

Hickson, G. B., Clayton, E. W., Githens, P. B., & Sloan, F. A. (1992). Factors that prompted families to file medical malpractice claims following perinatal injuries. *Journal of General Internal Medicine*, 267, 1359–1363.

Hobgood, C., Tamayo-Sarver, J. H., Elms, A., & Weiner, B. (2005). Parental preferences for error disclosure, reporting, and legal action after medical error in the care of their children. *Pediatrics*, 116, 1276–1286.

Hobgood, C., Xie, J., Weiner, B., & Hooker, J. (2004). Error identification, disclosure, and reporting: Practice patterns of three emergency medicine provider types. *Academic Emergency Medicine*, 11, 196–199.

Kohn, L. T., Corrigan, J., Donaldson, M. S. (Eds.). (2000). *To err is human: Building a safer health system*. Washington, DC: National Academy Press.

Leape, L. L., Brennan, T. A., Laird, N., Lawthers, A. G., Localio, A. R., Barnes, B. A., . . . Hiatt, H. (1991). The nature of adverse events in hospitalized patients: Results of the Harvard Medical Practice Study II. *New England Journal of Medicine*, 324, 377–384.

Leung, A., Luu, S., Regehr, G., Murnaghan, M. L., Gallinger, S., & Moulton, C. A. (2012). "First, do no harm": Balancing competing priorities in surgical practice. *Academic Medicine*, 87, 1368–1374.

Mazor, K. M., Simon, S. R., Yood, R. A., Martinson, B. C., Gunter, M. J., Reed, G. W., & Gurwitz, J. H. (2004). Health plan members' views about disclosure of medical errors. *Annals of Internal Medicine*, 140, 409–418.

Moskop, J. C., Derse, A. R., Geiderman, J. M., Larkin, G. L., & Marco, C. A. (2005). From Hippocrates to HIPAA: Privacy and confidentiality in emergency medicine – part I: Conceptual, moral, and legal foundations. *Annals of Emergency Medicine*, 45, 53–59.

Moskop, J. C., Geiderman, J. M., Hobgood, C. D., & Larkin, G. L. (2006). Emergency physicians and disclosure of medical errors. *Annals of Emergency Medicine*, 48, 523–531.

O'Shaughnessy, J. (2007). Disclosing the errors of other physicians. *Annals of Emergency Medicine*, 49, 826–827.

Quality Interagency Coordination Task Force. (2000). *Doing what counts for patient safety: Federal actions to reduce medical errors and their impact*. Report of the Quality Interagency Coordination Task Force (QuIC) to the President, February 2000, Washington, DC. http://archive.ahrq.gov/quic/report/errors6.pdf

Studdert, D. M., Mello, M. M., Gawande, A. A., Brennan, T. A., & Wang, Y. C. (2002). Disclosure of medical injury to patients: An improbable risk management strategy. *Health Affairs*, 26, 215–226.

Truog, R. D., Browning, D. M., Johnson, J. A., & Gallagher, T. H. (2011). *Talking with patients and families about medical error: A guide for education and practice*. Baltimore, MD: Johns Hopkins University Press.

Wu, A. J., Cavanaugh, T. A., McPhee, S. J., Lo, B., & Micco, G. P. (1997). To tell the truth: Ethical and practical issues in disclosing medical mistakes to patients. *Journal of General Internal Medicine*, 12, 770–775.

15

Expert Witness Testimony

ROBERT C. SOLOMON, MD

THE ROLE OF THE EXPERT WITNESS

In the U.S. judicial system, it is common to characterize a witness as a "fact witness" or an "expert witness." A fact witness, as the term suggests, testifies about matters of fact being introduced into evidence in a trial, typically based on direct knowledge. By contrast, an expert witness is asked questions that call for an opinion to help the judge or jury to understand and interpret the facts presented to them in court. An expert witness must be qualified by knowledge, skill, experience, training, or education in an area of scientific, technical, or other specialized knowledge. The expert is declared qualified as such by the presiding judge for the case at hand.

When testifying in a case of alleged medical malpractice, the most important role of the expert witness is helping the judge and jury to define the standard of care and arrive at a judgment about whether the defendants' actions were in accord with it.

The expert witness must form opinions based on sufficient data (the "facts of the case") using reliable methods of interpretation of the data. In some situations, the expert may be called upon to help determine facts. For example, it may be difficult for members of a lay jury to determine, from the information contained in a medical record, what happened in the course of management of a patient. Fact witnesses will likely be asked to elaborate upon the record, but an expert may also be asked to help the jury to interpret information whose meaning is not plain to a layperson, to understand why certain information is important, and even to understand the possible implications when information is missing.

The data on which an expert's opinions are based may include direct observation as a treating physician or as one who conducted an independent medical examination. More commonly, opinions are based on information contained in medical records, including test results and narrative accounts, and on the statements and testimony provided by fact witnesses. Opinions should be formulated by reasonable inferences from the facts of the case, application of relevant scientific literature, and the expert's own knowledge and experience.

BASIS FOR EXPERT OPINIONS: SIGNIFICANT CASES

Frye v. United States (1923)

Frye established the principle of "general acceptance." The decision focused on the "systolic blood pressure [SBP] deception test." The defendant passed the test (lack of rise in SBP when questioned about a murder), and it was used as a basis for his claim of innocence. The appellate court (DC Circuit) held that the test had "not yet gained such standing and scientific recognition among physiological and psychological authorities as would justify the courts in admitting expert testimony deduced from the discovery, development, and experiments thus far made." Based on *Frye*, a novel scientific technique, no matter how convincingly demonstrated, might be disallowed for evidentiary purposes if it had not yet gained general acceptance. This principle also offers insight into the attorney's questioning of an expert witness about whether he believes others in the field would concur with his opinions.

Daubert v. Merrell-Dow (1993)

Seventy years later, the Supreme Court of the United States decided that the principle of general acceptance in *Frye* was not as liberal or flexible as the Federal Rules of Evidence, enacted by Congress half a century after *Frye*, envisioned. Rule 402 generously allows all "relevant evidence." Rule 702 on the role of expert witnesses says, broadly, "If scientific, technical, or other specialized knowledge will assist the trier of fact to understand the evidence or to determine a fact in issue, a witness qualified as an expert by knowledge, skill, experience, training, or education, may testify thereto in the form of an opinion or otherwise."

The Daubert case involved Bendectin (doxylamine), Merrell-Dow's drug for nausea and vomiting in pregnancy. In the absence of epidemiologic data supporting the plaintiff's allegation that the drug caused birth defects, experts testified about animal studies and unpublished human studies, which testimony was ruled inadmissible by lower courts based on *Frye* (general acceptance). The Supreme Court ruled that "general acceptance" was too restrictive under the Federal Rules of Evidence. While thus calling for broader admissibility of expert opinion than "general acceptance" might allow, the high court in *Daubert* also charged trial judges with screening expert testimony for relevance, scientific validity, and reliability. In fulfilling this gatekeeper role, a judge is expected to consider whether an expert's opinion relies on a theory that has undergone empirical testing; been published or subject to peer review; or gained broad acceptance or, instead, been rejected by the scientific community. A judge may elect to conduct a "Daubert hearing" to determine the admissibility of expert testimony. *Daubert* is now followed in most state courts.

General Electric v. Joiner (1997)

Joiner was an electrician who was exposed on the job to polychlorinated biphenyls (PCBs) and sued General Electric, claiming the company was liable for contributing to his development of lung cancer. Expert testimony for the plaintiff relied heavily on animal studies. Lower courts excluded this testimony because the authors of the published studies had themselves declined to suggest a link between exposure to PCBs and lung cancer in humans. The Supreme Court upheld that reasoning and concluded that lower courts did not abuse their discretion in excluding this opinion: "nothing in either Daubert or the Federal Rules of Evidence requires a district court to admit opinion evidence which is connected to existing data only by the ipse dixit [unproven dictum] of the expert. A court may conclude that there is simply too great an analytical gap between the data and the opinion proffered."

Kumho Tire v. Carmichael (1999)

Carmichael, while driving a minivan, experienced a catastrophic tire blow-out. An expert for the plaintiff opined that this was caused by a manufacturing defect and based this opinion on inspection of the tire and his own experience. This visual inspection method, according to lower court rulings, had not been validated by published research and was not used by other industry experts. The Supreme Court upheld the lower court's exclusion of this expert opinion (and reversed an appellate court ruling), rejecting Carmichael's claim that *Daubert* should not apply to technical (rather than scientific) opinion. An important element of this case is the concurring opinion by Justice Scalia that not only was the lower court not abusing its discretion by applying *Daubert*, but "failure to apply one or another of them [*Daubert* factors] may be unreasonable, and hence an abuse of discretion."

According to Scalia, "it is discretion to choose among reasonable means of excluding expertise that is fausse and science that is junky." (Perhaps only Antonin Scalia would use the feminine form of "faux" in recognition that the gender of the word "expertise" is feminine.)

TRUTH IN EXPERT WITNESS TESTIMONY

Given that lying under oath is known as perjury and regarded as a serious matter, one would think untruthful expert witness testimony would be distinctly uncommon. But expert witnesses render opinions, and identifying opinion as falsehood is problematic. We might instead say that sometimes testimony is provided that the expert knows, or should know, is faulty, which makes it unethical.

REASONS FOR UNETHICAL TESTIMONY

Most experts have had no formal training for this role. The attorneys who procure their services on behalf of clients are typically seeking not fair and impartial authorities who will facilitate the court's search for the truth, but advocates for a client's position. Expert witnesses who insist on rigorously adhering to principles of impartiality, thereby limiting their effectiveness as advocates, are likely to find themselves receiving very few queries from members of the bar.

Nonstandard Facts

The facts of a given case are unique, which means standardization of opinion is difficult. Or, looking at it the other way, nonstandard opinions are practically invited. Cases revolving around clinical controversies will necessarily invite varying opinions. Unfortunately, experts on either side typically are used to convince a lay jury that one way of looking at the scientific evidence is correct and another is not because admitting that there is legitimate disagreement among experts is likely to undermine the position of one side or the other (more commonly the plaintiff who is asserting that a standard of care was violated).

Lack of Standard Qualifications

State law is quite variable. Many states have no expert witness qualifications, leaving that to the discretion of the judge, case by case. Expert witnesses are typically not required to be in the same specialty as a physician defendant. A witness may not have to be licensed in the state where testimony is given, or even in any state. The expert may not have to be in active practice, with professional endeavors instead being limited to teaching, research, or administration, or the expert may be retired, deriving professional income only from expert witness work.

Lack of Guidelines for Formulating Opinions

This is an area that some medical professional organizations have sought to address. The American College of Emergency Physicians (ACEP) has established a set of guidelines for ethical conduct as an expert witness. However, adherence to these guidelines is required only by ACEP and only for its own members, and the only mechanism for enforcement is disciplinary action against one's membership, which can occur only in response to a complaint by another member through a detailed procedure that safeguards the due process rights of the expert who is the subject of the complaint.

Lack of Genuine Expertise

Given the lack of any requirements that an expert witness be a currently practicing clinician in the same specialty as a physician defendant, as well as the absence of any standard to which an expert might be held regarding knowledge of contemporary scientific literature, it can hardly come as a surprise that some expert witness testimony lacks accuracy, reliability, or scientific validity. If the physician defendant is in the specialty of emergency medicine and the plaintiff's expert is a retired family practitioner, defense counsel will be in a position of using that status to discredit, in the minds of the jury, a witness who reminds them of their own long-time, kindly, and beloved GP.

Partisanship

Experts are commonly advocates for one side or the other because it is the attorneys on either side of a case who procure their services. This may be taken even further, however, if an expert develops some degree of emotional investment in a case, leading to distortion of testimony through exaggeration and emotion-laden language to sway a jury toward the desired verdict. Whereas the popular view of courtroom behavior encompasses such behavior on the part of counsel, occasionally expert witnesses may also be swept up in the poignant or affecting aspects of a case.

Financial Incentives

Like attorneys, expert witnesses bill for their services by the hour (or fractions thereof). Rates are invariably higher than what an emergency physician would earn by spending that time caring for patients, and they may amount to several-fold clinical compensation. The expert who is a successful advocate will find himself in much greater demand than one who strives to be fair-minded, although the latter may be sought by defense counsel or by plaintiff's counsel in search of a sound opinion on weaknesses in a case. The market favors the expert who is effective in convincing a jury of the merit of a plaintiff's case.

Given what experienced expert witnesses know about the desire of plaintiffs' counsel for advocacy, this may even produce a preliminary opinion that a case has merit when it does not, leading to the filing of lawsuits ultimately characterized as "frivolous."

Absence of Disincentives

Outside of the potential for disciplinary action by an organization such as ACEP, disincentives for advocacy rather than fair, impartial conduct as an expert witness do not exist. State medical boards generally do not recognize expert witness work as the practice of medicine or entertain complaints against licensed physicians based on their conduct in this role. Courts allow wide latitude for experts in rendering opinions – which, unlike statements of fact, do not lend themselves to accusations of perjury, no matter how unsupportable they may seem to a physician defendant.

The view of the legal system on this point was captured by U.S. Supreme Court Associate Justice Byron White in *Imbler v. Pachtman* (1976), and his concurring opinion is worth considering in some detail:

> The ability of courts, under carefully developed procedures, to separate truth from falsity, and the importance of accurately resolving factual disputes in criminal (and civil) cases are such that those involved in judicial proceedings should be "given every encouragement to make a full disclosure of all pertinent information within their knowledge." For a witness, this means he must be permitted to testify without fear of being sued if his testimony is disbelieved. For a lawyer, it means that he

must be permitted to call witnesses without fear of being sued if the witness is disbelieved and it is alleged that the lawyer knew or should have known that the witness' testimony was false. Of course, witnesses should not be encouraged to testify falsely nor lawyers encouraged to call witnesses who testify falsely. However, if the risk of having to defend a civil damage suit is added to the deterrent against such conduct already provided by criminal laws against perjury and subornation of perjury, the risk of self-censorship becomes too great. This is particularly so because it is very difficult if not impossible for attorneys to be absolutely certain of the objective truth or falsity of the testimony which they present. A prosecutor faced with a decision whether or not to call a witness whom he believes, but whose credibility he knows will be in doubt and whose testimony may be disbelieved by the jury, should be given every incentive to submit that witness' testimony to the crucible of the judicial process so that the fact finder may consider it, after cross-examination, together with the other evidence in the case to determine where the truth lies.

EXPERT WITNESSES DO LIE

Although much of the conduct by expert witnesses that might be considered questionable can be explained (or rationalized) as opinion, expert witnesses do tell outright lies in court. They may, for purposes of bolstering credibility in the eyes of jurors, make false statements regarding board certification, education and training, clinical practice experience, academic positions held, membership or leadership roles in professional organizations, and authorship of publications. Less blatantly, they may err in attributing statements about medical science to authoritative references, incorrectly describe data or conclusions from published studies, or fail to acknowledge that there are other schools of thought that contradict their views. Testimony on a given point may be inconsistent from question to question as counsel probes the logic of an expert's opinion.

One of the most common examples of lying occurs when an expert is asked a pointed question about the standard of care. This is a phrase that has a well-understood meaning in medical negligence cases, and it refers to what any prudent practitioner would do under the same or similar circumstances. An expert may make a statement regarding what he would have done in the case at hand, and the jury may be led to believe that this is a statement regarding the standard of care. A skillful attorney will address this question directly, and the expert witness may respond by claiming that his statement of what he would have done, and therefore believes the physician defendant should have done, is a genuine statement of the standard of care, knowing that it is no such thing because practice among prudent practitioners under the same or similar circumstances would, in truth, be significantly variable.

MANAGING THE EXPERT WITNESS ADVOCATE

The expert witness who serves as an advocate for the side of the case paying his fees and expenses seems, unfortunately, more common than the expert who strives to be fair and impartial. The ACEP has a statement that may be used to remind an expert of his duty to act ethically. An expert can be asked by counsel to sign this statement affirming willingness and intent to behave ethically:

As a member of the medical profession and the American College of Emergency Physicians, I hereby affirm my duty, when giving evidence or testifying as an expert witness, to do so solely in accordance with the merits of the case.

Furthermore, I declare that I will uphold the following professional principles in providing expert evidence or expert witness testimony:

1. I will always be truthful, and I will abide by the principles of Ethics of the American College of Emergency Physicians.
2. I will conduct a thorough, fair and impartial review of the facts and the medical care provided, including any and all relevant information.
3. I will provide evidence or testify only in matters in which I have recent clinical experience and knowledge in the areas of medicine that are the subject of the case or proceeding.
4. I will evaluate the medical care provided in light of generally accepted clinical standards, neither condemning performance that falls within generally accepted practice standards nor condoning performance that falls below these standards.
5. I will evaluate the medical care provided in light of the generally accepted standards that prevailed at the time of the occurrence giving rise to the case.
6. I will provide evidence or testimony that is complete, objective, scientifically based, and likely to assist in achieving a just resolution of the proceeding.
7. I will make a clear distinction in my testimony between a departure from accepted practice standards and an untoward outcome.

8. I will make every effort to determine and to specify whether I believe there is a causal relationship between any substandard practice and the medical outcome.
9. I will submit my testimony to peer review, if requested by a professional organization to which I belong.
10. I will not accept compensation that is contingent upon the outcome of the litigation.

The expert who signs the statement yet does not act in accord with it, and the expert who refuses to sign it, are both subject to having their credibility impugned by skillful counsel.

THE *DAUBERT* CHALLENGE

Under *Daubert*, a judge may use discretion in determining the admissibility of an expert opinion. A hearing may be held on specific questions about the relevance, accuracy, reliability, and validity of expert testimony. In the view of Associate Justice Scalia, judges have a responsibility to use this discretion. However, judges typically have little knowledge of medical science and are ill-equipped to evaluate the admissibility of complex medical testimony. Thus, they have a low threshold for allowing questionable evidence, instead relying on the process unfolding in the courtroom to guide the jury (finders of fact) toward the truth or at least toward sensible decisions about how much credence to lend to the expert opinions presented.

CROSS-EXAMINATION

The most effective way to address the merit of the opinions being expressed by a witness is the cross-examination. A good cross-examination requires knowledgeable counsel with substantial insight into the fine points of the medical care at issue. Such counsel can be greatly aided by thorough preparation, and detailed consultation with his own expert(s) can very constructive. Experts on either side, especially if they are seasoned, are likely to know what those on the other side are apt to say in support of the opposing theory of the case. They are also likely to be able to identify any flaws in that theory, to have suggestions on how to expose them, to know what opposing experts are likely to say in response to probing questions that expose such flaws, and to have recommendations on how to follow up on those responses effectively. For defense counsel, sometimes a knowledgeable physician defendant can also be quite helpful in preparing effective cross-examination.

THE FRIVOLOUS LAWSUIT

We all think we know a frivolous lawsuit when we see one. There is a widely held opinion that plaintiff's counsel should be held accountable for bringing such a lawsuit. Doing so is seen as an abuse of the judicial process and is analogous to malicious prosecution in the criminal arena, where such an allegation would be based on action by a prosecutor that proceeded without probable cause.

However, the *presence* of expert opinion, no matter how flawed, supporting the notion that a plaintiff's case may have merit makes it extremely difficult to show *absence* of probable cause.

Other terms that sometimes come up in discussion of perceived misconduct by counsel and expert witnesses include legal malpractice, defamation, fraud, and perjury.

Legal malpractice implies an attorney–client relationship with a breach of duty in that relationship. Because there is no such relationship between counsel on one side and client on the other, this becomes inapplicable.

Defamation applies only to statements of fact, not to opinions, which are generally regarded as protected by "witness privilege." Even for statements of fact, proving they were "knowingly false" is quite difficult.

Fraud would require the same sort of crossing of sides as legal malpractice: for example, an attorney or expert must make a false statement, knowing that it is false, with the intent that the opposing side rely on the truth of the statement. That reliance would then have to lead the victim of the fraud to take action to his own detriment and suffer damages as a result of that action. Thus, the legal definition of fraud, unlike the common-sense meaning of the word, is very unlikely to apply.

Perjury is the making of a false statement under oath. The false statement must be made knowingly, and the standard of proof is "beyond a reasonable doubt" – a high standard to apply to the making of statements that are almost certain to be cast as opinions rather than statements of fact. Prosecutors have shown great reluctance to bring charges of perjury against expert witnesses.

ACTION BY A STATE MEDICAL BOARD

Few state medical boards consider the provision of expert witness testimony to constitute the practice of medicine, which is what they govern. A board that does so regard this activity may assert jurisdiction over it. The North Carolina Medical Board took disciplinary action against neurosurgeon Gary Lustgarten, who testified that another neurosurgeon had made entries in the medical record that were factually inaccurate. Defense attorneys tried valiantly to pin him down by asking him if he was asserting that the neurosurgeon who made those entries was falsifying the medical record. Lustgarten was artfully evasive, instead asserting why he thought the content of those entries was very unlikely to be accurate and saying the jury should draw its own conclusions.

The Medical Board drew its own conclusions and suspended Lustgarten's license. Lustgarten then appealed the Board's ruling to Superior Court, which upheld the ruling. Subsequently (in 2006), the North Carolina Court of Appeals reversed the Superior Court's ruling, but that reversal was based on a review of the facts of the malpractice case and Lustgarten's testimony. The Court of Appeals did not question the Medical Board's authority to take disciplinary action against Lustgarten for unethical conduct as an expert witness. Rather, it concluded that Lustgarten's artful avoidance of defense counsel's efforts to get him to use the words "lying" or "falsifying the record" was sufficient to show that his characterization of those entries in the record was not a "bad faith accusation."

The Lustgarten case illustrates the challenge of taking legal action against an expert witness who makes statements in a court of law that the physician defendant likely considered unsupportable, egregious, and outrageous.

ACTION BY A MEDICAL PROFESSIONAL ASSOCIATION

If a medical professional association takes disciplinary action against a member for unethical conduct (which may include unethical conduct as an expert witness), such disciplinary action may, depending on the nature of the action, be reported publicly, including to the National Practitioner Data Bank. The ACEP has taken disciplinary action in a number of cases based on complaints of unethical expert witness conduct. Some professional societies fear liability because there exists the potential for (expensive) litigation by a physician who has been disciplined. Such a physician may assert damages to professional reputation and to income, especially if there is an adverse effect on his ability to earn compensation as an expert witness.

Neurosurgeon Donald Austin was disciplined (six-month suspension) by the American Association of Neurological Surgeons (AANS) for what it deemed unethical conduct as an expert witness for the plaintiff in a medical malpractice case involving a surgical complication. Austin subsequently sued AANS, alleging economic damages (decline in expert witness income). In 2001, the Seventh Circuit Court of Appeals ruled for the AANS, and the opinion includes these salient statements: "[T]here is little doubt that his testimony was irresponsible and that it violated a number of sensible-seeming provisions of the Association's ethical code." And: "Although Dr. Austin did not treat the malpractice plaintiff for whom he testified, his testimony at her trial was a type of medical service and if the quality of his testimony reflected the quality of his medical judgment, he is probably a poor physician." To the reader interested in such matters, the relatively short, cogent, and skillfully written opinion[7] by Judge Richard Posner is highly commended.

GUIDELINES

The ACEP has developed guidelines for serving as an expert witness in cases of alleged medical malpractice. These guidelines have been in place for nearly two decades and were most recently revised in 2010:

> Expert witnesses are asked to render opinions as to assess the requisite standard of care pertaining to emergency physicians in cases of alleged medical malpractice and peer review. Because medical expert witness testimony has demonstrated the potential to establish standards of medical care, and because physician expert witnesses hold themselves out as qualified to render an opinion by virtue of a medical degree, such testimony is considered by the American College of Emergency Physicians (ACEP) to constitute the practice of medicine.
>
> In order to qualify as an expert witness in the specialty of emergency medicine, a physician should:
>
> - Be currently licensed in a state, territory, or area constituting legal jurisdiction of the United States as a doctor of medicine or osteopathic medicine;
> - Be certified by a recognized certifying body in emergency medicine
> - Be in the active clinical practice of emergency medicine for three years immediately preceding the date of the event giving rise to the case
> - Abide by the following guidelines:
>   * The expert witness should possess current experience and ongoing knowledge in the area in which he or she is asked to testify.
>   * The expert witness should not provide expert medical testimony that is false, misleading, or without medical foundation. The key

to this process is a thorough review of available and appropriate medical records and contemporaneous literature concerning the case being examined.

* A medical expert's opinion should reflect the state of medical knowledge at the time of the event giving rise to the case.
* The expert witness should review the medical facts in a thorough, fair, and objective manner and should not exclude any relevant information to create a view favoring either the plaintiff or the defendant.
* Expert witnesses should be chosen on the basis of their experience in the area in which they are providing testimony, and not on the basis of offices or positions held in medical specialty societies, unless such positions are material to the expertise of the witness.
* An emergency physician should not engage in advertising or solicit employment as an expert witness where such advertising or solicitation contains false or deceptive representations about the physician's qualifications, experience, titles or background.
* The expert witness should be willing to submit the transcripts of depositions and testimony to peer review.
* An expert witness should never accept any compensation arrangement that is contingent on the outcome of litigation.
* Misconduct as an expert, including the provision of false, fraudulent, or misleading testimony, may expose the physician to disciplinary action.

When an emergency physician accepts membership in ACEP, he agrees to abide by the organization's Code of Ethics. This encompasses a compendium of policies in the realm of ethics. This compendium is annually reviewed by the Ethics Committee and approved by the Board of Directors. The expert witness guidelines are in that compendium, and so an alleged violation of the guidelines can become the basis of an ethics complaint by one member of the College against another. Such complaints are considered by the Ethics Committee and the Board of Directors through a highly developed procedure that safeguards due process rights for all concerned.

Critics of such an approach by a medical professional organization claim that guidelines are intended to inhibit those who might serve as experts for the plaintiff, noting that complaints are much more likely to be made against experts for the plaintiff than for the defense. The record of complaints sent to ACEP supports that claim of distribution, although not the claim of intent. But this criticism raises the question of who, exactly, is inhibited by guidelines that recognize the importance of a fair-minded, impartial review of the facts of a case. When this author has received correspondence from plaintiffs' attorneys about possibly reviewing a case, the response indicates a willingness to conduct a review and an intention to do so according to the cited guidelines, with special attention to fairness and impartiality and a disinclination to serve in the role of an advocate. Thus far, without exception, such a response has marked the end of the correspondence. In a legal system for addressing claims of medical negligence that has been described as a "battle of the experts," counsel for the plaintiff wants an expert who will pick up the lance and the shield, not one who prefers to don the cloak of the philosopher.

PATHS TO IMPROVEMENT

Many recommendations have been advanced for improving the process through which expert witnesses testify in cases of alleged medical malpractice. One of these is certification of expert witnesses based on medical education, training, experience, specialty, and possibly specialized education and even a certifying examination to assure special competence to serve in this role. Some advocate having experts appointed by and serving the court rather than selected and paid by either side in the case. Some jurisdictions require a certificate of merit from an expert for a case to proceed. Given that this requirement is subject to the tendency toward advocacy that plagues testimony in deposition and in the courtroom, replacement of this mechanism with a certification of (potential) merit by a court-appoint panel of experts has many supporters. A process akin to *voir dire* for jurors has been suggested, so that experts could be questioned in advance by counsel and the judge to ascertain qualifications, knowledge, and sources of bias. Education of judges, with assignment of medical negligence cases selectively to judges with demonstrated expertise and qualifications, especially in the judgment of the quality of evidence and opinion that is to be presented to jurors, might serve the system well. All of these improvements could be incorporated into a specialized system of health courts in which expert panels might even replace lay juries.

RECOMMENDATIONS FOR TODAY'S EXPERT WITNESS

Be objective: the expert's role is to educate the finders of fact (judge, jury); it is the role of counsel to advocate.

Stay within your expertise: if asked to provide an opinion that strays over the line into another medical speciality, don't yield to temptation just because patients with conditions within that specialty are often seen in your domain. Make sure the question is about the appropriate care that should be provided by a practitioner of your specialty. It may also be prudent to resist opining about standards of care for other health care workers. An emergency physician may be knowledgeable about standards of practice in emergency nursing, but an expert from emergency nursing may well be a better choice.

Remember what standard of care means. It is defined by what a reasonable and prudent practitioner would do under the same or similar circumstances. Do not substitute for this what you think you would have done.

Your opinion is not the focus. The jurors are interested in your opinion. They are (or should be) more interested in how the facts of the case and the medical science support your opinion.

Avoid overstatement and favor understatement. An opinion is better expressed in a way that would be approved by your professional peers than one that might grab the attention not only of a jury but also of opposing counsel, who will relish the opportunity to force you to defend every intemperately chosen word or phrase.

Change your opinion. If new information comes to light during a trial, an admission that it alters your perspective will better serve the process, not to mention gain greater respect from judge, jury, and counsel, than will rigid adherence to your original position. An expert who clearly places integrity at the top of the hierarchy of values is one the jury will, and should, believe.

ETHICS TAKEOUT TIPS

- The role of the expert witness is to educate judge and jury in a fair, impartial, objective manner, using knowledge of contemporaneous medical literature and clinical experience.
- There should be standard expert witness qualifications that include being in the same speciality as a physician defendant and being engaged in active clinical practice.
- A judge has a responsibility to serve as a gatekeeper, assuring the relevance and reliability of expert testimony.
- There are guidelines for ethical conduct as an expert witness. They should be well-disseminated and scrupulously followed.
- Our system of adjudicating claims of medical negligence would be better served by having experts who serve the court rather than being retained by either side in the case.

FOR FURTHER READING

ACEP Expert Witness Guidelines: www.acep.org/Clinical-Practice-Management/
Expert-Witness-Guidelines-for-the-Specialty-of-Emergency-Medicine/
Byron White on the dangers of self-censorship by attorneys and witnesses: www.
oyez.org/cases/1970-1979/1975/1975_74_5435
On *Austin v. AANS*: caselaw.findlaw.com/us-7th-circuit/1429913.html
On *Daubert v. Merrell-Dow*: www.law.harvard.edu/publications/evidenceiii/cases/
daubert.htm
On *Frye v. United States*: www.law.harvard.edu/publications/evidenceiii/cases/
frye.htm
On *General Electric v. Joiner*: www.law.harvard.edu/publications/evidenceiii/
cases/joiner.htm
On *Kumho Tire v. Carmichael*: www.law.harvard.edu/publications/evidenceiii/
cases/kumho.htm
On *Lustgarten v. North Carolina State Medical Board*: www.aoc.state.nc.us/www/
public/coa/opinions/2006/050891-1.htm

16

Values and Responsibilities in Professional Practice

GREGORY L. HENRY, MD, AND KARTIK RAO, DO

INTRODUCTION

Emergency medicine in its "fact-based pursuit of health" is a science. In actual practice, it is a complex interaction of ever-changing facts, cultural norms, often illogical distribution of resources, and hopefully humane management of diverse family groupings. All pure science is mathematically based, but any implementation of a diagnostic or treatment modality is a philosophical process based on the belief systems of both the physician and the patient unit being treated. Science questions are always "how" or "what" questions. Philosophic questions always ask "why." In the Western tradition of understanding meaning, it is still reasonable to build on Aristotle's four causes of existence to explain not only the way things are, but also why they exist and how we are to judge our response to them. Our actions are based on both anticipated results for the individual as well as on how that individual relates in his or her larger societal context.

As emergency medicine further becomes the central hub of clinical decision-making, increasingly more value-laden situations will come under the immediate action agenda of emergency physicians. Ethical issues of practice become dilemmas only when there are conflicting clashes at the level of actual decision-making.

CHAPTER OBJECTIVES

The objectives of this chapter are (1) to understand the ancient and historical basis of medical ethics, (2) to examine the morale and legal duty of the emergency practitioner to the ethical principles of medicine, (3) to initiate a personal value system that reflects the traditions of medical ethics, and (4) to encourage the practitioner to practice a system of actions

and attitudes that provide protection for both the patient and the traditions
of medicine.

BACKGROUND

Our current predicament is generated by the following tenets:

- Our technological abilities and virtuosities in the maintenance of life
  have moved far ahead of our wisdom to know when to apply such
  time-consuming and expensive technology. We have no consensus
  has to when "enough is enough."
- Authority for making life-and-death decisions is often unresolved,
  and clashes of authority fall prey to the legal system for mediation and
  resolution despite obvious predicted known outcomes. Patient's
  families are often determined to have their rights, wants, and desires
  put ahead of the society at large, thus ignoring normal fiduciary
  constructs.
- Physicians are placed between the legitimate need to control resource
  utilization and a family's expectations. Physicians are now the stewards of society's most expensive but limited resource pool.
- The public knowledge of medicine and it limitations has diminished.
  Once-private matters between the patient and the doctor have, by
  virtue of the media, the law, and third-party payers, become a not
  always intelligent public process.
- Emergency medicine functions in the tyranny of the immediate. Full
  understanding of all facts is rarely if ever available to the emergency
  physician who must act now: "we can be wrong but never in doubt."

ETHICAL PRINCIPLES

Ethics can be defined as a group of moral precepts or values governing the
behavior of members of the profession. Clinical ethics, the kind experienced by emergency physicians every day, are the rules that govern our
actions for the patients presenting before us at any given moment in time.

There is no single universally accepted moral or ethical base on which
all physicians agree, but traditions sends us back to both the Greeks and the
utilitarians and deontological exponents of the eighteenth and nineteenth
centuries.

Jeremy Bentham (1748–1832) and John Stuart Mill (1806–1876) are
referenced elsewhere in this book with regard to utilitarian thinking. Mill

wrote "actions are right in proportion as they tend to promote happiness; wrong as they tend to produce the reverse of happiness." In other words, the greatest benefit for the greatest number of people. Taking all things into account, utilitarianism seeks the greatest net happiness.

Immanuel Kant (1724–1804) expressed the belief that rightness of an act is based on intent, sense of duty, and the intricate character of that act and not upon its consequences. Kant's categorical imperative sets the base for all decisions and actions: "I ought never to act except in such a way that I can also will that my maxim shall become a universal law." In other words, we do for the patient and their families only those things we would do for the people we love and care about.

ISSUES AND CONTROVERSIES

Bernard Gert, a contemporary moral philosopher, combines these schools of thought in a list of the ten moral concepts that are driving medical ethics today. In his book *A New Justification of Moral Rules*, he lists behaviors that he feels we would be wise to obey. If you need to break these rules, justifications must be provided:

1. Do not kill.
2. Do not cause pain.
3. Do not disable.
4. Do not deprive anyone of freedom or opportunity.
5. Do not deprive anyone of pleasure.

The second five moral rules, if violated, would increase the probability that someone will come to harm:

6. Do not deceive.
7. Keep your promises.
8. Do not steal.
9. Obey the law.
10. Do your professional duty.

The direct application of these rules to clinical practice are obvious. All of these maxims have logical and defendable exceptions, but, in general, they form the base of an ethical career. These rules and the need to violate such rules on occasion is the practice of emergency medicine. It is this cost–benefit analysis that determines what we do on a daily basis. Restraining intoxicated patients restricts freedom but to a higher end. Starting IVs and giving injections gives pain but with the hope and expectations of a better outcome. The ultimate question is, does your violation of any rule pass the test of public scrutiny? Could you defend the action to outside bodies such as media and various review boards? More importantly, can you defend such violations to yourself and your own conscience?

MORAL PRECEPTS

Clouser and Gert have pointed out that these moral rules do not, in and of themselves, comprise a complete philosophical system, but it is still these various rules boiled down to the four basic ethical concepts that are recognized by most professional ethicists today.

1. *Concept of respect for autonomy.* In this context, we are referring to the right of patients to be self-governing and make their own decisions. One hundred years ago, Justice Benjamin Cardozo expressed this belief in a famous New York Supreme Court case when he concluded "Every human being of adult years and sound mind has a right to determine what shall be done with his body." Lack of controlling influences is the key. Human beings have both ethical and constitutionally defendable rights to self-determination.

2. *Concept of nonmaleficence.* Nonmaleficence is the duty of all of us not to inflict evil or harm. The physicians' Latin motto, *Primum non nocere* (above all do no harm), best describes this charge to the profession. When complexity of both diagnosis and treatment have minimal advantages, these must all be taken into account when dealing with the individual patient.

3. *Concept of beneficence.* Beneficence is more than just nonmaleficence. It is our duty to not only prevent harm but to promote the good. These judgments require us to take into account the viewpoint of the patient. It's not just what is right to us but what is right to them. This prevails throughout the entire doctor–patient relationship. The Hippocratic Oath summarizes the role of the provider and reminds us that it is the patient who ultimately has the problem to be solved, the needs that need to be serviced. The common error of the medical community is to take the paternalistic view that "doctor knows best." *Paternalism*, in its most positive sense, is a medical tradition recognizing that we hold the scientific knowledge in our hands. But it is to aid the patient and family in making informed judgments, not to define the final goal of care for them.

4. *Concept of justice.* Finally, justice overlays the entire process that looks at the distribution of resources in light of the ethereal ideas of fairness and decency. This is a relatively newer process, one that recognizes a unity of man and the limitations of our abundance. These concepts are discussed elsewhere in the book, but should be understood as part of all our decision-making.

Many views of justice exist, but all recognize unlimited human expectations and limited resources as the central issue of economics. Adam Smith, author of *Inquiries into the Nature of the Wealth of Nations* (1776) was a professor of moral philosophy who understood these inherent human conflicts. Universal care, no matter what system in the world is being referenced, should never support the provision of futile care. Emergency departments (EDs) are the new location where the needs of the individual and the demands of the society most closely come into conflict. An emergency physician must be expert at knowing these concepts and then walking the fine line between such competing forces.

ETHICAL PRACTICE

Ethical practice is the difficult final common pathway linking philosophical abstracts to the practical, humane management of all patients who present for care. Seldom does the tyranny of the immediate that is the daily scenario of the ED allow for the quiet deliberations of the hospital ethics committee: it's yes or no, and frequently families and patients do not understand the complex thought processes that go into "calling the code" or allowing the debilitated and demented patient to expire. The importance of physician virtue cannot be overemphasized in this forum and needs to be the principle upon which decisions are based.

AREAS OF CONCERN

The problems of valid consent or refusal of care, competence, historical truth, and innate paternalism must all function under the "faithful servant" doctrine. All these situations require a rational resort to autonomy and justice for the "good of the patient" to be served. Rationality of a decision is always based on one's perspective. Perfectly competent people can make perfectly irrational decisions that are harmful. Both the stock market and the entire gambling industry are based on this truism. There is conflicting data on the results of many of our therapies (i.e. TPA and stroke), so either taking or not taking medication may represent a rational decision on the part of the patient. The shifting trend toward joint decision-making is often difficult for physicians to accept. Overriding a patient's grossly irrational decision with regard to his care is fraught with medical legal danger for the physician, and strict adherence to hospital-approved process may be the best protection for all parties involved.

For the emergency physician, purposeful deception should be viewed as a "last resort" and a potentially harmful concept to furthering excellent doctor–patient relationships. Not telling the truth about serious or hopeless illness, over- or underemphasizing the risk and results of proposed treatments, and use of placebos all may have unexpected consequences. Honesty is generally the most appreciated and defensible policy.

Nowhere are the dilemmas of treatment more evident than in management of the terminal or near-terminal patient. Physicians have no ethical duty to provide care that has not been proved to work despite the fervent demands of patients and their families. This problem sphere is aided by the Internet and social media, which are replete with medical misinformation. It is not unusual for the emergency physician to need to counter such fallacies as family units are confronted with these difficult moral decision. With a provision of adequate and timely palliative care, requests for active euthanasia should be a rare event for emergency physicians. Aggressive pain management in the dying, suffering patient is a cornerstone of current care. No dying patient should be consigned to ending his or her life in pain.

FIXED DUTIES

Ethical duties to the general physician community follow long-standing traditions that include improving everyone's knowledge base through teaching, courteous behavior, and a duty to recognize and rehabilitate impaired physicians. The removal of impaired and incompetent physicians is both an obligation to the profession and the general society.

DUTY TO SOCIETY

Defense of the patient is still the emergency physician's first priority. Reporting statutes vary slightly from state to state, but all function under the belief that emergency physicians have the clearest view of the soft underbelly of society and its cultural problems. When a patient clearly constitutes a danger to self or others, the physician is obligated to act in defense of the wider society. Similarly, whenever a physician detects the reasonable possibility of an abuse to our most defenseless (i.e. the young, the old, the infirm), the obligation to report under the legal protection of the state is mandatory. Duty to third parties either named or unnamed but anticipated frequently forms the basis for our actions in the ED.

Last, knowledge of ethical, moral, and legal principles forms only a platform for our actions. Most situations clarify themselves under invocation of the "Favorite Uncle Louie Rule." If it was your Favorite Uncle Louie, someone you cared about, what would you do? If an emergency physician can answer this question, almost all ethical conundrums dissolve.

Selected Examples

Case 1: The Children with an Intoxicated Parent
A mother presents on Christmas Eve shortly before midnight. She has with her three small children. The patient has never been married, and there is no current partner with whom she has a relationship. The mother is clearly intoxicated. She brings the children in to be examined as a group for fever. The physician's exam of the children shows they are somewhat disheveled, physically dirty, and suffering what are probably viral illnesses. The mother has slurred speech and ataxia. It is 4 degrees below zero outside and snowing.

The moral and ethical decisions are difficult. Should the emergency physician call social services? Is the emergency physician willing to sign the papers necessary to have the children removed from the home? To what extent is the physician liable should the mother proceed to further neglect these children or some untoward event happens? Is it a reasonable use of resources to admit the children? Any discussion of this case must revolve around the fact that there are more than the immediate physical health of the children involved. The mother in an intoxicated state could certainly have a motor vehicle accident. The emergency physician has a duty not only to the children who are presented for care, but to the mother herself, who could be injured. The interaction with social services is not only an option, but in many states would be considered mandatory due to the fact that children at risk are presenting to the emergency physician. Separation of children from their natural parents is always an emotionally distressing situation. The search for other reasonable relatives who may become involved in the care of such children and possible intervention steps by child protective services (CPS) test the balance between autonomy and beneficence.

Case 1: Discussion

Inherent to any scenario used to discuss ethical questions are many complicating factors at hand. The effectiveness and potential drawbacks of the child protective system and foster care is a confounding factor in this situation, for example. Our duty and moral obligation is not in the role of judge, jury, and executioner. The emergency physician's role is limited in the society that we live in. As in most decisions in this field, risk versus benefit is the scale on which we base our choices. In this scenario, we are faced with a mother who is putting herself and her children at real risk if driving while intoxicated. The potential drawbacks of activating the CPS system, although from this vantage point only theoretical, are still very real; these drawbacks, however, are superseded by the imminent danger of doing nothing. Always act like it was a member of your own family, then think through the options.

Case 1: Resolution

As would be expected, the entire situation was run by the police department and CPS. An alternative living situation was arranged.

Case 2: An Elderly Immigrant Women with an Extremely Aggressive Family Member

The emergency physician is presented with a seventy-eight-year-old Lithuanian woman who was brought in by her son. The patient has only a moderate understanding of English, and, although the son's English is good, it is not perfect. The son has instructed the emergency physician that he wants all communication about the woman's health care to go through him. His statement is, "she is too old and fragile and that bad news would only upset her." Because of her chronic cough and failing health, the emergency physician performs a chest x-ray that shows an obvious mass in which the differential diagnosis would be headed by cancer. The son does not want this mentioned to the women.

Case 2: Discussion

Even if discussed in the setting of no cultural and language barriers, this scenario is still an appropriate example of an ethical challenge. I think the addition of the cultural aspect actually simplifies the conundrum. At face value in this scenario, it seems that, although the physician may have fulfilled the minimum requirements of care to his patient, the question remains whether or not she will receive the appropriate follow-up and care. The dilemma here exists because the cultural paradigm that this patient lives in is different from our own. In acting according to the regulations regarding patients with language barriers, the physician has determined that this woman is of sound mind and has made the decision to allow medical decision-making to proceed through the filter of her son through an unbiased third-party translator. Any further question that exists as to the moral and ethical implications here should call into question the paternalistic nature of our own practice, as well as the cultural norms witnessed here. To violate their wishes would likely disrupt not only the present doctor–patient relationship, but also potentially any future one as well. It is not our place to impose our own cultural, personal, or societal norms on our patients. This is not to say that our responsibilities do not reach beyond in the setting where abuse or neglect may be suspected; but, in a scenario such as this, any further action on the physician's part against what both patient and son have expressed would lead to real deterioration of the doctor–patient relationship versus a theoretical possibility of poor follow-up. The ethical dilemma here is to determine who the physician is obligated to inform. It would be beyond the pale to assume that no one needs instruction, but is it required that the physician speak only to the son? The debate about right to know must be coupled with the equal premise of the right not to know. In a sense, the emergency physician is required to speak to this woman through whatever means possible, which may include the family. Current rules and regulations requiring translators are to be ignored at the peril of the physician. Through a translating service, the emergency service asked the patient if she wished to be in charge and hear all of the medical information or if she would rather that be handled by her son. The woman, being an Old World traditionalist, gave the emergency physician permission to speak openly with her son and said she personally felt she could not deal with the information. The emergency physician then spoke directly to her adult son, explaining the reasonable differential and the required workup for the disease. A third phone conversation was held with the woman's primary care physician who had not seen her for eight months. A visit within the next two days and further workup studies were ordered. Has the emergency physician truly met his obligation to the family? Will this woman get the evaluation and care that she needs? Should any further actions be taken at that moment in time to fulfil the physician's ethical obligations to this patient?

Case 2: Resolution

The patient was asked whether she wanted to carry on the discussion with the physician herself or whether she wished the physician to carry on the actual discussion with her son. The patient preferred that her son handle all information about and aspects of her care.

Case 3: A Fifteen-Year-Old Girl with a Positive Pregnancy Test

A fifteen-year-old girl presents in the company of her mother with nausea and vomiting. During the history taking, the patient relates that she is approximately four weeks late for her menstrual period but says this happens on a not infrequent basis. The girl, in front of her mother, denies the possibility of pregnancy. Anticipating the possibility of infection, a urine sample has already been obtained by the nursing staff. The physician then asks if he might have some individual time with the patient and requests that the mother step out of the room for a few moments. The mother flatly refuses and becomes angry with the physician for even suggesting that her daughter could be pregnant or involved with drugs. The mother says she will sue the physician and the hospital if pregnancy or drug testing is performed. The mother also threatens to leave against medical advice if the child is not simply treated for her nausea and vomiting.

Case 3: Discussion

The physician in this example committed no ethical fault, but no style points should be awarded either. This is clearly a scenario in which the best possible encounter will occur with the patient alone in the room, without her mother present. The narrative clearly describes a situation in which tension is high, and the mother's violent reaction is not entirely a surprise. Therefore, it falls on the physician's shoulders to more preemptively diffuse the situation. Under the legal precedent that exists to protect the patient's rights concerning pregnancy, the physician has a responsibility to the patient to speak to her privately. De-escalation of the tension in this encounter is unquestionably challenging because the emergency physician knows that the urine drug screen is negative and the urine pregnancy test, which was started prior to his seeing the patient, is positive. In this case, there are at least three levels of obligation on the part of the physician to this family unit: (1) there is an obligation to the patient's mother because the child is a minor and therefore under the control of her guardianship; (2) there is also some obligation to the unborn child, although this obligation is both mitigated and mediated through the patient, and (3) there is an absolute obligation to notify the patient that she is pregnant. Decisions need to be made with regarding health care behavior, alcohol use, smoking, and the like and her further plans and desires with regard to the pregnancy.

Parents do not own their children; they are merely guardians who are recognized by the state as having usual parental jurisdiction. The patient's mother cannot prevent a fifteen-year-old from interacting with a physician with regard to her health care needs and those of her unborn child. Virtually all states have laws that designate pregnant women as the guardians and decision-makers with regard to their health care for pregnancies. By virtue of pregnancy, this patient functions under the status of an emancipated minor despite her living conditions, income support level, or current activities.

Case 3: Resolution

The physician asks the girl whether she wishes to speak with him privately or with the mother in the room. The patient, obviously under some duress, decides to have her mother stay. Both are informed of the pregnancy, at which time the mother begins to hit the child. Local authorities are called in to quell the disturbance. The physician, along with confirming the pregnancy, sets up an obstetrics visit within the next week and enlists social services to deal with the intrafamily violence taking place. The various levels of obligation to inform and protect are both activated and documented.

Case 4: A Two-Year-Old with a Spiral Fracture

A mother enters the ED with her crying two-year-old son stating that he will not stand up to walk. On history taking, this is a single mother who has a boyfriend living in the house. The mother is unaware of any trauma, but, over the past eight hours, the boy has been in the care of the boyfriend. There is no history of a fall or any other trauma. During the workup, an x-ray is obtained that shows a spiral fracture of the right tibia. The emergency physician notifies the mother that, at this time, without other history of trauma, he will be "notifying the authorities" for further discussion and intervention because a spiral fracture is unusual in a child of this age without child abuse being a strong consideration. While the physician is at the desk making the call, the mother and child leave the ED. The physician then must decide what actions to take. He notifies the local police of the possibility of an abused child, and authorities are dispatched to the home. The child is returned to the ED. The mother is crying, angry, and fighting with the boyfriend, who is now taken into custody. The obligations of the physician are further extended into completing paperwork in which he acts as the agent of the state to begin an investigation into child abuse.

Case 4: Discussion

As with the previous case, this example illustrates the challenging social aspects that face the emergency physician when there is a paucity of insight and planning. The fleeing mother not only endangers the child because he has not received appropriate care for his injuries, but she also is placing him at risk by returning him to an environment with a possible abuser. If a campus officer had been placed outside the room or protective services brought in sooner, the risk of flight may have been prevented.

The emergency physician is often placed in the position of being a quasi-member of the municipal authorities. It is mandated in all fifty states that elder abuse, child abuse, and crimes of violence are mandatorily reported to authorities. In many states, it is a requirement to report suspicion of transient loss of consciousness (i.e. seizures) that may interfere with a patient who has a driver's license. Although the particulars vary from state to state in situations that range from communicable disease to violence to incapacitation, the physician has a role that is broader than his relationship with an individual patient. Society, which has both educated and licensed the physician, has needs that also must be met, and these include protecting the society at large and those members of that society who cannot protect themselves. The need to become involved in dysfunctional family situations is the norm in emergency medicine. A truism learned by all emergency physicians is that all families are dysfunctional in their own unique way. Such involvement constitutes one of the true difficulties in the practice of emergency medicine.

Case 4: Resolution

Protective services became involved, and it was found that the mother's boyfriend was responsible for the injuries. The boyfriend was arrested and is now serving time. Careful supervision of the family is being undertaken by protective services.

Case 5: Duty to Third Parties

A sixteen-year-old male has been beaten in a fight at the local high school. As he is sitting on the cot, the emergency physician sees him pounding his first and exclaiming, "I hope you are here this afternoon Dr. Jones because you are going to see Jimmy Smith come in here dead." The physician's evaluation of the patient finds minimal abrasions and contusions but nothing requiring hospitalization or intervention by a surgical specialist. The patient is ready for release.

Case 5: Discussion

The duty to report is a well-established responsibility. As discussed earlier, there is a legal precedent obligating the emergency physician to do so when there are parties that may be harmed. How far that line extends, however, is not well established.

As the new movement of anti-vaccine parenting propagates, we face an additional infectious disease threat in the setting of drug-resistant super bugs, novel viral species, and the spread of Ebola. There is no question regarding the vitality of proper vaccinations in the medical community; however, we sit idly as record numbers of outbreaks of preventable and nearly extinct illnesses strike innocent children both vaccinated and unvaccinated. Do we not have a responsibility to the nonconsenting children of scientifically illiterate parents? Or, even more importantly, to the greater majority of responsible parents who vaccinate their kids for the greater benefit of society? There is undeniable research showing the risk of not vaccinating. Therefore, in the interest of public health, is there not an onus to report those who refuse to do so or to require adherence to a reasonable vaccination schedule to attend school? The question that now presents itself is that of a duty to a third party. Two types of third parties are recognized under law. There are known third parties (i.e. where the victim or the intended victim is known). And there are also unnamed but anticipated third parties. Our liability to these unnamed third parties is assumed every time a patient with diminished capacity is discharged and every time a prescription is given for a narcotic medication that presents the possibility that the patient will take a toxic amount of the drug, drive, and injure innocent others. Such third parties are impossible to identify before the event but are predicted. This makes it imperative to make sure the patient with diminished capacity is under the supervision of a reliable other and why patients taking certain medications are warned to restrict certain activities.

Known third parties present a more difficult situation. Whenever a sexually transmitted disease is identified, a third-party situation by definition exists. The patients need to be informed that the health department will be contacting them, and they have an obligation to identify their sexual contacts. When, as in our case, a named party is identified who may be the victim of violence, the physician has an obligation to notify authorities. In the famous California case of *Tarasoff v. The Regents of the University of California*, just such a situation was identified, and the physician was found guilty of negligence for not informing authorities of a potential harm to a known potential third-party victim. The physician's responsibility to the patient not yet injured is well recognized throughout the medical/legal community.

Case 5: Resolution
Proper notification through the police department resulted in the arrest of Jimmy Smith on assault charges and a full discussion with the patient that essentially put him on notice that any acts of revenge would be not looked on favorably by the police department.

Case 6: The Arresting Patient
The emergency physician enters the room to see an eighty-two-year-old patient from a local nursing home in which active cardiopulmonary resuscitation (CPR) is being performed. The EMTs on the scene have intubated the patient and started an IV line. There are intermittent runs of idioventricular rhythm. The pupils are fixed and dilated. Upon obtaining more history, the physician learns that the patient has severe Alzheimer's disease, has had contractures and dementia, and has been fed through a feeding tube for the past eighteen months. The patient has not actually recognized anyone for about that same period of time. A decision must be made as to further medical treatment. Family members are not present, and no current Do Not Resuscitate (DNR) form is available.

Case 6: Discussion
End-of-life management is one of the most significant ethical challenges facing health care providers in this country today. Despite being a universal constant, we exist in a society that avoids death seemingly at any cost. In landmark case reviews that examined the end-of-life wishes of physicians compared to lay people, the desires of most people were similar: to die without pain, surrounded by family, with dignity. The discrepancy lies in how that translated into end-of-life wishes. Are ethical dilemmas surrounding end-of-life care a problem with misinformation and a lack on the medical community's part in educating the public, or is a paradigm shift truly necessary, one that recognizes that life without quality is worse than the mortality that we all face? This is the quintessential case of emergency medicine in this era. When to put a stop to activity in terminal or near-terminal patients can be a quandary. There is no obligation in any state for a physician to provide futile care. The return of a heartbeat is not the return of a person. The emergency physician should use all reasonable

attempts to involve a designated family member in what decisions need to be made, but, on a larger societal scale, the emergency physician is also the steward of health care resources. The exact reason why such a patient underwent CPR at the nursing home is the larger and much darker question that surrounds this situation – one that is becoming daily routine in the ED.

Case 6: Resolution
The emergency physician informed the family that resuscitative efforts would be futile, and the patient was pronounced dead.

CONCLUSION
ETHICS TAKEOUT TIPS
- You are a health care advisor, not a dictator.
- People come to us for care, not for judgment.
- We are involved and responsible for the family unit, not just the patient.
- The medical degree is a license to heal, not to cause needless pain or suffering.
- The competent patient has the right to decide about his or her own health care.
- Honesty is the best policy.
- Keep your promises to the patient.
- You are the steward of the patient's and the society's resources – don't steal.
- You are an agent of the state in protecting both the patient and society.
- You have a professional duty at all times to the patient.

FOR FURTHER READING

Gillon, R. (1985). An introduction to philosophical medical ethics: The Arthur case. *British Medical Journal*, 290(6475), 1117–1119.

Hansson, S. O. (2005). Extended antipaternalism. *Journal of Medical Ethics*, 31, 97–100.

Henningfeld, D. A. (2011). *Medical ethics*. Detroit, MI: Greenhaven.

Holbrook, D. (1985). Medical ethics and the potentialities of the living being. *British Medical Journal*, 291(6493), 459–462.

Hope, R. A. (2004). *Medical ethics: A very short introduction*. Oxford, UK: Oxford University Press.

Kant, I. (1964). Groundwork of the metaphysic of morals. In H. J. Paton (Ed.), *The moral law*. London: Hutchinson University Library.

Mill, J. S. (1974). Utilitarianism. In M. Warnock (Ed.). *Utilitarianism, on liberty, essay on Bentham: Together with selected writings of Jeremy Bentham and John Austin* (p. 268). Glasgow: Fontana.

Pence, G. E. (2015). *Medical ethics accounts of ground-breaking cases* (7th ed.). New York: McGraw-Hill.

Rourke, K. (1989). *Medical ethics: Common ground for understanding*. St Louis, MO: Catholic Health Association of the United States.

17

The Ethics of Disasters

PAUL P. REGA, MD, FACEP

INTRODUCTION

Emergency medicine, bridging emergency medical services (EMS) and hospitals, is the vanguard of disaster preparedness and response. The emergency physician, by virtue of temperament, experience, knowledge base, adaptability, flexibility of thought, availability, and skill set, is uniquely qualified to manage current mass casualty incidents (MCIs) and those that loom more ominously in the future. Worldwide, the incidence of natural disasters has increased sixfold in the past fifty years and the twenty-first century shows no signs of disaster abatement, natural or otherwise. Climate change, global terrorism, international conflicts (refugees), emerging infectious diseases (Ebola [EVD], SARS, H1N1, Chikungunya, MERS-CoV, etc.), nuclear proliferation, and population overgrowth are well-publicized threats. Additionally, future situations may arise that will be the result of a confluence of events that few could have predicted or planned for (e.g. the Fukushima nuclear power plant collapse following a tsunami).

Therefore, the challenges for the emergency physician with regard to disasters will not dissipate, but worsen. When disasters metamorphose into catastrophes, decisions and actions could easily run counter to everyone's current frame of reference. There must therefore be an ethical weave sewn into the tapestry of a community that will guide it through the most treacherous and mutating of landscapes. That may be easier said than done.

MICROETHICS AND MACROETHICS

The emergency physician is committed to the care and well-being of the patient: the patient–doctor relationship (so-called *microethics*). Parallel to that exists a set of ethics safeguarded by public health that looks to the safety and well-being of the community (*macroethics*).

Traditionally, both concepts work synergistically and complement one another. What is beneficial for the individual should enhance the well-being of the society in which he or she lives. Conflict between the two is rare, and processes are in place within the community's infrastructure to adjudicate whatever perceived conflicts may arise (consider Typhoid Mary and tubercular Andrew Speaker).

However, as disasters grow in complexity, what may be good for society may conflict with the emergency physician's best efforts for the individual patient – not only passively but actively. The American College of Emergency Physicians (ACEP)'s Code of Ethics addresses this issue in a general fashion, but, as is often the case, general concepts are difficult to translate when a real issue arises that requires an immediate resolution. "[T]he emergency physician has duties to allocate resources justly... and promote the public health that sometimes transcend duties to individual patients."

With ethics, there is no absolute. An ethical framework may be difficult, if not impossible, to achieve in an increasingly pluralistic society. It is a constantly evolving process that needs to be re-examined often. This conundrum has become glaringly obvious with the ongoing global EVD outbreak. Using this outbreak as an example, the macroethical issues include initial global indifference about a strictly African issue, a dearth of EVD vaccine research and development, disproportionate quarantine measures, international border closures, and current vaccine research that pits randomized controlled trials against compassionate use guidelines. The microethical issues include altered standards-of-care proposals based primarily on providers' fears, refusals to report for patient-care duty, and lackadaisical personal protective equipment (PPE) training mandates.

Therefore, the purpose of this chapter is to explore the various ethical issues associated with disasters in general, but more specifically as they pertain to catastrophic disasters where conflicts between micro- and macroethics are more transparent and more fractious (e.g. pandemics, nuclear cataclysms). Fortunately or unfortunately, the current EVD outbreak, which is far from catastrophic, has become a showcase for the inclusion of an ethical framework in any type of disaster.

DISASTER 101

To understand more fully the ethical issues associated with disasters, one must understand the nature of disasters (an inherent imbalance between victims and resources). (3)

Disasters can be classified as simple, complex, or catastrophic. At each level, an ethical framework is required and, as the level of complexity grows, so does the need for a strong ethical foundation.

The *simple disaster* is limited in time, victims, and expanse. The vast majority of disasters in the United States are simple disasters. The simple disaster's key component is that the local infrastructure remains intact. The initial response may be temporarily overwhelmed, but fire, EMS, law enforcement, local mutual aid, and the hospital system will rebound, usually within hours or at most days.

The major ethical issue centers on *triage*: the sorting of victims based on level of criticality. The history of triage began with Napoleon's chief medical officer, Dominique Jean Larrey and his "*ambulance volantes*" who, under fire, retrieved the wounded and ministered to them regardless of rank, friend or foe. Later, in the 1840s, British Naval Surgeon John Wilson expanded triage in that care should be tiered based on the severity of the victim's condition; resources should be expended on those with the greatest chance for survival. Today's triage system is founded on these principles (a utilitarian-egalitarian hybrid), reinforced with objective physiologic parameters (i.e. pulse, respiration, mentation).

This system allows the appropriate distribution of scarce resources to those who need it the most. In this classic example of utilitarianism, care is not denied. It is simply apportioned to those who require it immediately and then redistributed equally as the influx of resources catches up. The intent is that all will eventually receive full medical attention consistent with traditional American medicine (egalitarian).

Most triage systems in the world employ these concepts. One system has arguably become the standard in this country and also enjoys a foothold in other countries: the START (Simple Triage and Rapid Treatment) system. This triage system, like others, has not been scientifically field-validated.

While current triage precepts are a hybrid of well-established egalitarian and utilitarian concepts ("the greatest good for the greatest number"), can exceptions be made for special populations, thereby forfeiting the purity of egalitarianism?

Although certain triage guidelines address pediatric issues (e.g. JumpSTART), there has been little clarity about prioritizing children with respect to adults in a large MCI. Pediatric physiologic maintenance capabilities can be so deceptively innocuous that an unskilled first responder, misinterpreting the child's vital signs, may fail to identify an occult life threat. Therefore, it is justifiable both medically and ethically to upgrade a child's triage status based solely on age regardless of the apparent stability of the vital signs and the lack of severe clinical manifestations. This pediatric prioritization will also maximize the child's mental well-being and lessen first responder mental stress.

Similarly, a female pregnant with a viable fetus may also be an automatic upgrade to "Red" regardless of the mother's traumatic or medical issues. Responders are dealing with two victims but can only fully assess one. Here again, based on sound evidence-based medicine, upgrading these two types of victims can be morally, ethically, and medically justifiable.

Can the case be made to upgrade automatically elderly victims based solely on age, given their propensity for greater morbidity and mortality when assaulted with adversity? Historically, that has not been the case. Since their complaints and manifestations are more readily apparent to the traditional first responder, it is ethically reasonable to assess them with the general population at risk and not automatically resort to "ageism" to make triage decisions.

A final special population is the injured or ill responder. Should that individual, given his or her status as a health care provider, automatically receive higher priority in triage and transport regardless of complaint or injury severity? If it will help with the morale and efficiency of that victim's colleagues to know that their comrade is being cared for, then an argument can be made that would be ethically acceptable because it would fall under the precept of "the greatest good for the greatest number." The one condition that must remain inviolate is that the actions specifically taken for the responder do not jeopardize the care of another.

Another ethical quagmire also requires evaluation in most triage systems. Classically, there are four basic patient categories:

1. *Red*: Critical; first priority for extrication, care, and transport
2. *Yellow*: Urgent; no immediate life/limb threat; second priority
3. *Green*: Delayed; no immediate or potential life/limb threat; last priority
4. *Black*: Dead (without any vital signs); these victims receive no care, no attempts at resuscitation

However, there are some victims who have obviously nonsurvivable conditions but still maintain some semblance of life. These are the "Expectant." If tagged "Red," severely limited resources could be wasted on these victims when they could have been allocated to viable victims. If tagged "Black," then other victims will receive the maximum benefit of those precious resources. Meanwhile, this victim, tagged "Black," by definition and practice will receive no further evaluation, no palliative care, and no emotional and spiritual sustenance at the terminus of his or her life.

This ethical conundrum has at least been addressed in one of the latest triage iterations. Recognizing that no triage system is perfect or has been fully scientifically validated, subject matter experts, under the umbrella of federal and nongovernmental disaster management entities developed the SALT triage system: Sort, Assess, Life-threat, Transport. In addition to certain modifications and therapeutic additions, the group classifies the "expectant" victim as "Gray." Although this victim will be excluded from the use of scant resources, they could still benefit from emotional/ spiritual support and/or palliative care. In addition, should a sudden influx of resources arrive, that "gray" victim can now be upgraded to "Red."

The second category is the *complex disaster*, which comprises two subcategories: the *expansive event* and the *novel event*. For both, the number of unknowns looms large. In the expansive event, the unknowns can include geographical dimension, number of immediate and potential victims, and response and recovery duration. In this event, the local infrastructure has been so crippled that surge capacity must originate from state and federal resources. Examples include Hurricane Andrew (1992), the Northridge earthquake (1994), the Hanshu-Awaji earthquake (1995), and Hurricane Katrina (2005).

Patients are victimized not only by the direct impact of the incident, but also by its indirect effects, such as various environmental exposures, exacerbation of chronic comorbidities, infectious disease threats, psychobehavioral adversities, and socioeconomic disruption. Therefore, in a complex disaster, a victim is subject to the acute as well as the long-term effects of myriad stressors.

The *novel event* under the complex disaster umbrella requires the highly specific resources, expertise, and capabilities of external agencies. This specialized assistance will be for both short- and long-term (months to years) activities. Consider a hypothetical airborne dissemination of anthrax spores over Chicago. In order to save thousands of lives, a mass prophylaxis campaign (antibiotics/vaccination) within forty-eight hours has been proposed (Kyriacou, 2012).

Because a complex disaster has ill-defined characteristics that veer into unchartered waters, it conjures up both real and imagined threats to the health care worker and his or her loved ones. The ethical focus here is on the caregiver's duty. Health care providers may simply not show up to serve. The emergency physician, by the very nature of emergency medicine, must confront an ethical dilemma that is more onerous than that faced by other professions and specialties.

SARS is illustrative of the problem. In Toronto, slightly fewer than half of the cases involved health care workers. As a consequence, many of these professionals refused to come to work. Health care worker abandonment was also documented in Taiwan and Hong Kong. This same issue has been in evidence during both the on-going MERS-CoV and EVD outbreaks. According to ACEP precepts, it is incumbent on the emergency physician to assume certain risks in caring for patients. However, the physician's duty to render care may not be absolute. The issue centers on motive: (1) is there an exceedingly high risk to oneself to care for victims of a disaster? (2)Are there two or more conflicting obligations requiring an abandonment of one to serve the other (e.g. duty to family)?

When considering an action that may be perceived as unethical or contrary to the community's expectations, the emergency physician should consider the following:

- *Expressed consent*: A formal agreement that mandates the physician to care for any and all patients presenting to the ED
- *Implied consent*: An understanding that emergency physicians would automatically respond to any and all emergencies presenting in the hospital
- *Special training*: An understanding that emergency physicians possess a unique skill set that cannot be acquired elsewhere
- *Reciprocity (social contract)*: An obligation to render aid because part of the emergency physician's training has been subsidized by the public
- *Professional oaths and codes*: Language within the emergency physicians' professional organizations that commits the doctor to assuming a greater amount of risk than is usual

The American Medical Association (AMA)'s Code of Ethics asks physicians to balance the needs of the present patient with the ability to care for patients in the future. Here, the implication is that one may refuse to care for the immediate emergency, not out of concern for oneself or one's family, but to fulfill a social necessity for caring for potential patients at a time when the health care infrastructure may be in disarray.

Regardless of the moral and ethical considerations, the physician must understand his or her legal rights and obligations. Spontaneous, ill-tempered decisions may expose one either to unnecessary exposure medicolegally and professionally or to needless morbidity or even death.

Nothing is absolute. Decisions are made relative to the crisis, and the needs of the physician, the physician's family, and the community. These needs cannot be predicted. However, to minimize one's ethical conflicts about a future crisis, the physician as well as the community's health care institutions and infrastructure must recognize that ethical dilemmas will exist in the future and that they are bound to address these issues now. There is an ethical duty on the part of the physician to respond to a crisis, but there also exists a duty on the part of the health care infrastructure to provide the necessary support and training to mitigate individual fears and potential conflicts of interest as much as possible.

A physician obligations are that he or she:

- Perform a hazards assessment and personal/family risk assessment based on the hazards.
- Institute a family disaster plan that addresses food, water, transportation, and communication issues.
- Receive basic education on atypical disaster situations that go beyond patient care issues.
- Receive formal PPE education.

The health care institution's obligations are that it:

- Provide compulsory education on complex/catastrophic disasters, including hospital evacuations. In one study, 200 of 1,000 senior U.S. physicians would not expose themselves to the risk of caring for a patient with a potentially lethal exposure to an unknown agent. Only 33 percent would care for a known smallpox victim.
- Provide and mandate PPE education and fit-testing.
- Execute tabletop and functional exercises with particular emphasis on atypical or complex disasters.
- Identify operations or functions that may be managed at home for those who are unable for one reason or another to come to work.
- Develop a family care network to assist staff and employees with their familial obligations.

It remains to be seen how many health care providers and institutions assumed these ethical obligations during the current EVD outbreak.

The EVD ethical crises are not unique. Consider two recent complex disasters: the SARS outbreak in Toronto and Hurricane Katrina in New Orleans. Each provides both insight and forewarning concerning ethical issues that could mushroom should a catastrophic disaster achieve global proportions.

With SARS in Toronto, some of the issues included enforced quarantine (including health care workplace quarantine), duty to care versus personal fears and familial obligations, and altered standards of medical practice. With Hurricane Katrina in New Orleans, the issues included arbitrary triage reprioritization (e.g. DNR patients designated the last to be evacuated) and euthanasia considerations (allegedly practiced at one institution). In both these instances, there was little precedent to draw from. Planning for the unusual was not considered. Much of the response, individual and agency, was arbitrary and inconsistent, based on a failure of leadership, training, communication, and unique stressors.

The final category, *catastrophic disaster*, is one in which the national infrastructure, even the global infrastructure, has been rendered incapable of caring for its citizens. State and federal assets are nonexistent or significantly limited, possibly for years into the future.

When the catastrophe is limited to one or more nations, unaffected foreign governmental and nongovernmental organizations (NGOs) will assist (e.g. the Haitian earthquake). However, if the catastrophe is global, then a fundamental and long-lasting – maybe even permanent – alteration in man's relationship to one another, to the community, and to the current way of life may develop.

The direct and indirect medical assaults on victims will be measured in years, possibly decades. Every nation's political, cultural, sociological, and medical network will struggle to harness any resources and allocate them in a manner that sustains and preserves their community. This is where the macroethics of population health will supersede the microethics of the physician–patient contract – the preservation of society over the preservation of a patient.

Two occurrences can force civilization into those uncharted waters: pandemics and a global nuclear war. Of the two, a pandemic is the more nebulous. Will it start, how it will start, where will it start, how long will it last, and how severe will it be (e.g. an H1N1 pandemic or a 1918 influenza pandemic)?

The relatively mild H1N1 pandemic revealed population health inadequacies in many nations, including industrialized ones. However, public health and medical leaders ultimately look to the 1918 influenza pandemic for insight into planning for and responding to a worst-case scenario.

The great influenza A(H1N1) pandemic of 1918 killed anywhere from 50 to 300 million people worldwide. U.S. deaths have been estimated to be anywhere from 500,000 to 700,000, a morbidity rate of up to 53 percent of the population. It is feared that a pandemic on the level of 1918 at its height could infect 30 percent of the U.S. population, cause a 40 percent worker absenteeism rate, and kill upward of 2 million people.

During the initial wave, in the absence of any control measures (i.e. vaccines and drugs), it has been estimated that, in the United States, even a medium-level pandemic could cause 89,000–207,000 deaths; between 314,000 and 734,000 hospitalizations; 18 million to 42 million outpatient visits; and another 20 million to 47 million people fallen ill.

Between 15 and 35 percent of the U.S. population could be affected by an influenza pandemic, and the economic impact could range between $71.3 and $166.5 billion.

A more severe 1918-like pandemic in the United States would result in 90 million symptomatic cases, 45 million outpatient visits, and 9.9 million hospitalizations. More than 360 percent of the intensive care unit (ICU) beds that are currently in place would be required and more than 200 percent of the existing ventilators.

State and federal surge capacity will be crippled. Communities, unable to rely on state and federal assets, will shift from patient-directed health care (microethics) to population-based health care (macroethics). This shift will be imperceptible initially, but as the severity of the pandemic becomes more palpable, the survival of the community will be the primary goal. The tenets of traditional medicine will inexorably be replaced by catastrophic medicine and altered standards of care.

In the early stages, much of that transition will be societal in nature and have no direct repercussions on the emergency physician. It will involve activation of alternative care sites (ACS), points of distribution (PODs), social distancing measures, and deferral of unessential services so as to maintain basic services and optimize medical care without overwhelming the hospital-based infrastructure. Many of the ethical decisions with regard to these measures will have no immediate bearing on the emergency physician's doctor–patient relationships.

However, as the pandemic's severity becomes more evident, the medical infrastructure will recognize that its initial measures will not suffice, and resources will be rapidly exhausted. Whatever altered standards of care may be in place will be replaced by even more draconian measures: "catastrophic medical care," a time of allocation of scarce resources and prioritization of patient care. Here is when the community's ethical framework, hopefully already developed, disseminated, and agreed upon, becomes the foundation for future deliberations and decisions. Otherwise, fear, loss of trust, poor morale, and misinformation will prevail.

An ethical framework was considered vital after the SARS outbreak in Canada. "Stand on Guard for Thee" laid out the ethical dynamics, and this document has become the model for subsequent discussions, debates, and guidelines. It established ten ethical substantive values and five procedural ones that should be considered in pandemic planning and response. "Stand on Guard for Thee" can serve as a model for any other catastrophic event. The substantive values are:

1. *Individual liberty*: May be restricted for the good of the community
2. *Public protection from harm*: Potential restriction of individual liberty
3. *Proportionality*: Any applied measure should be as minimal as possible in keeping with the immediate threat
4. *Privacy*: May be superseded for the public good
5. *Duty*: An obligation to provide medical care versus competing obligations to oneself, family, and friends
6. *Reciprocity*: The community must recognize the disproportionate burdens that its members must undertake to preserve the community and should attempt to minimize those burdens as much as possible
7. *Equity*: Normally, everyone has an equal claim to essential health services; however, this may be modified to provide the most essential services and defer others
8. *Trust*: As care becomes continually altered to adapt to the pandemic's course, trust must be nurtured among the individual, the health care professional, and the health care infrastructure
9. *Solidarity*: Every infrastructural-political entity, while confronting the same threat, should intensely collaborate with regard to strategy and tactics in order to control the evolving situation
10. *Stewardship*: Community leaders, while struggling to make difficult decisions, must strive to balance the best outcome for both the individual and the community

Decisions will be difficult in pandemic situations, but for them to be understood and accepted by the community, these five procedural values should be adopted:

1. *Reasonable*: The decisions should be made by leaders who are skillful and credible.
2. *Transparency*: The decisions and the basis for making those decisions must be subject to public scrutiny.

3. *Inclusive*: Every member of the community must have the opportunity to be part of the decision-making process.
4. *Responsive*: No decision is fixed; steps and processes can be altered as events change.
5. *Accountable*: Decision-makers should be held accountable for actions and inactions that have occurred during the emergency.

These fifteen principles should serve as a guide for community leaders, including emergency physicians, when considering everything from positioning of alternative care sites and PODs, mass fatality managements, constituent/patient prioritization, and allocation of scarce resources.

The two main areas that are of particular concern to the emergency physician are duty and pandemic (catastrophic) triage. Whereas duty was addressed under the section on complex disaster response, it is a more omnipresent burden during a pandemic. There is no discernable endpoint, and every contact with anyone might result in the transmission of the deadly microorganism to a vulnerable loved one. Any decision can have significant personal and professional repercussions. Ultimately, it will be a simple matter of personal risk assessment intertwined with an individual's value system.

Apart from the emergency physician's specific duty to care at this catastrophic stage, the area that will intimately involve the emergency physician's expertise, scope of practice, and intense involvement will be with pandemic triage (patient prioritization and allocation of scarce resources). Triage under such circumstances will require (1) establishment of inclusion criteria for those who may benefit by admission to a critical care area for respiratory support and hemodynamic resuscitation and (2) establishment of exclusion criteria for those who are not candidates for a critical care admission because they have a poor prognosis despite intensive care (withdrawal of care), require nonexistent resources for survival, or have comorbidities that could exacerbate the likelihood of death. The emergency physician, as the EMS medical director, must evaluate and develop these criteria that will have to be established in the pre-hospital arena. Patient triage will change drastically as the pandemic peaks, and patient calls for assistance multiply in conjunction with a 30–40 percent EMS absenteeism rate. The EMS medical director must gauge the stage of the pandemic and the level of current resources and personnel and then decide on a limited response, a severely restricted response, or no response whatsoever. Because many communities have multiple EMS agencies, it is imperative that their respective medical directors agree on the same responses.

The inclusion criteria for hospital/ICU admission based on hemodynamic and respiratory measures are essentially noncontroversial, both medically and ethically. Controversy will arise as the pandemic assumes catastrophic proportions and the exclusion criteria are more aggressively applied. That application may be done as EMS personnel assess the patient in person. It may even be accomplished telephonically when there are no resources to respond to each call for assistance. EMS will have few objective tools available such as Sequential Organ Failure Assessment (SOFA), modified Sequential Organ Failure Assessment (mSOFA), and Pediatric Index of Mortality (PIM2) scores to assist with triage decisions, especially if triage is by long-distance. Patients will no longer be transported to an overwhelmed hospital but now will be directed to ACSs for basic or merely palliative care.

The proposed exclusion criteria are separated into "hard" categories that are readily identifiable and understood by most practitioners (e.g. second- and third-degree burns 90 percent total body surface area) and "soft" criteria that are less obvious (e.g. liver failure).

In the emergency department (ED), adoption of inclusion and exclusion criteria is facilitated by the ability to utilize certain triage tools. Currently, SOFA and modified SOFA (mSOFA) scores are the tools most often cited to assist with inclusion in and exclusion from the ICU. However, they are meant to limit patient access to critical care areas of the hospital to those who have a reasonable chance of survival. Guidance as to arranging disposition of patients who are not deemed good candidates for critical care is nebulous. The emergency physician must then decide alternative care options: non-ICU admission, a nontraditional ACS, discharge to home, or hospice. The physician is still ethically bound to provide the best alternative care when traditional provisions of care are exhausted. That process can be arduous and time-consuming unless it is addressed well before catastrophic conditions develop. Therefore, it is important for the emergency physician to have significant input regarding the specific patient characteristics that would make up the exclusion criteria and ensure that the ED staff can accept the criteria.

Withdrawal of care is an issue that is alien to most health care providers. However, it will have to be considered in pandemic planning. There will be ICU patients who will have no improvement or even worsening of their SOFA scores at 48 and 120 hours post-admission. A Hospital Pandemic Triage Team may decide that it is both medically and macroethically proper to remove such patients from ventilator support so as to make this very scarce resource available to another with a greater likelihood of survival. This would be at the nadir of a pandemic: not merely limiting care, but withdrawing care that is actively in place. This aspect affects the emergency physician in several ways, including requesting a ventilator for a new patient in the ED who meets the inclusion criteria, assisting with withdrawal-of-care guidelines, and writing orders to withdraw care as part of a hospital team.

Although some may argue that this action is another aspect of resource allocation, others may find that actively removing a patient from a lifeline ("primum non nocere") is vastly different from trying to provide some type of care to a patient regardless of its intensity.

However, SOFA scores and other iterations are not perfect. They have not been validated in pandemics, they are not meant to be applied to children, and they are insensitive. According to recent studies, actual patients on ventilators who would have been removed from them in a theoretical pandemic based on SOFA sores actually survived to discharge. A single-system strategy that utilizes an imperfect instrument and could potentially discriminate against age, functionality, and social worth would not be viable. Employing the "multiplier" principle would minimize an attempt to be selective and potentially discriminatory. Such a method could include a number of factors:

- SOFA score (or its variations)
- *Instrumental value*: Different from social worth, it selects those whose survival would improve the survivability of others
- *Maximization of life-years*: Number of life-years saved via medical intervention
- *Life cycle*: An attempt to give everyone a fair opportunity to advance through all the stages of life

The published ethics regarding patient prioritization and allocation of scarce resources is limited extensively to pre-hospital and hospital activities. Those in chronic and extended-care facilities are excluded from these criteria until they, too, develop an acute problem and must enter the system. More specifically, there has been no concerted effort made to remove this type of patient from a ventilator so as to provide this resource to a more viable candidate. However, it is also ethically incumbent upon the medical staff at these chronic and extended-care institutions to provide a more intense level of care so as to minimize their patients' transportation to an overloaded hospital.

CATASTROPHIC NUCLEAR EVENT RESPONSE

With a blinding flash of light and a mushroom cloud, traditional medicine could immediately devolve into catastrophic medicine. There is no time to ponder the alternative strategies and tactical maneuvers that may be contemplated with the slowly developing pandemic. Consider the detonation of a 10-kT improvised nuclear device (IND) over Washington, DC:

- *Physical damage*: Extensive building collapse; 250 major fires within a three-quarter-mile radius; loss of electrical power, most electronics, and communication within three-quarters of a mile. In the outer ring, shattered glass and auto crashes that could cause thousands of injuries.
- *Fallout*: Extending into Virginia, Maryland, and environs.
- *Casualties*: 9,000 instantaneous deaths; 19,000 injured from blast, burns, trauma, and radiation (6,000 dead in <24 hours; 13,000 acutely injured survivors).
- *Injuries and illness*: An additional 120,000 victims exposed to significant fallout, with acute radiation syndrome (ARS) over one to fourteen days.
- *Hospital capacity:*
  * Within a twenty-mile radius: four of forty-nine hospitals destroyed or nonfunctional; the estimated surge capacity of forty-five other hospitals in the area is 3,500 beds.
  * Within a 100-mile radius: Approximately 14,000 surge beds and 2,000 ICU beds could be available within twenty-four hours.
- *Communications*: Most modes of communication will be disrupted.

Then consider the ramifications of global nuclear war involving the destruction of major population centers across the industrial world. In addition to loss of assets seen with a pandemic crisis, there could also be vaporization and radiological contamination of the community's physical footprint that would last for decades.

Despite more than seventy years of scientific and medical data with regard to acute and long-term radiation injuries and their management (http://orise.orau.gov/reacts/resources/radiation-accident-management. aspx), a level of insecurity about acute management issues prevails. In order to make an effective and ethical response to this horrific event, a basic level of education is required and is readily available. After this first step, an understanding of how the federal government will respond is also critical.

Should the surviving emergency physician not abandon societal expectations and obligations, then nuclear triage will need to occur immediately – both for those living in the unscathed community and those displaced by the detonation. The medical mechanics of nuclear triage is abetted by the well-known clinical manifestations that are related to the amount of radiation exposure and the likelihood of survivability based on radiation levels absorbed and degree of trauma. *Biodosimetry* (e.g. absolute lymphocyte count) will reinforce triage decisions. These tools are ubiquitous, but given the possibility that the Internet will be unavailable, hard copies should be added to the hospital disaster plan.

SOCIO-POLITICAL ISSUES

Finally, an avocation that many emergency physicians share is involvement in global health care and international disaster response. However, the socio-moral climate of one region of the world may conflict with the ethics of NGO medical personnel and agencies. In the early 1980s, a Norwegian Red Cross hospital in Cambodia closed because a political appointee controlled the keys to the pharmacy and allowed medications to be given only to patients of a certain political persuasion. In another instance, when a Swedish medical team protested the political machinations that allowed a delay in care to cause the death of a child, the team was placed under house arrest. Therefore, when considering a global mission, knowing the socio-political climate of a country first may provide the emergency physician with sufficient information about whether the ethics of a country are compatible with the medical provider's.

CONCLUSION

The specialty of emergency medicine will be center stage on this "proscenium of disasters." Its physicians can be major actors ensuring that medical plans and guidelines will be ethically sound. Or, they can be passive participants who will accept the dictates of well-meaning but largely ignorant bureaucrats. The emergency physician can either choose to react to the situation or proactively engage in the challenges well before a disaster manifests itself.

Community leaders, private/public stakeholders, and the lay public all need to address these concepts. Because these constituents and agencies will be coming from diverse backgrounds and points of view, there needs to be that one ethical framework that is accepted by all and that will be the foundation on which all these difficult decisions will have to be made.

Unless this is properly approached well before the advent of a disaster or catastrophe, response decisions may become arbitrary, opaque, and excessive. It will further undermine the faith, confidence, and obedience of the public. The emergency physician has an obligation to ensure that this does not happen. The public needs to know that emergency medicine will always strive to balance the needs of the individual with that of society within an accepted ethical framework.

ETHICS TAKEOUT TIPS

- Encourage the adoption of the SALT triage system in order to provide more appropriate care to those with nonsurvivable injuries.
- Ensure inclusion of emergency medicine representation at community disaster planning and preparedness venues.
- Partner with local health care institutions to develop ongoing educational programs devoted specifically to catastrophic medical care within the framework of disaster medicine.
- Identify and attempt to resolve any personal/family issues that may conflict with one's duty to serve in times of disaster.
- Ensure that, prior to deployment to a global catastrophe, the ethical tenets of the nation in crisis are compatible with one's own ethical framework.
- Review published iterations of inclusion/exclusion criteria in a catastrophe.
- Review published withdrawal-of-care criteria in a catastrophe.
- Review SOFA and mSOFA scales and their employment during catastrophes.
- Initiate within the health care institution a pandemic cohort within the existing disaster committee.

FOR FURTHER READING

American College for Emergency Physicians. (n.d.). *Code of ethics for emergency physicians.* www.acep.org/Clinical-Practice-Management/Code-of-Ethics-for-Emergency-Physicians/
Center for Biosecurity of UPMC. (2009). *The next challenge in healthcare preparedness: Catastrophic health events.* Prepared for the U.S. Department of Health

and Human Services under Contract No. HHSO100200700038C. Baltimore, MD: Author.

Coleman, C. N., Weinstock, D. M., Casagrande, R., Hick, J. L., Bader, J. L., Chang, F., ... Knebel, A. R. (2011). Triage and treatment tools for use in a scarce resources-crisis standards of care setting after a nuclear detonation. *Disaster Medicine and Public Health Preparedness, 5,* S111–S121.

Devereaux, A. V., Dichter, J. R., Christian, M. D., Dubler, N. N., Sandrock, C. E., Hick, J. L., ... Rubinson, L. (2008). Definitive care for the critically ill during a disaster: A framework for allocation of scarce resources in mass critical care. *Chest, 133,* 51S–66S.

Fink, S. (2013). *Five days at Memorial, life and death in a storm-ravaged hospital.* New York: Crown Publishers.

Grissom, C. K., Brown, S. M., Kuttler, K. G., Boltax, J. P., Jones, J., Jephson, A. R., & Orme, J. F. (2010). A modified sequential organ failure assessment score for critical care triage. *Disaster Medicine and Public Health Preparedness, 4,* 277–284.

Hrdina, C. M., Coleman, C. N., Bogucki, S., Bader, J. L., Hayhurst, R. E., Forsha, J. D., ... Knebel, A. R. (2009). The "RTR" medical response system for nuclear and radiological mass-casualty incidents: A functional TRiage-TReatment-TRansport medical response model. *Prehospital and Disaster Medicine, 24*(3), 167–178.

Iserson, K. V., Heine, C. E., Larkin, G. L., Moskop, J. C., Baruch, J., & Aswegan, A. L. (2008). Fight or flight: The ethics of emergency physician disaster response. *Annals of Emergency Medicine, 51,* 345–353.

Kyriacou, D. N., Dobrez, D., Parada, J. P., Steinberg, J. M., Kahn, A., Bennett, C. L., & Schmitt, B. P. (2012). Cost-effectiveness comparison of response strategies to a large-scale anthrax attack on the Chicago metropolitan area: Impact of timing and surge capacity. *Biosecur Bioterror, 10*(3), 264–279.

Lerner, E. B., Schwartz, R. B., Coule, P. L., Weinstein, E. S., Cone, D. C., Hunt, R. C., ... O'Connor, R. E. (2008). Mass casualty triage: An evaluation of the data and development of a proposed national guideline. *Disaster Medicine and Public Health Preparedness, 2*(Suppl. 1), S25–S34.

Malm, H., May, T., Francis, L. P., Omer, S. B., Salmon, D. A., & Hood R. (2008). Ethics, pandemics, and the duty to treat. *American Journal of Bioethics, 8*(8), 4–19.

Sztajnkrycer, M. D., Madsen, B. E., & Baez, A. A. (2006). Unstable ethical plateaus and disaster triage. *Emergency Medical Clinics of North America, 24,* 749–768.

University of Toronto Joint Centre for Bioethics. (2005). *Stand on guard for thee – ethical considerations in preparedness planning for pandemic influenza.* http://jointcentreforbioethics.ca/people/documents/upshur_stand_guard.pdf

U.S. Department of Transportation. (2007). *Preparing for pandemic influenza: Recommendations for protocol development for 9-1-1 personnel and Public Safety Answering Points (PSAPs).* www.az-apco-nena.org/Pandemic.htm

Velji, A., & Bryant, J. H. (2014). Global health ethics. In W. Markle, M. Fisher, & R. Smego (Eds.), *Understanding global health* (2nd ed., pp. 463–487). New York: McGraw-Hill Education.

White, D. B., Katz, M. H., Luce, J. M., & Lo, B. (2009). Who should receive life support during a public health emergency? Using ethical principles to improve allocation decisions. *Annals of Internal Medicine, 150,* 132–138.

18

Stewardship of Health Care Resources

SHELLIE ASHER, MD

Stewardship is defined by the American Medical Association as the "obligation to provide effective medical care through prudent management of the public and private health resources with which physicians are entrusted" (Douglas, 2012). The American College of Emergency Physicians (ACEP) describes stewardship as "the provision of quality emergency care through the prudent management of public and private resources" (American College of Emergency Physicians [ACEP], 2001). The Accreditation Council for Graduate Medical Education (ACGME) includes resource utilization in the milestones to be assessed in emergency medicine training programs as an integral part of patient care (see Table 18.1). The emergency physician must "work within the institution to develop hospital systems that enhance safe patient disposition and maximize resource utilization."

Within this framework, what is the responsibility of the individual emergency physician to steward limited resources? Why is stewardship important? Although the political and economic influences on stewardship decisions are vast and important, we will focus on the concept of stewardship through the lens of health care ethics, around a framework of universality, affordability and allocation, quality, and responsibility (Freeman & McDonnell, 2001).

UNIVERSALITY

What is the basis for a moral "right" to health care? Arguments supporting a right to health care may be general or specific. One general argument for a right to health care is collective social protection: similar to needs protected by the government, such as police, fire, and clean water, government has an obligation to provide other essential services, such as basic health care. Additionally, investment in health care benefits society via returns on that

TABLE 18.1. *Related ACGME emergency medicine milestones*

Patient Care 7: Establishes and implements a comprehensive disposition plan that uses appropriate consultation resources; patient education regarding diagnosis; medications; and time and location specific disposition instructions.	**Systems-Based Practice 2:** Participates in strategies to improve health care delivery and flow. Demonstrates an awareness of and responsiveness to the larger context and system of health care.
Level 1: Describes basic resources available for care of the emergency department (ED) patient	Level 2: Mobilizes institutional resources to assist in patient care
Level 2: Formulates a specific follow-up plan for common ED complaints with appropriate resource utilization	Level 3: Practices cost-effective care
Level 3: Involves appropriate resources (e.g. PCP, consultants, social work, PT/OT, financial aid, care coordinators) in a timely manner	Level 3: Demonstrates the ability to call effectively on other resources in the system to provide optimal health care
Level 4: Engages patient or surrogate to effectively implement a discharge plan	Level 4: Recommends strategies by which patients' access to care can be improved
Level 5: Works within the institution to develop hospital systems that enhance safe patient disposition and maximize resource utilization	Level 4: Coordinates system resources to optimize a patient's care for complicated medical situations
	Level 5: Develops internal and external departmental solutions to process and operational problems

investment in related education and research, which further serves to improve the health of the population. Other general arguments for a right to health care include benefits to society as a whole (healthy citizens contribute to society, which provides a benefit for all), fair-opportunity (all citizens have access to the same level of basic resources regardless of their personal circumstances), and a moral duty to address suffering.

Prior to the Patient Protection and Affordable Care Act (PPACA) of 2010, 18 percent of the nonelderly population in the United States were without health insurance, and many were uninsurable due to preexisting conditions. In addition, individuals obtaining coverage in the open market paid much higher premiums than those who qualified for group coverage through their employer or another organization. At this time, it remains to be seen what impact the PPACA will have on accessibility of coverage, affordability, and, subsequently, emergency department (ED) utilization.

Resources may be adequate to address the needs of the majority of the U.S. population but not necessarily every desire of every individual. Possible solutions include "middle ground" scenarios in which a "decent minimum" set of basic services (socially enforced basic or catastrophic coverage, in addition to the ED and other safety net services currently available) may be available to everyone, with additional resources to cover other needs and desires available to those with the resources to purchase them. A two-tier system with universal basic coverage and private insurance for uncovered costs is another possibility but may result in disparate care and the same ethical issues currently faced. In addition, there exists significant controversy over the definition of "basic" or "decent minimum" coverage.

Societal values, and hence policy, in the United States prioritizes care for the young, elderly, pregnant, and patients with chronic renal failure over all others, whereas market forces predominantly benefit wealthy, white, urban men. What is the best way to address unfair distribution of access for poor, rural, female, non-white members of society? Does this discrepancy need to be addressed? What is the best way to determine whether a system of resource allocation is "fair?"

The Emergency Medical Treatment and Active Labor Act (EMTALA) of 1986 mandates provision of emergency services as a "safety net" for health care, but it has been criticized as an unfunded mandate, with many hospitals struggling to provide this care without adequate reimbursement to meet expenses. EMTALA does not entirely prevent transfers to other institutions for financial reasons, nor does it address the impact on current patients if the needs of patients transferred exceed available resources.

An ethical system for the provision of universal health care in the United States would need to address these issues on the ethical basis supporting universal coverage, equitable access for all populations, and financing.

AFFORDABILITY AND ALLOCATION

What are the specific entitlements accorded to or limits of a "right to health care?" What does "basic" health care entail? Equal access to health care involves development of a system that does not prevent individuals from obtaining health care. On the other hand, it does not necessarily confer that others must provide or equitably distribute that care. Should every person have access to the same level of health care? As a society, there is considerable debate over uneven distribution of and unequal access to health care resources but less so over other goods and services (food, clothing, and shelter) – should access for all be the same regardless of personal circumstances?

The concept of *distributive justice* suggests that a fair system should be applied so that every individual has the same opportunity to acquire access to health care, if not exactly the same resources. There is a wide variation of opinion about how to go about achieving a just system, from a libertarian perspective (in which the market sorts out the level of resources each individual can access) to a communitarian one (in which each person has access to the same range of health care resources to use when those resources are required; this is the basis for many universal health care systems outside the United States).

Allocation of resources can be considered on a macrolevel and a microlevel. At the macrolevel, a society must consider what funds will be expended and what goods will be made available. At the highest policy level, budget allocations determine how much of a particular resource (generally money) to devote to a particular purpose (health care, military, education, nutrition, public health, etc.). Within the health care infrastructure, *macroallocation* is the system by which it is determined how much to spend within each area of health care, including direct medical care, public health, education, and research. In addition, macroallocation addresses issues such as what kinds of health care will exist in a society, who will receive them and on what basis, who will deliver them, how the burdens of financing will be distributed, and how control of these services will be distributed. Macroallocation is generally determined by a budgeting process with the viewpoint of health care for a population.

Whereas macroallocation may direct or develop policies to direct allocation of resources to certain populations, *microallocation* is the means by which it is determined which individuals will receive particular scarce resources. For example, which patients will get into difficult-to-arrange follow-up appointments, or who will be placed on ventilators in a severe flu pandemic? Microallocation can also be considered rationing. Although the term has developed an unsavory reputation, rationing in U.S. health care exists on a daily basis. No community has an infinite supply of any resource, and rationing occurs in multiple settings: insurer decisions regarding reimbursement, limitations on payments to providers, limitations on the resources providers or hospitals can obtain, limitations on interventions available. In fact, rationing happens every day in the ED via the triage process. From French, meaning "sorting" or "choosing," *triage* is the means by which scarce resources (ED providers) are allocated to individual patients on the basis of need.

Microallocation can be approached via a utilitarian (maximal benefit) or egalitarian (fair opportunity, equal worth) strategy. First, one must develop criteria and procedures to determine the qualifying pool of potential recipients. This can be based on constituency (categories of people who may potentially benefit), scientific progress (research participants most likely to advance knowledge), or the prospect of success (using resources for those with reasonable chances of benefit). If the latter, questions of medical utility (which patients will get the most benefit?) versus social utility (which recipients would contribute the most to society?) must also be considered.

Once the pool of potential recipients is determined, one must develop criteria and procedures for the final selection of recipients. This can be based on medical utility, social utility, or impersonal mechanisms such as lotteries and waiting lists. For example, allocation of intensive care unit resources in most hospitals is determined on a first-come-first-served basis; U.S. citizens are "entitled" to dialysis for end-stage renal disease (ESRD), but there are a limited number of dialysis slots for those patients to go to; Medicaid patients are "entitled" to long-term skilled nursing care, but a limited number of funded beds are available; distribution of organs for transplantation is based on a combination of medical need and time waiting. In disaster settings, triage generally does not take into account social worth, with certain exceptions (vaccinations for health care workers, prioritization for those needed to maintain essential services, etc.).

In most current systems, resources are allocated based on an assessment of medical utility followed by an impersonal system for those with roughly equal need. Social utility is occasionally considered if favored individuals will contribute to better overall outcome for the population. In this way, egalitarian and utilitarian strategies are used in conjunction to make decisions for both populations and individuals.

Macroallocation decisions affect microallocation decisions and vice versa. Criteria to determine allocation of resources are generally not explicit, but implicit factors include location of resources, access constraints such as transportation, finances, and administrative factors.

Should physicians explicitly make decisions regarding allocation based on the needs of the overall community over the needs of the individual patient? If so, at what level? Local community? State? Country? World? Resource limitations and the necessity of this type of decision-making may have significant impacts on the physician–patient relationship.

All health care comes with costs, and resources to provide health care are not unlimited. Costs must be paid for – by public entities such as state and federal government, private entities such as individuals, private insurance, or private subsidies such as grants or community funding. Health care provided should be cost-efficient, using the smallest amount of resources possible to achieve the desired outcome. Drivers of cost include high administrative costs; an aging population with an increasing prevalence of chronic medical conditions; liability costs; patient expectations; the high prices of pharmaceuticals, devices, and services; use of new technologies; and the intensity of services provided. Some of these factors can be affected by individual providers although many cannot.

In modern U.S. society, autonomy (individual choice) has been the ethical principle valued over justice (fair distribution), beneficence (do good), or nonmaleficence (do no harm). Without a radical shift in societal values and/or expectations, how can the emergency physician have an impact on the fair stewardship of limited resources? "Autonomy" does not mean offering a limitless list of choices that don't make sense for the clinical situation (i.e. head CT for an ankle injury, antibiotics for viral infection). Patient and family requests for interventions of marginal benefit should generate a discussion regarding the goals of care and how to best achieve said goals, and autonomy can be respected by communicating with and educating the patient so that he or she can make appropriately informed decisions.

Emergency physicians should speak out for the fair allocation of burdens and benefits of limited resources on all facets of society, not preferentially serving benefits to one constituency and burdens to another. In fact, emergency physicians function in the ideal setting of providing the same care for all who present regardless of income, contribution, or other individual factors. As the first line for many patients and gatekeepers to the health care system, emergency physicians are in a position to connect individual patients with the resources they need to maximize their health (and future contributions to society).

Outside of individual considerations in the distribution of health care resources, other societal factors should also be considered in making decisions at the policy level regarding health care access. What does society lack access to because of health care spending? Resources currently devoted to health care could be used to fund research, education, or public health initiatives that may be a better investment in societal health overall than current patterns of funding and spending.

In setting priorities for resource allocation, policy makers (and individuals) should consider first the clinical effectiveness of the intervention being considered. Interventions with little chance for clinical effectiveness (achieving the desired outcome) should not be offered. Other considerations include cost-effectiveness and social value or impact.

One of the pitfalls of public conversations about distribution of resources is the tendency of society to prioritize "identifiable lives" over "statistical lives." People are more willing to utilize resources to rescue one individual trapped under a bridge than to repair a bridge that may collapse and injure five or ten people. Although individuals may conceptually agree that there should be limits on health care spending, when the rubber meets the road and decisions need to be made, they want to be free to make whatever choice best fits their values and sense of entitlement, regardless of the sustainability of those choices as applied to an entire population.

QUALITY

Quality health care should be simple, understandable, and navigable. There is currently a mismatch between the cost of health care in the United States and the quality of care provided, with the highest health care expenditures per capita in the world, but without concomitant gains in longevity for this investment. Interventions should be based on evidence of effectiveness for care provided, with preference for low-cost interventions that have been shown to be effective.

There are several barriers to cost-effective, quality health care in the United States. There is an emphasis placed on costly of end-of-life care, which may have limited benefit to the patient. Provider fear of liability precipitates defensive medicine and results in increased costs without increased benefit. Health care payment is fraught with conflicts of interest, in which tests and procedures that may not benefit the patient result in higher reimbursement. Physicians are often ignorant of the costs of care provided, and health care is coordinated via complex systems with multiple decision-makers and a lack of communication between interested parties. In addition, determination of "quality" is subject to government oversight rather than peer review, and "quality measures" imposed by government may serve to drive up health care costs rather than have a positive impact on patients. Other pay-for-performance measures, such as patient satisfaction, may also result in an increase in unnecessary tests or interventions without improving overall health. Interventions such as the Choosing Wisely campaign and protection afforded by specialty society guidelines may serve to ameliorate some of these issues, but their impact remains uncertain. In order to improve health care quality, reimbursement should be based on outcomes – the health of the patient and/or population – rather than fee-for-service for tests and procedures.

In recent years, there has also been an increased emphasis placed on shared decision-making. Rather than an entirely autonomy-based approach or frank paternalism, providers are increasingly assisting patients in making educated choices about their health care. Continued patient engagement and provider education may increase quality and decrease costs. The importance of this is reflected in the ACGME milestone "engages patient of surrogate to effectively implement a discharge plan." In addition, the emergency physician's dedication to quality care and prudent expenditure of resources based on medical benefit and patient preference may set the tone for further care provided by other physicians, thus resulting in even greater impact than what can be seen in the ED.

RESPONSIBILITY

The existence of rights for one person confers a concomitant duty or responsibility on another person and/or society to make provisions to fulfill those rights. The U.S. Declaration of Independence defines certain "inalienable rights," but on what basis are those rights derived? Religion? Social contract? Moral law? If one person has a "right" to health care, then upon who does the duty to provide it rest?

Who should be held accountable for an individual's health? If one posits that there should be a basic level of health care available to all individuals, does that confer on those individuals a responsibility to avail themselves of those resources? Should lifestyle factors affect an individual's access to certain services (e.g. alcoholics and liver transplants, intravenous drug users and heart valve replacement)? Freedom and choice are core values in American society, but who should bear responsibility for the consequences of those freedoms? Is it "fair" for society to cover individuals who voluntarily engage in risky behaviors? Should the actions of risk-taking individuals (who paradoxically may consume fewer health care resources) reduce their opportunity to access services or require them to pay more? If so, who should provide accountability or determine causality? Will individuals abuse a resource if it is provided to them free of charge (other than through general taxes)?

Physicians and society have a responsibility to the health of each individual patient and also to the welfare of the overall community. At what point does the responsibility of the society become the responsibility of the individual provider? How should the legitimate interests of third parties (providers, hospitals, payers, society) influence decisions made regarding the care of individual patients?

CONCLUSION

In most cases, medical need and patient preferences via shared decision-making should be the primary driving factors in making medical decisions for individual patients, with the well-being of those patients at the focus. Physicians also have an obligation to promote public health and access to care. This obligation requires physicians to be prudent stewards of the shared resources with which they are entrusted. Managing health care resources responsibly is compatible with physicians' primary obligation to serve the interests of individual patients, with a resultant benefit for society. The overall health of a population should also be considered at the policy level, with the goals being improved health, a quality patient experience, and judicious use of resources.

To fulfill their obligation to be prudent stewards of health care resources, physicians should base recommendations and decisions on patients' medical needs, use scientifically grounded evidence to inform professional decisions when available, help patients articulate their health care goals, help patients and their families form realistic expectations regarding likely outcomes, endorse recommendations that offer reasonable likelihood of achieving the patient's health care goals, choose the course of action that requires fewer resources when alternative courses of action offer similar likelihood and degree of anticipated benefit, be transparent about alternatives, disclose when resource constraints play a role in decision-making, and participate in efforts to resolve persistent disagreement about whether a costly intervention is worthwhile, which may include consulting other physicians, an ethics committee, or other appropriate resources.

Although this is certainly a daunting task, it is the responsibility of the emergency physician to advocate with all the resources available to her for the health of her patients and community. Different solutions may present themselves depending on the emphasis placed on liberty, equality, utility, or community. Ideally, a just system for health care distribution should provide unobstructed access to a decent minimum standard of health care, acceptable incentives for providers and consumers that promote health rather than expenditure, and a fair system of resource macro- and micro-allocation. In such a system, the emergency physician would truly be free to provide "quality emergency care through the prudent management of public and private resources" (ACEP, 2001).

CASES TO STIMULATE FURTHER THOUGHT AND DISCUSSION

You are working in the ED and pick up a patient with low back pain. He does not have any clinical indications for emergent magnetic resonance imaging (MRI), but he is demanding that one be done immediately. Your hospital's policy is that MRIs only be done for certain clinical indications. The patient is wealthy and states that he will pay for the MRI out of pocket. What is the physician's ethical response? Although the direct cost may be covered by the patient in this case, there are other costs and potential consequences associated with this decision. An incidental finding on the MRI that would not have impacted the patient's health might be discovered, which could potentially lead to negative consequences for the patient through further testing or unnecessary interventions. In addition, unnecessary utilization of resources for this patient may negatively impact access to resources (either directly or indirectly) for other patients who legitimately require them.

A flu pandemic strikes your town, and thirty-two patients are in need of ventilators. You currently have thirty ventilators in the hospital. How do you decide who gets a ventilator? In most cases, institutions should have a policy and procedure for utilization of resources in the setting of a pandemic illness. In most cases, medical condition and chances for improvement should define a group of patients eligible to have access to those resources, followed by an objective system such as a lottery to determine which of those individuals will receive the resources.

Your hospital's ICU is at capacity, including two patients aged more than ninety years on vents with a poor prognosis. Two younger patients arrive in the ED with critical care needs and have a good prognosis if those needs are met. In addition, your hospital does not have capacity to take ICU-level transfers from community hospitals while the ED is holding ICU patients. In this situation, the hospital has several conflicting responsibilities – to its current ICU patients, the ED patients (those awaiting ICU beds and others), and the community. The hospital should have policies and procedures in place to take care of all these constituencies to the best of its ability, with contingency plans for an approach when its resources are exceeded. These policies and procedures should be communicated clearly so that decision-making is transparent to all involved.

ETHICS TAKEOUT TIPS

- The ACEP defines stewardship as applied to emergency medicine as "the provision of quality emergency care through the prudent management of public and private resources" (ACEP, 2001).
- Stewardship of resources and the health of a population is a shared responsibility among individual patients, providers, and society as a whole.
- There are multiple ethical arguments supporting a moral right to health care, but there is much controversy regarding the minimum level of this care and the funding for it.
- Recent legislation in the United States is likely to increase the number of individuals with health care coverage, but the impact on ED care is as of yet unclear.
- Health care resources are allocated on macro (system) and micro (individual) levels. Macroallocation decisions are determined on the policy level – selection of populations eligible for resources, funding decisions, and the like. Microallocation decisions are generally based on prioritization of medical need and some element of impersonal mechanisms such as lotteries or waiting time.
- Drivers of high health care costs in the United States are multifactorial and should be considered primarily at the policy level. Individual providers should keep costs in mind as they assist in making decisions based on what is best for the patient's health and preferences, making every effort to provide the highest quality care at the lowest possible cost.
- In most cases, medical need and patient preferences via shared decision-making should be the primary driving factors in making medical decisions for individual patients, with the well-being of those patients at the focus.
- Physicians also have an obligation to promote public health and access to care. This obligation requires physicians to be prudent stewards of the shared resources with which they are entrusted.

FOR FURTHER READING

American College of Emergency Physicians. (2001). *Emergency physician stewardship of finite resources.* www.acep.org/Content.aspx?id=29422
Beauchamp, T., & Childress, J. (2001). *Principles of biomedical ethics* (5th ed.). New York: Oxford University Press.

Combes, J. R., & Arespacochaga, E. (2013). *Appropriate use of medical resources.* American Hospital Association's Physician Leadership Forum, Chicago, IL. www.aha.org/advocacy-issues/appropuse/index.shtml

Douglas, S. (2012). *Physician stewardship of health care resources.* American Medical Association Council on Ethical and Judicial Affairs. www.ama-assn. org/resources/doc/ethics/ceja-1a12.pdf

Freeman, J., & McDonnell, K. (2001). *Tough decisions: Cases in medical ethics.* New York: Oxford University Press.

Furrow, B., Greaney, T., Johnson, S., Jost, T., & Schwartz, R. (2004). *Bioethics: Health care law and ethics* (5th ed.). St. Paul, MN: Thomson West.

Jonsen, A., Sigler, M., & Winslade, W. (1992) *Clinical ethics* (3rd ed.). New York: McGraw-Hill.

Robert Wood Johnson Foundation. (2013). *Strengthening affordability and quality in America's health care system.* www.rwjf.org/content/dam/farm/reports/reports/2013/rwjf405432

19

Education in Emergency Medicine

WALTER LIMEHOUSE, MD, AND CATHERINE A. MARCO, MD, FACEP

TRAINING IN EMERGENCY MEDICINE

Education in emergency medicine is essential to the provision of quality emergency care. Emergency medicine was established as the twenty-third recognized medical specialty by the American Board of Medical Specialties (ABMS) in 1979. Since that time, the Accreditation Council on Graduate Medical Education (ACGME) has approved graduate medical education in emergency medicine. The number of programs, residents in training, and graduates has continued to gradually increase. As of 2015, there are 167 accredited U.S. categorical emergency medicine residency programs in the United States.

This rapid growth in training has served important functions in the training of emergency physicians and the growth and recognition of emergency medicine as a specialty. However, with growth, several ethical issues of training should be recognized.

Roles and Responsibilities of Learners

The ACGME oversees training in emergency medicine to ensure an optimal learning environment. Of greater importance, learners must assume responsibility for their education and acquisition of the knowledge, skills, and abilities necessary to safely and effectively deliver quality emergency care to their patients. For example, the ACGME sets a minimum standard of five hours per week of planned didactic experiences. The value of these planned didactic experiences depends on faculty planning and, most importantly, resident preparation, participation, and application of concepts addressed in didactics.

Medical knowledge is an essential milestone of emergency medicine training as defined by the ACGME Milestone 15: Medical Knowledge

(MK): "Demonstrates appropriate medical knowledge in the care of emergency medicine patients. Individual commitment to acquisition of medical knowledge is essential to successful knowledge development and clinical application."

Ethical Responsibilities of Faculty

The Hippocratic oath addresses the responsibility of physicians to educate: "to teach them this art; and that by my teaching, I will impart a knowledge of this art to my own sons, and to my teacher's sons, and to disciples bound by an indenture and oath according to the medical laws, and no others."

Faculty in emergency medicine carry important responsibilities for the education and mentorship of residents in training. Mentorship carries an important responsibility to demonstrate ethical and professional conduct. Faculty must recognize the stressors that occur during residency training and mentor residents to achieve the healthiest and most productive goals of residency training.

Faculty should ensure the wellness of residents. Signs of fatigue, mental illness, or substance abuse should be addressed and remediated if necessary. Faculty are in a unique position of working closely with and identifying personal or professional challenges with individual residents.

Faculty should support resident duty hour regulations during training. The ACGME has implemented standards on duty hours and supervision since 2003, with several revisions. A maximum of eighty hours of duty per week is required in all specialties. Emergency medicine has additional duty hour requirements during ED rotations, including a maximum of twelve continuous scheduled hours, a maximum of sixty scheduled hours per week seeing patients in the ED, and no more than seventy-two duty hours per week.

Faculty share the responsibility to ensure a safe, productive, educational, and fair learning environment. If learners identify a potential breach in the appropriate learning environment, the American Medical Association (AMA) Code of Ethics states: "Clear policies for handling complaints from medical students, resident physicians, and other staff should be established. These policies should include adequate provisions for protecting the confidentiality of complainants whenever possible."

Faculty are responsible for the appropriate supervision of learners. The ACGME Program Requirements in Emergency Medicine states that "Supervision in the setting of graduate medical education has the goals of assuring the provision of safe and effective care to the individual patient;

assuring each resident's development of the skills, knowledge, and attitudes required to enter the unsupervised practice of medicine; and establishing a foundation for continued professional growth."

Education in Ethical and Professional Responsibilities

Education in ethical and professional responsibilities should be as high a priority as education in clinical emergency medicine. Ethics and professionalism are taught through a variety of mechanisms, including modeling, mentoring, didactic experiences, simulated experiences, and personal study and application of ethical principles.

The Liaison Committee on Medical Education accreditation standard ED-23 requires instruction in medical ethics and human values, such that medical students demonstrate ethical principles during patient care and in relating to patients' families and care team members. The Emergency Medicine Milestone Project, a joint initiative of the ACGME and the American Board of Emergency Medicine, specifies curricular goals for residency levels that imply that the resident substantially demonstrates the milestones at a given level, as well as those at lower levels. Milestone 30 is Professional Values (PROF1): "Demonstrates compassion, integrity, and respect for others as well as adherence to the ethical principles relevant to the practice of medicine."

The five defined milestones within Professional Values include:

- *Level 1* (expected of incoming resident): Demonstrates behavior that conveys caring, honesty, genuine interest, and tolerance when interacting with a diverse population of patients and families
- *Level 2* (advancing resident, not yet mid-residency level): Demonstrates an understanding of the importance of compassion, integrity, respect, sensitivity, and responsiveness and exhibits these attitudes consistently in common/uncomplicated situations and with diverse population
- *Level 3* (advancing resident, demonstrates majority of milestones for this category): Recognizes how own personal beliefs and values impact medical care. Consistently manages own values and beliefs to optimize relationships and medical care. Develops alternate care plans when patients' personal decisions/beliefs preclude the use of commonly accepted practices
- *Level 4* (resident meets graduation targets for this category): Develops and applies a consistent and appropriate approach to evaluating

appropriate care, possible barriers, and strategies to intervene that consistently prioritizes the patient's best interest in all relationships and situations. Effectively analyzes and manages ethical issues in complicated and challenging clinical situations

- *Level 5* (resident demonstrates aspirational goals more typical of post-graduation): Develops institutional and organizational strategies to protect and maintain professional and bioethical principles

Remediation

Ideally, learners would act professionally and responsibly at all times, study diligently, and prepare and develop the knowledge, skills, and abilities necessary to be a capable emergency physician. However, some learners may require mentorship, counseling, remediation, probation, or dismissal. Remediation can be a challenging process for faculty and for residents. Emotions may lead to counterproductive feelings of anger, denial, or diminished self-worth. It is crucial that remediation be conducted in an environment of support and encouragement, with a goal of progress and improvement.

The ACGME requires evaluation of resident performance in a timely manner during each rotation. For residents who require remediation, progress and improvement must be monitored at a minimum of every three months.

Teacher–Learner Relationships

Physician educators should serve as mentors of professionalism, ethical behavior, and high-quality caregivers. Faculty hold a power differential compared to learners, and this may introduce vulnerability on the part of learners. Hence, when working with learners at any level, professional boundaries should be respected. Exploitation of learners based on training status, gender, ethnicity, or any other personal attribute must be avoided. Mentoring and modeling of quality patient care, application of medical ethics, and professional behavior should be the primary goals of educators.

The Society for Academic Emergency Medicine (SAEM) encourages teachers to abide by its code of conduct to "be considerate, forthright, and just in all my dealings with patients and colleagues regardless of their power, position, or station in life." Recognizing learner vulnerability within academics, the SAEM code further pledges: "I will advance the ideals of the

profession, and I will not abuse the privilege of my knowledge or position."
The academic emergency physician also pledges:

As a teacher of emergency medicine, I vow:

1. Altruism, generously sharing the art and science of emergency medicine for the betterment of others and the honor of the calling.
2. A commitment to excellence, maintaining my technical expertise and moral sensitivity through continued study and practice.
3. Respect, giving all who seek to learn emergency medicine the dignity due a colleague.
4. Fairness, treating all students and fellow teachers equitably, in a manner free of prejudice, abuse, or coercion.
5. Honesty, imparting truth and uncertainty openly, and identifying clearly for my patients all trainees and students involved in their care.
6. Mentorship, nurturing and encouraging the requisite technical, intellectual, and moral virtues of the profession in students of every kind through my words and deeds.

LIFELONG LEARNING

Lifelong learning is an essential aspiration in emergency medicine. Knowledge of and skills encompassing current diagnostic and treatment modalities provide the best quality clinical care. Physicians should consider lifelong learning an essential professional obligation.

Maintenance of Certification

The ABMS now requires all recognized specialty boards to require maintenance of certification (MOC) programs. MOC includes four components: professional standing, including an unrestricted license to practice medicine; lifelong learning and self-assessment (LLSA); demonstrated cognitive expertise; and assessment of practice performance (APP). ABEM implemented the Emergency Medicine Continuous Certification Program (now referred to as the ABEM MOC Program) in 2004. MOC is associated with improved quality of clinical practice and lower cost, more efficient medical care.

Continuing medical education (CME) is an important component of lifelong learning. Many professional societies and organizations provide CME activities relating to clinical, educational, research, and administration skills.

Faculty Development

Faculty development is an important component of career development in academic emergency medicine. Faculty development is a requirements of the common ACGME program requirements that require program directors (PDs) to document the faculty development program for each residency. Faculty development is key to promote an education and learning environment for residents and fellows, to encourage academic productivity, and to promote faculty career satisfaction. Faculty development may include a broad range of academic activities, such as professional leadership and clinical, instructional, research, organizational, and administrative skills. A proactive individual plan of goals and objectives, with regular assessments, can be an important pathway to faculty development.

ETHICS TAKEOUT TIPS

- Education in emergency medicine is essential to the provision of safe, effective, quality emergency care.
- Residents in emergency medicine training are responsible for their education and should actively seek to improve medical knowledge, procedural skills, and all knowledge, skills, and abilities essential to the practice of emergency medicine.
- Faculty in emergency medicine have important responsibilities to mentor, model, and educate learners about the principles of emergency care and ethical and professional responsibilities.
- All emergency physicians should aspire to lifelong learning and MOC.

FOR FURTHER READING

Accreditation Council for Graduate Medical Education. (n.d.). *Program requirements for graduate medical education in emergency medicine.* https://www.acgme.org/acgmeweb/Portals/0/PFAssets/2013-PR-FAQ-PIF/110_emergency_medicine_07012013.pdf

American Association of Colleges in Nursing (AACN), & American Association of Medical Colleges (AAMC). (2010). *Lifelong learning in medicine and nursing: Final conference report* (pp. 1–92). Washington, DC: Authors.

American Board of Medical Specialties. (2015). *MOC standards.* www.abms.org/media/1109/standards-for-the-abms-program-for-moc-final.pdf

American Medical Association. (n.d.). *Code of medical ethics* www.ama-assn.org/ama/pub/physician-resources/medical-ethics/code-medical-ethics.page

Counselman, F. L., Borenstein, M. A., Chisholm, C. D., Epter, M. L., Khandelwal, S., Kraus, C. K., . . . Keehbauch, J. N. (2014). The 2013 model of the clinical practice of emergency medicine. *Academic Emergency Medicine*, 21, 574–598.

Houry, D., Shockley, L. W., & Markovchick, V. (2000). Wellness issues and the emergency medicine resident. *Annals of Emergency Medicine*, 35(4), 394–397.

Larkin, G. L., for the SAEM Ethics Committee. (1999). A code of conduct for academic emergency medicine. *Academic Emergency Medicine*, 6, 45.

Larkin, G. L., & Mello, M. J. (2010). Commentary: Doctors without boundaries: The ethics of teacher-student relationships in academic medicine. *Academic Medicine*, 85(5), 752–755.

Marco, C. A., Lu, D. W., Stettner, E., Sokolove, P. E., Ufberg, J. W., & Noeller, T. P. (2011). Ethics curriculum for emergency medicine graduate medical education. *Journal of Emergency Medicine*, 40(5), 550–556.

Marco, C. A., & Perina, D. G. (2004). Mentoring in emergency medicine: Challenges and future directions. *Academic Emergency Medicine*, 11, 1329–1330.

Miller, S. H. (2005). American Board of Medical Specialties and repositioning for excellence on lifelong learning: Maintenance of certification. *Journal of Continuing Education in Health Professions*, 25, 151–156.

Mohr, N. M., Moreno-Walton, L., Mills, A. M., Brunett, P. H., Promes, S. B., on behalf of the SAEM Aging & Generational Issues in Academic Emergency Medicine Task Force. (2011). Generational influences in academic emergency medicine: Teaching & learning, mentoring, & technology (Part I). *Academic Emergency Medicine*, 18(2), 190–199.

Smith-Coggins, R., Baren, J. M., Beeson, M. S., Counselman, F. L., Kowalenko, T., Marco, C. A., . . . Korte, R. C. (2014). American Board of Emergency Medicine report on residency training information (2013–2014), American Board of Emergency Medicine. *Annals of Emergency Medicine*, 63, 637–645.

Wagner, M. J., Wolf, S., Promes, S., McGee, D., Hobgood, C., Doty, C., . . . Muelleman, R. (2010). Duty hours in emergency medicine: Balancing patient safety, resident wellness, and the resident training experience: A consensus response to the 2008 institute of medicine resident duty hours recommendations. *Academic Emergency Medicine*, 17(9), 1004–1011.

Yeung, M., Nuth, J., & Stiell, I. G. (2010). Mentoring in emergency medicine: The art and the evidence. *Canadian Journal of Emergency Medicine*, 12(2), 143–149.

20

Suicide Attempts

JENNIFER NELSON, MD, AND ARVIND VENKAT, MD, FACEP

INTRODUCTION

Attempted suicide represents an epidemic, one with medical, financial, emotional, and ethical burdens. According to the Centers for Disease Control and Prevention, suicide now causes more deaths than motor vehicle accidents in the United States. It is estimated that approximately 1 million adults attempt suicide annually. Together, suicide and suicide attempts lead to approximately $41.2 billion in direct health care costs and lost productivity annually. As of 2011, approximately 487,000 individuals were treated in U.S. emergency departments (EDs) for suicide attempts or self-inflicted injuries. These figures do not include the emotional and psychological toll on patients and families when a suicide attempt occurs. As a result, health care providers, medical societies, and government agencies have devoted considerable resources to evaluating the causes of and preventing suicide attempts.

At the same time, patients, physicians, ethicists, and governments have outlined circumstances where suicide may be justified with the assistance of health care providers. In the United States, Oregon, Vermont, and Washington have statutes that allow patients to request a physician prescription of medications for the purposes of suicide where an individual has a terminal condition and is free of any condition that impairs judgment. Montana has legalized this approach via court decision. Even with safeguards in place and evidence that these laws have not disproportionately affected underserved or vulnerable minorities or the elderly, professional medical societies such as the American Medical Association have taken positions that physician-assisted suicide represents a fundamental ethical violation of the physician's obligation to do no harm. Internationally, countries such as the Netherlands and Switzerland have legal frameworks that permit euthanasia, and Belgium recently passed legislation allowing this procedure in minors.

From this variation, it is clear that suicide attempts represent an ethically challenging situation for physicians and other health care providers. For emergency physicians and ED staff, the ethical difficulties are compounded by the acute nature of the care provided and the limited information available at the time of patient presentation. It is common for emergency physicians to have little knowledge about the underlying illnesses in their patients and, in the context of a suicide attempt, the personal motivations or psychological circumstances that may have led to the patient's presentation. Further complications arise when a patient or his surrogate decision-maker present evidence through an advanced directive document or actionable medical order (e.g. Do Not Resuscitate [DNR] order) that resuscitative measures would not be desired. Together, these logistical barriers make treating patients following a suicide attempt in the ED profoundly challenging.

A simplistic response for ED and acute care health care providers would be to presume that every suicide attempt is evidence of an impairment in decision-making capacity and that a physician's obligation to treat patients in need should lead to aggressive treatment. However, such a default pathway may have the same ethical concerns as a path that presumes that a suicide attempt may be a rational ethical choice. For example, aggressive resuscitation may lead to futile care measures, unnecessary resource expenditure, and willful ignoring of the life circumstances of the patient that led to the suicide attempt.

In this chapter, we provide an overview of the ethical, legal, and medical issues that can affect the assessment of a patient following a suicide attempt. From this overview, we will outline a medical and ethical pathway to evaluate and treat these individuals and an ethical framework based on the principle of proportionality for determining the extent to which resuscitative measures should be put into effect. We conclude by providing case examples of how this ethical framework can be applied at the bedside in the ED and acute care setting.

ETHICAL PARADIGMS

Earlier chapters in this text provided an overview of the common ethical paradigms used in emergency medical practice and acute hospitalizations. All provide insight into the assessment of patients following a suicide attempt, but none provides a definitive response. Ethical theory provides a framework for assessing the clinical situation, but, as all health care providers are aware, case nuances rarely follow textbook theory. It behooves the emergency physician to first garner the clinical facts prior to making ethical judgments. If "good facts make good ethics," then understanding case nuances are a necessary prerequisite to quality ethical decision-making.

At the same time, ethical theories, whether principlist, virtue-, or narrative-based, provide insights for analyzing clinical situations. When evaluating a patient following a suicide attempt, we would suggest that knowledge of these theories can help emergency physicians make ethical judgments on how to proceed. For example, a principlist approach might weigh an evaluation of the presence of autonomous decision-making capacity in a chronically ill patient who attempted suicide versus the provider's obligation to provide beneficent care. A virtue approach might emphasize the specialized knowledge of the emergency physician and the professionally imposed obligation to apply that knowledge to care for the patient. Narrative theory might suggest further exploration of the social-cultural-personal milieu that may have led the patient to attempt suicide.

None of these theories in isolation is likely to provide an overarching approach that can address all patients following a suicide attempt and how the emergency physician should respond. Rather, the combination of these theories coupled with case-based assessment can lead to an appropriate ethical response when coupled with the larger principle of proportionality. *Proportionality*, at its most basic level, suggests that our reaction to a situation should be congruent with the consequences of not taking action or the results of the response itself. As we will discuss, in the case of a suicide attempt, understanding the surrounding facts and placing them in context can aid in developing an ethically proportionate ethical response that respects both the patient's circumstances, the emergency physician's professional responsibilities, and the medical consequences of the courses of action.

LEGAL FACTORS AND ADVANCED PLANNING DOCUMENTS IN THE CONTEXT OF SUICIDE ATTEMPTS

The legal framework concerning suicide attempts has evolved tremendously both in the United States and internationally. Until the mid-twentieth century, suicide attempts legally fell under criminal statutes that could theoretically result in prosecution, although that rarely occurred. However, since that time, all U.S. states have removed criminal laws against suicide attempts. At the same time, statutes in all states commonly view suicidal ideation as a rationale to force psychiatric evaluation. This fits within the larger state interest to preserve life and for medical professionals to exercise their skills to prevent the harm of a suicide attempt. For emergency physicians, these legal provisions commonly lead to the need to acutely stabilize patients with suicidal ideation and transfer them to more definitive psychiatric care, often with significant logistical difficulty.

Today, multiple jurisdictions have passed legislation to permit physician-assisted suicide. In the United States, Oregon, Vermont, and Washington have statutes that permit terminally ill patients to request a prescription from a physician to allow suicide, while Montana allows the same based on judicial precedent. These laws include provisions for certification of the prognosis of the patient by more than one licensed physician, that there is no evidence of psychological impairment, and that the choice to pursue this option is not coerced. Similarly, physician-assisted suicide is legal in the Netherlands and Switzerland under somewhat looser circumstances than those in the United States. As a result, media reports have noted that a type of suicide tourism has arisen in which individuals travel to these countries to receive medical assistance in ending their lives through suicide. Uniquely, Belgium has passed an amendment to its statute on euthanasia to allow this procedure in minors with chronic or terminal illnesses who experience unbearable suffering. Under the law, the minor him- or herself must initiate this request with parental consent and health care provider evaluation of the patient to discern the nature of their illness. Together, these changes in laws in a variety of jurisdictions suggest that, in the case of terminal illness and significant pain or loss of dignity, there may be legal approval for suicide.

However, in the vast majority of locales, although suicide is not illegal, it is viewed as a situation to be avoided. For emergency physicians, this will generally lead to medical treatment of patients who present following a suicide attempt. This treatment can appear to be in contradiction to patient statements, suicide notes, and other often eloquent documentation that the patient had apparent reasons for attempting suicide and not wanting resuscitation. However, it is important to remember that suicide attempts are commonly an impulsive, rather than contemplatively planned, gesture. In this circumstance, it is difficult to conceive that patient statements or notes can be viewed as meeting the conditions for informed refusal of treatment. Informed refusal in its truest form requires an ability to understand alternatives and state within a coherent moral framework why a particular choice of treatment is made. In contrast, a suicide note or statement at a time of impulse does not allow that consideration of alternatives and therefore should not be viewed as forcing emergency physicians to abdicate their professional responsibilities to aid patients in times of crisis.

Where a more difficult issue arises is when a patient arrives following a suicide attempt with an advanced directive document or actionable medical order that limits life-sustaining treatment (e.g. DNR order or Physician Orders for Life-Sustaining Treatment [POLST] form). These documents are presumed to be valid based on patient or surrogate decision-maker discussion with a health care provider and executed to reflect patient wishes. However, it is reasonable for an emergency physician to evaluate their application in the context of a suicide attempt. In the case of an advanced directive that might indicate a patient's wish to avoid life-sustaining treatment when he or she is in an end-stage condition or permanently unconscious, it is rare that in the ED these conditions can be definitively established. That uncertainty plus a presumption to preserve life where possible suggests that a presented living will document or advanced directive would not be dispositive on the medical course of action after a suicide attempt. There is an additional consideration that, given the commonly impulsive nature of suicide attempts and that with treatment, the underlying impairments that led to such attempts can be addressed, it is ethically muddled at best whether an advanced directive written to address a hypothetical future medical condition is applicable. In this context, it is largely untenable to conclude that, ethically, an advanced directive would provide significant guidance for or constraint on emergency medical care following a suicide attempt.

Actionable medical orders, such as DNR or POLST forms, represent more significant ethical dilemmas in the context of attempted suicide when compared to advanced directives. These documents are meant to be used in the context of a patient with a degenerative, progressive, or terminal ailment. For example, a patient diagnosed with metastatic cancer can, in collaboration with his or her oncologist, use a POLST form to document the course of treatment desired at times of acute medical crisis. Should a patient with a DNR order or POLST form present following a suicide attempt, the issue that arises is whether the manner in which a patient develops an acute medical crisis is relevant to whether a physician follows the terms of these forms. Legally, there is little to no precedent or statutory interpretation that provides guidance. As we discuss later, the ethical judgment largely will be dependent on the case-specific circumstances and a reference to proportionality. Again, however, the typical hurried nature of emergency care suggests that, in the absence of definitive evidence on all the case circumstances, it would behoove the emergency physician to move to resuscitate patients given that without immediate action, the patient who attempted suicide may die.

INITIAL EVALUATION OF THE PATIENT
WHO HAS ATTEMPTED SUICIDE

In the context of the ethical and legal factors presented, how should emergency physicians approach the initial evaluation of the patient who has attempted suicide? In a patient presenting in extremis, where there is little opportunity for exploration of the context in which the attempt took place, it would seem logical and ethical to take measures to preserve the life of the patient by taking commonly used interventions such as intubation and antidote treatments. Even in the presence of an actionable medical order, there is enough uncertainty as to their application in the context of a suicide attempt that it would behoove an emergency physician to save the patient and explore the circumstances over time. It is far easier and ethically appropriate to withdraw life-sustaining treatment after an evaluation rather than lose the patient without a chance to have this discussion.

If the patient is not in distress, there is the opportunity for the emergency physician to assess the context under which the suicide attempt took place. Some of the factors that are relevant include the past medical and social history of the patient, the context of the suicide attempt, the physiologic state in which the patient arrives, the prognosis for recovery with treatment of both a physical and psychological nature, and the likely decision-making capacity or lack thereof of the patient at the time of the suicide attempt. These factors together provide the context in which to determine the proportionate response to the clinical situation.

For past medical and social history, key information points include whether the patient had a degenerative or terminal condition at the time of the attempt. Examples might include the presence of metastatic cancer, amyotrophic lateral sclerosis, or dementia. Given the presence of a terminal condition, there may be an ethical justification to determine that aggressive treatment measures to forestall death by suicide may present little benefit if death will occur shortly thereafter due to the underlying disease process. Here, the focus is largely a utilitarian one, where the resources expended will make little difference in the outcome of the patient. In contrast, a suicide attempt in a patient without such conditions or with solely social stressors provides a context in which an emergency physician would rightly determine that, on a utilitarian level, medical treatment is likely to be beneficial and allow further exploration of how the patient can be helped in the long-term.

The context of the suicide attempt also becomes relevant when considering how treatment should proceed and to whom the emergency physician should turn for surrogate decision-making. For example, a suicide attempt that contextually is triggered from disagreement or conflict with the patient's next of kin may raise the question as to whether the relative can rightly represent the best interests of the patient. Similarly, a suicide attempt in a patient with untreated depression who leaves a note requesting no resuscitative measures should lead to questions about the validity of that patient statement. In contrast, a suicide attempt in a patient with a terminal illness who lives in a jurisdiction where physician-assisted suicide is legally permitted, used the resultant prescription but did not die, and presents with respiratory depression and coma may appropriately not receive resuscitative measures in the ED.

The physiologic state of the patient following a suicide attempt is also an important factor in the initial ED evaluation. However, there is a nuance that makes this assessment quite challenging. Given that patients present to the ED with limited historical information and in the initial stages of an acute disease process, it may be difficult for the emergency physician to determine the prognosis of the patient over the near term. It is in this context that most emergency physicians will presume that the patient following a suicide attempt is salvageable and should receive acute resuscitative treatment. However, there may be cases where the emergency physician has relevant background medical history (e.g. end-stage amyotrophic lateral sclerosis) in combination with acute parameters (e.g. profound respiratory acidosis despite ventilator support) that suggests further life-sustaining treatments may be futile.

Another difficulty related to the physiologic state of the patient is that after the initial ED resuscitation, there may only be a short period of time where withdrawal of critical care treatments will result in the patient experiencing a peaceful demise – a so-called window of opportunity for discussions on goals of therapy. After this time period has passed, it is very possible that removal or continuation of life-sustaining therapies will have the same result – a debilitated, medically dependent patient with little chance of meaningful recovery. An example includes a patient who may have attempted suicide by using a medication that causes respiratory depression and a profound anoxic injury. At the time of initial resuscitation, the patient showed little to no respiratory effort, and withholding or withdrawal of life-sustaining treatment would have resulted in his demise. However, after forty-eight hours of care, the medication has been sufficiently metabolized such that respiratory depression is not likely to occur after extubation, but with little benefit to the patient given the hypoxic insult he encountered. The ethical dilemma that arises is whether emergency physicians can or should consider this potential for poor outcome when deciding on initial treatment.

There also should be consideration during the initial presentation or shortly thereafter as to the patient's prognosis for recovery from a psychological perspective if the suicide attempt was related to mental illness. Emergency physicians regularly support this concern when invoking legal provisions to force psychiatric evaluation in the presence of suicidal ideation. It may be as important for the acute care provider to evaluate whether, along with aggressive treatment of the medical consequences of the suicide attempt, there is an opportunity for psychiatric treatment that can prevent such attempts in the future. As we previously noted, the vast majority of suicide attempts are impulsive in nature, and it is well-established that there is an ethical, medical, and legal obligation to try to identify and prevent such attempts. What is less clear is how the prospect for effective psychiatric treatment should weigh on decisions on continued medical treatment to save a patient who attempted suicide. For example, does the likelihood of effective psychiatric treatment weigh ethically in favor of continuing intensive care treatment rather than allowing a patient or surrogate decision-maker to withdraw life-sustaining measures? Again, the specifics of the case and an evaluation in the context of proportionality would seem to provide a framework for addressing how far medical treatment should extend in a patient following a suicide attempt in the hopes of providing subsequent psychiatric treatment.

A final consideration is what the nature of the patient's decision-making capacity was at the time of the suicide attempt and thereafter. It seems prudent in the immediate presentation period of the patient following a suicide attempt to have great skepticism of statements or suicide notes that contend that resuscitative treatment should be withheld. To not have that skepticism would too quickly foreswear the professional obligations of physicians to care for patients in acute need and the likely desire of a rational patient to be treated and given the opportunity to recover. This is an example of the application of the best interest standard, in which health care providers attempt to assess what a reasonable person would want in a particular situation where the patient cannot express this for him- or herself. However, after the initial treatment period, the question arises as to whether or when a patient can begin to make decisions for him- or herself following a suicide attempt. Even with formal psychiatric certification that the patient has intact decision-making capacity, it is understandable that a health care provider would be wary of allowing a patient following a suicide attempt to make a decision to forego curative treatment. On the other hand, if a suicide attempt is generally an impulsive gesture or decision, there may be support for allowing a patient after initial treatment to resume his or her presumptive right to make medical decisions in an autonomous manner. When that should take place, again, is a judgment based on the specifics of the case.

APPLYING PROPORTIONALITY

Proportionality is an ethical principle whereby the individual judges her response to a situation based on two factors. First, what are the consequences of not taking action in this situation? Second, what are the consequences of the action itself relative to the current course of events? Both these judgments, by necessity, are grounded in the particulars of the case. Without reference to these particulars, judgments on consequences are theoretical at best.

In the case of a suicide attempt, proportionality allows a three-step process for assessing how emergency physicians and acute care providers can ethically evaluate the treatment options available and how to incorporate patient statements into this decision-making process. As an initial step, when a patient presents to the ED following a suicide attempt, in the absence of complete information, the consequences of inaction appear quite profound (patient demise) whereas the consequences of action seem less concerning by comparison. This creates a strong presumption for emergency physicians to aggressively treat a patient following a suicide attempt regardless of patient statements or suicide notes.

The next step in applying proportionality is a relatively rapid assessment of the circumstances of the suicide attempt. Here, the patient's background, medical condition, and personal narrative merit consideration. Judgments can then be made as to the consequences of continued medical treatments or initiating new ones. It is important to remember that, from an ethical perspective, there is little difference between withholding and withdrawing treatment measures. Both require medical knowledge and professional judgments on effectiveness, consequences, and outcomes. As such, an initial decision to resuscitate a patient following a suicide attempt does not ethically bind a health care provider to continue that course of treatment under the proportionality standard.

Finally, an appeal to proportionality allows health care providers to judge when continued treatment in the context of a suicide attempt is crossing into a realm of not providing beneficial care, given the patient's likely outcome. This is a discomforting notion because it is natural for health care providers to not want to feel or be perceived as acquiescing or assisting in the completion of a suicide attempt. However, reference to the facts of the case will allow consideration of whether, after a good faith attempt at resuscitation, further treatment measures are not likely to aid the patient but rather result in a debilitated or dependent patient with little chance of meaningful physical or psychological recovery. Given the issue with the "window-of-opportunity," some authors have suggested that seventy-two hours of treatment is a reasonable period of time at which to make the decision on whether continued aggressive treatment measures are reasonable. These authors contend that after this time period, the perceived stigma of allowing the completion of the suicide attempt is expunged and that the patient should be viewed as others with similar physiologic parameters. We would caution that seventy-two hours is, at best, a rule of thumb and that particular case circumstances will govern when this third stage is reached.

There is a fair criticism that applying proportionality leads to a type of paternalism because judgments on consequences largely reside with health care providers as opposed to the patient. Clearly, emergency physicians and other health care providers must show humility in their ability to draw definitive conclusions based on the information available at the time and after patient presentation. However, health care providers are held accountable in this process in a manner that perhaps other parties are not. Physicians face scrutiny from administrative (institutional credentialing), governmental (licensure), and medico legal (malpractice) authorities. In contrast, patients following a suicide attempt may not have full insight into the consequences of their actions or decisions. This suggests that it may be appropriate for health care providers to have more of a role in determining how proportionality is applied to the management of a patient following a suicide attempt, certainly early in the clinical course.

CASE EXAMPLES

To show how case particulars and proportionality can be applied, we present three case examples related to attempted suicide to allow the reader to apply our discussion to the clinical environment. We do not provide an outcome because the cases are meant to stimulate thought and discussion rather than suggest that a particular path is the correct one. These and additional cases are also presented in the accompanying multimedia presentation.

Elderly Patient

A ninety-five-year-old woman presents to the ED following an attempted suicide through a salicylate overdose. She is unconscious upon arrival to the ED and is quickly intubated and begun on sodium bicarbonate treatment. Over the next twelve hours, the patient develops profound metabolic acidosis and hypotension. Her daughter states that the patient had experienced significant depression since her husband had died six months prior and that her physical health had also declined recently following a fall leading to her needing to use a walker in an independent living facility. The daughter requests that the patient be extubated and allowed to die under palliative care measures, without the initiation of pressors or dialysis. The daughter states that the patient would not want continued life-sustaining treatment given her grave condition.

In addressing this case, it is fair to ask whether a ninety-five-year-old in poor health and now with acute critical illness should at least have a trial of potentially curative treatments such as dialysis. At the same time, what is the true recovery potential of this patient from either a physical or psychological perspective? It is also worth considering the concern for the "window of opportunity," where a decision to withdraw life-sustaining treatment would make a difference in patient outcome. A proportionate response given these case facts might suggest either a trial of further aggressive therapeutic measures, the withholding of dialysis, or withdrawal of life-sustaining therapy.

Chronic Pain

A thirty-five-year-old man with ongoing chronic low back pain presents to the ED following an overdose of oxycodone and acetaminophen. He states that his primary care physician has involuntarily separated from continuing to treat him due to perceived concerns with addiction and that his insurance will not cover management by a pain specialist. He expresses deep regret for his suicide attempt and states that what he really wants is help with managing his pain. He readily acquiesces to all treatment measures and inpatient hospitalization. At the end of the hospitalization, psychiatry concurs that this was largely an impulsive gesture and that the patient is not a significant threat to attempt suicide again should he receive long-term pain management. The treatment team has arranged that follow-up, but the appointment is not for six weeks, and the patient requests a prescription of narcotic pain medications until that time.

In this case, the proportionality issue is how to weigh the potential consequences of not prescribing narcotic medication versus those of prescribing. Clearly, pain management is complex from an ethical and medical perspective. Emergency physicians and acute care providers are commonly confronted by the limitations of their knowledge of the patient and how to optimally manage the patient's pain and the logistical barriers to effective long-term pain care. In the case of a suicide attempt, the decision on how the manage the patient's pain is more fraught given that the prescription to treat the patient's pain can also be the instrument for a new suicide attempt. Some proportionate responses might be a short prescription with interim psychiatric and primary care follow-up, the signing of a formal pain management contract, alternative treatment modalities (e.g. acupuncture or physical therapy), and agreements on testing and pill counts to ensure compliance with the prescribed pain regimen. At the same time, a decision to withhold narcotic pain medications should not be viewed as a benign one given the course of events that led to the patient's suicide attempt.

Attempted Suicide with a POLST

A seventy-two-year-old woman with recently diagnosed dementia presents to the ED following a suicide attempt through an overdose of a beta-blocker. She presents hypotensive and bradycardic but conscious and has a POLST form she had executed a few weeks prior asking for do-not-resuscitate, comfort-measures-only status. The patient states that she does not want to lose her independence through progression of her dementia and is ready to die. She asks that her POLST form be respected in its provisions, and that includes not placing a central line, transvenous pacemaker, or other life-sustaining/aggressive measures. The patient is completely coherent and not apparently debilitated at this point from her dementia, which is in its early stages.

The tension between the ethical and legal are apparent in this case. On the one hand, the POLST is meant to be actionable upon presentation to the health care provider. On the other side is a clearly salvageable patient who may have taken a decision in haste and without insight. Her actions suggest the possibility of untreated depression and psychiatric impairment in the context of her recent dementia diagnosis. In the acute setting, it may not be possible to explore all of these issues in a timely manner. A proportionate response might include temporizing measures such as medical therapy with glucagon and hyperinsulin-glucose infusion. Similarly, a lack of action may result in the patient's rapid demise without allowing time to further explore the patient's potential for physical and psychological recovery. Proportionality would also require an assessment of how to initiate therapy in a manner causing the least discomfort and alienation of the patient from her care. Physical restraints to allow therapy may in this context be quite extreme versus more patient discussion with her and deliberate step-by-step care. However, the POLST form by itself is likely not dispositive given the factual context presented by this case, in which rapid medical therapy may avoid the need for the more aggressive therapies that the patient states she wishes to not have performed.

CONCLUSION

Suicide attempts represent an area of profound medical, ethical, and legal controversy. Although there is a general presumption to treat patients in a manner to preserve life following a suicide attempt, the particulars of the case may raise the issue of whether that is a proportionate ethical response. Factors that should be considered include the medical and social history of the patient, the context of the suicide attempt, the physiologic state in which the patient arrives, the prognosis for both physical and psychological treatment and recovery, and the decision-making capacity of the patient at the time of the attempt, upon presentation, and in the course of acute care. Emergency physicians should approach these cases with humility and understand that patient specifics and an ethical framework of proportionality can allow for the effective and ethical treatment of patients following the distressing event of a suicide attempt.

ETHICS TAKEOUT TIPS

- Attempted suicide represents an area of profound medical, ethical, and legal controversy.
- Suicide attempts are commonly impulsive and stem from immediate social stressors and underlying disease processes.

- The general approach in the ED is to treat the patient to preserve life.
- However, case-specific factors and the principle of proportionality will allow consideration of how to resolve these difficult cases.
- In the setting of attempted suicide, advance planning documents are relevant to the extent that clinical and case-specific circumstances allow.
- Be humble and understand that these judgments may need to evolve as the patient's circumstances change.

FOR FURTHER READING

American Medical Association. (1996). *Opinion 2.211 – Physician-assisted suicide.* Chicago, IL: Author.

Battin, M., van der Heide, A., Ganzini, L., van der Wal, G., & Onwuteaka-Philipsen, B. (2007). Legal physician-assisted dying in Oregon and the Netherlands: Evidence concerning the impact on patients in "vulnerable" groups. *Journal of Medical Ethics*, 33, 591–597.

Blackall, G., Volpe, R., & Green, M. (2013). After the suicide attempt: Offering patients another chance. *American Journal of Bioethics*, 13, 13–16.

Brown, S., Elliott, C., & Paine, R. (2013). Withdrawal of nonfutile life support after attempted suicide. *American Journal of Bioethics*, 13, 3–12.

Centers for Disease Control and Prevention. (2012). Suicide: Facts at a glance. www.cdc.gov/violenceprevention/pdf/Suicide-DataSheet-a.pdf

Hermeren, G. (2012). The principle of proportionality: Interpretations and applications. *Medical Health Care Philosophy*, 15, 373–382.

Jacobs, D., & Brewer, M. (2006). Application of the APA Practice Guidelines on Suicide to Clinical Practice. *CNS Spectrums*, 11, 447–454.

Jesus, J., Geiderman, J., Venkat, A., Limehouse, W. E., Jr., Derse, A. R., & Larkin G. L. (2014). Physician Orders for Life-Sustaining Treatment and emergency medicine: Ethical considerations, legal issues, and emerging trends. *Annals of Emergency Medicine*, 64, 140–144.

National Center for Injury Prevention and Control, & Centers for Disease Control and Prevention. (2010). Web-based Injury Statistics Query and Reporting System (WISQARS). www.cdc.gov/injury/wisqars/leading_causes_death.html

Siegel, A., Sisti, D., & Caplan, A. (2014). Pediatric euthanasia in Belgium: Disturbing developments. *Journal of the American Medical Association*, 311, 1963–1964.

Spike, J. (2013). The distinction between completing a suicide and assisting one: Why treating a suicide attempt does not require closing the "window of opportunity." *American Journal of Bioethics*, 13, 26–27.

Terman, S. (2013). Is the principle of proportionality sufficient to guide physicians' decisions regarding withholding/withdrawing life-sustaining treatment after suicide attempts? *American Journal of Bioethics*, 13, 22–24.

Venkat, A. (2012). Surrogate medical decision making on behalf of a never-competent, profoundly intellectually disabled adult who is acutely ill. *Journal of Clinical Ethics*, 23, 71–78.

Venkat, A., & Drori, J. (2014, Winter). When to say when: Responding to a suicide attempt in the acute care setting. *Narrative Inquiry in Bioethics*, 4(3), 263–270.

Venkat, A., Fromm, C., Isaacs, E., & Ibarra, J. (2013). An ethical framework for the management of pain in the emergency department. *Academic Emergency Medicine*, 20, 716–723.

21

Geriatric Emergency Medicine

V. RAMANA FEESER, MD

In 2007, it was estimated that 11 percent of the world's population was age sixty or older, and this age group is projected to account for 22 percent of the worldwide population in 2050. In the United States, the 2010 census estimated that more than 40 million people were age sixty-five or older, and this segment of the population is projected to be 47 million in 2016 and 62 million in 2025. Between 2000 and 2010, the population aged sixty-five and older increased at a faster rate than the total U.S. population. This census data also demonstrated that the population aged eighty-five and older is growing at a rate almost three times the general population. Because nearly all countries of the world are experiencing a growing proportion of older adults, there is reason to expect an increased demand for emergency physicians to gain specific knowledge, training, and experience geared toward providing optimal quality services to the geriatric patient. The expertise that the emergency department (ED) staff can bring to an encounter with a geriatric patient has the opportunity to "set the stage" for the subsequent inpatient and outpatient care that is provided. More accurate diagnoses and improved treatments can not only expedite and improve care and outcomes, but also can guide resource allocation in a patient population that utilizes significantly more resources per event than younger populations.

The geriatric population constitutes a unique group of patients who seek emergency care. The medical, psychological, social, and ethical issues involved in their care are complex and challenging. A first step is identifying trends in geriatric emergency medicine and establishing standards of care in practice. Four of eleven proposed standards of care in geriatric practice have been proposed that pertain specifically to ethics: respect for decisional capacity and justice, effective end-of-life care, effective palliative care, and coordination with hospice care. As the number of older people increases worldwide, the role of the emergency physician and others involved in the care of the geriatric patient will depend on the ability to generate new standards of care as dictated by our better understanding of the scientific, social, and ethical aspects of care of older people. Recently, geriatric emergency medicine clinicians, educators, and researchers from the American College of Emergency Physicians (ACEP), the American Geriatrics Society, the Emergency Nurses Association, and the Society of Academic Emergency Medicine collaborated to develop geriatric ED guideline recommendations that represent best evidence and best practice-based research and consensus. Finally, patient assessments are complicated, and this can be minimized through professional competence to acquire the knowledge and skill sets to meet the health care needs of older adults and through comprehensive assessments by use of specialized multidisciplinary providers. This chapter identifies some of the special ethical concerns that arise in the care of the geriatric emergency patient and provides a framework for recognition, analysis, and resolution, with the ultimate goal of improving the care of the geriatric patient in the ED.

DETERMINATION OF DECISION-MAKING CAPACITY AND GOALS OF CARE

As noted, one of the standards of geriatric practice is respect for decisional capacity and justice. The physician should understand the basics of autonomy and decisional capacity and be familiar with the documents that can be executed to protect patient autonomy when decisional capacity is no longer present. Determining decision-making capacity is a critical step in the care of geriatric patients, and, the majority of times, this is done without difficulty. Capacity is the ability to receive and understand information and make choices based on this information. When dementia, delirium, medications, substance abuse, mental illness, and social issues arise in the geriatric patient, this determination may become more difficult. Different from legally determined competency, decision-making capacity may vary over time depending on the current state of the patient and the complexity of the situation and decision that needs to be made. It is important to limit determination of a patient's decisional capacity to a specific instance, and it is possible that patients can make decisions in one specific area even when capacity for decision-making is absent in others. A patient's decisional capacity can vary even during a brief period of time – even from hour to hour – and a decision for a medical procedure during one time should carry force during later periods in the stay when the patient may not have decisional capacity. Although patient choices are influenced by a multitude of factors, it is important to ensure that the patient has the ability to communicate his or her choice voluntarily and free from coercion. If possible, reversible causes of impaired capacity should be treated to determine if a patient may be able to participate in decision-making. Tests such as Mini-Mental Status Examination and Quick Confusion Scale can be used to standardize the process used to determine capacity. If refusal of care occurs, it is important to understand the reasons of refusal to know if any misperceptions or misinformation exists and to facilitate development of alternative treatment options. If patients can communicate alternatives and consequences of treatment or refusal of treatment, this generally suggests that decision-making capacity exists. Finally, documentation of the elements of capacity or its impairment in the medical record is crucial, especially when an intervention or lack of intervention carries significant risk. In emergency situations, implied consent is accepted practice. The emergency physician must treat the patient who has impaired capacity. When time allows, and the emergency physician determines capacity is impaired, a surrogate decision-maker should be identified. Patients have several ways to ensure their wishes are honored after they have lost decisional capacity, and physicians need to be knowledgeable about these legal documents. The *durable power of attorney for health care* and the *living will* are two written directives that carry the force of law even when the patient loses decision-making capacity. If written expressions are not available, the physician must rely on qualified surrogate decision-makers. Where the patient has identified a surrogate, consent should involve that individual. When a surrogate has not been pre-identified by the patient, most states have a next-of-kin order of decision-makers. If neither written instruments nor surrogate decision-makers are available, physicians alone or with consultation with an ethics consultation team will have to take on this responsibility, and, in rare circumstances, decision-making by courts may be necessary.

Another critical decision point in the care of any patient is the recognition of the patient's goals for treatment. The geriatric patient is different from the younger patient in that the usual imperative of maximal intervention in time of medical need may not be acceptable. Aggressive or painful treatments in order to prolong life and not necessarily to improve quality of life may not be acceptable to the patient. Some geriatric patients may desire aggressive interventions, and it is important that the provider not wrongly assume that all elderly patients wish to limit interventions. At the same time, patients may choose not to limit interventions because of fear that they will be refused treatment completely. The unique challenges of caring for the geriatric patient in the ED are complicated by the limited opportunity to establish a doctor–patient relationship; unfamiliarity with patient's values, beliefs, and wishes regarding resuscitation; little knowledge of the patient's medical history; and a need for rapid treatment. Compounding this dilemma is determining the goals of care when time is critical and adequate information is unavailable in an elderly individual with complex medical and psychosocial needs; in these situations, a carefully predetermined approach to ethical issues is invaluable to guiding what is "right and good ... here and now."

A number of ethical issues are relevant to geriatric emergency medicine. Basic ethical principles such as beneficence, nonmaleficence, autonomy, paternalism, use of family and other surrogates, and justice provide consistent guidelines that can be used in the ethical analysis and medical care of the geriatric emergency patient. The principle of beneficence is a physician's obligation to do what's best for a patient's needs. Particularly in the geriatric patient, the goal is to optimize health and function, to limit pain and disability, and to minimize patient losses rather than to maximize longevity at any cost. The principle of nonmaleficence refers to causing no harm to patients. In the geriatric patient, determining the specific goals of care for each individual, especially ones that promote quality of life over prolonging death, is important in achieving this principle. The principle of autonomy recognizes the patient's right to have treatment guided by the patient's beliefs or personal values, with decisions made freely based on adequate understanding of the medical circumstances and informed by recognition of the potential outcomes. Competence does not decide autonomy, so careful consideration needs to be taken when assessing autonomy, particularly in the geriatric patient. Some individuals are not competent to care for themselves or make financial decisions, yet they are autonomous enough to make decisions about aggressive medical interventions like intubation and resuscitation. In contrast, a fully competent individual may have impaired physical or communication abilities and may not be able to express autonomous decisions. For example, a wheelchair-bound patient can retain the power to have someone to carry out his wishes, especially in the setting of modern communication technology. This scenario may have the appearance of dependency and being in a wheelchair can be interpreted as loss of autonomy and lead to unethical behavior. Finally, even when a patient is

competent and able to communicate clearly, it is not uncommon for a
family member or a physician to override a patient's expressed wishes
because the individual is uncomfortable with the patient's decision. This
leads in to the principle of *paternalism*, which is beneficence unguided by
respect for individual autonomy. The practice of the physician knowing
what is best for the patient is presently a much less generally accepted
perspective than it once was. Particularly in the context of geriatric care,
paternalism has been replaced with respect for the patient's perspective as
an individual. Family members play a central role in the care of the
geriatric patient, especially when they provide basic daily care and
make routine financial and life decisions. As the geriatric patient becomes
more dependent on family, the patient has given up some autonomy. In
situations in which the patient's autonomy is limited, the physician can
turn to the family who know the patient's beliefs and values to promote
the patient's best interests and decision-making. *Distributive justice* is a
principle that may create an ethical dilemma in families. Family members
often assume a large obligation in the care of an elderly patient, and
sometimes this places unreasonable demands on the family. An example
of distributive justice is the determination of whether there is an appropriate balance between the benefit to the elderly patient of remaining
home with the family or if unreasonable burdens are being placed on the
family. Differing from distributive justice, the principle of *justice* is the
fair allocation of resources and equitable distribution of resources in a
finite health care system. Justice embraces the good of society as well as
the patient. At the end of life, the family may wish to use high-technology
procedures that may only prolong the act of dying. The physician must
balance the benefit the patient may receive from the diagnostics or
procedures with the potential for more general societal harm because of
inappropriate use of limited medical resources. In an acute crisis, each
patient deserves the intervention that will result in the greatest benefit for
that individual. Limitation of care in the geriatric patient may be acceptable only if it reflects the patient's wishes, as expressed through prior
instructions or family judgment, or when the burdens or risks imposed
on the patient by the medical intervention outweigh the potential benefits. This type of issue often is the focus when families wish to keep a
patient in the late stages of dementia with multisystem failure on a
respirator in the intensive care unit. Repeated and lengthy conversations
with the family, best begun with the patient's first visit, are the best way to
resolve these issues. Consultation with an ethics committee is another
option.

PRACTICAL APPLICATIONS OF ETHICAL PRINCIPLES

Advance Directives, Living Wills, and Physician Orders for Life-Sustaining Treatment (POLST)

These are instruments that allow an individual to express autonomous decisions about the use of specified medical interventions at a future time. When no advance directives have been made known, the emergency physician must make a determination of aggressive interventions with the patient first. The withholding of life-prolonging medical intervention when the competent patient refuses it is not only ethically permissible but morally required. When the patient is unable to decide, the principle of "substituted judgment" emphasizes the role of family. A pitfall associated with the increased use of advance directives and other such instruments is the potential to assume that the elderly patient who presents to the ED in extremis without such a directive desires full aggressive resuscitative efforts be undertaken. Most patients without advance directives have definite opinions regarding resuscitation and welcome the opportunity to discuss their wishes. Although not emphasized in the education and training of the emergency physician, there are many cases where dying should be accepted as part of the process, and palliative care, communication, and counseling with the patient and family may be of greater benefit than specific medical treatments. A landmark study on POLST in Oregon published by the *Journal of the American Geriatric Society* demonstrated that patients who specified comfort measures only or limited additional interventions are significantly less likely to die in a hospital. Just as importantly, patients with POLST forms indicating full treatment are significantly more likely to die in the hospital when compared to individuals without a POLST form.

Futile Cardiopulmonary Resuscitation (CPR)

In general, patients who are highly functional with fewer comorbidities and are hospitalized for a cardiac etiology and a witnessed arrest are more likely to benefit from CPR, and age alone does not appear to be a significant determinant of survival. Providers must take into account issues of advance directives and medical futility when formulating clinical decisions. Physicians may define futile interventions as those that carry an absolute impossibility of successful outcome, a low likelihood of success, a low likelihood of survival, or a low likelihood of meaningful quality of life. A difficult situation arises when the family makes unrealistic demands for resuscitation or futile interventions in geriatric patients who are terminally injured or ill. Many ethicists agree that physicians are not obligated to provide treatments that will render little or no benefit to the patient. In circumstances where CPR offers no hope for meaningful recovery, the physician is not morally or legally required to apply a useless intervention. The American Medical Association (AMA) Council on Ethical and Judicial Affairs asserted that futile CPR may be withheld from patients even if patients or families insist on its performance. Furthermore, an ACEP policy asserts that "physicians are under no ethical obligation to render treatment that they judge have no realistic likelihood of medical benefit to the patient." Decisions to provide, limit, or withhold treatments should be made by the emergency physician using an approach that combines professional judgment, well-established evidence-based medicine, and patient and family wishes.

Continued Treatment of the Fatally Ill/Injured for the Benefit of Others

Although the physician's priority is to address the best interests of the patient, there is an ethical obligation to consider the interests of the family in determining continuation of treatment. Although not medically indicated, and economic factors need to be factored in, the treatment of a fatally ill patient for the benefit of a third party may be morally justifiable if no additional suffering of the patient is incurred.

Privacy and Confidentiality

Based on the ethical principle of respect for autonomy, privacy is a fundamental right to one's dignity and freedom of self-determination and underlies a patient's right to choose how much of his or her personal information may be communicated to others. Confidentiality is based on the right to privacy and sets limits on the patient information that health care providers can share with others. While caring for the geriatric patient, emergency physicians often come into contact with family members, caregivers, and other people who are directly involved in the lives of their patients. Additionally, evaluation and treatment services provided to older adults are often multidisciplinary, involving a number of health care providers, which may foster an exchange of important information that can promote the care and treatment of patients but also increase the potential for violations of patient privacy. The ethical problem here concerns the invasion of the older person's privacy and autonomy. Identification of family members and treating professionals who can have access to confidential patient information should be clarified as early as possible. Before clinicians consult collateral sources of information regarding patient history, patients may be better served if confidentiality issues can be discussed in private to determine patients' wishes that may otherwise be unduly influenced by family members or others. A common problem in geriatric practice is the question of the physician's accountability: is it to the patient or to the family? In general, the patient is the priority; however, in the geriatric patient, the environment is complex, and this often includes the family. Assessing the burden on the patient caused by the illness includes how it affects the family looking after him or her. If the harm to the family significantly outweighs any benefit that the patient receives, an alternative solution may be justified to give priority to the family's needs.

Informed Consent

Informed consent in the medical setting originated in a New York State Supreme Court case in 1914, which determined that "every human being of adult years and sound mind has the right to determine what shall be done with his own body and a surgeon who performs an operation without his patient's consent commits an assault." The exception that arises often in the ED is "in the event of an emergency requiring immediate actions for the preservation of the life or health of the patient under circumstances in which it is impossible or impractical to obtain the patient's consent or the consent of anyone authorized to assume such responsibility." The bioethical principle of respect for autonomy addresses the right of patients to be fully informed about a proposed service and the possible impact it may have on their lives. Respect for patient autonomy requires that emergency physicians value a competent patient's capacity for self-determination, including the patient's right to refuse services. The basics of informed consent require adequate disclosure of information and a patient able to understand clearly and make a decision voluntarily. The patient should be provided the opportunity to ask questions and express any concerns. The informed consent process should be tailored to meet the unique needs of the patient, as well as the setting in which the service is performed. In the setting of the ED, the challenges to fulfill the fundamentals of informed consent become exaggerated in the elderly patient – even in previously competent patients – due to the acute stress and pace of the emergency situation. Individuals with impaired cognitive functioning may not be able to fully comprehend the purpose of the examination of ramifications of their participation, but the emergency physician maintains a responsibility to inform these patients, to the extent possible, about the nature and purpose of the proposed services, identify questions and concerns they may have, and seek their assent. For patients who have been determined to be incompetent to make health care decisions, the surrogate decision-maker should be fully informed and offered this same opportunity to have questions or concerns addressed. The question of informed consent in research studies in the elderly patient, particularly in the incompetent or partially incompetent patient, is a more difficult ethical issue.

Ethical Aspects of Aging Research

The main issues for ethical evaluation in geriatric research include the recruitment of older subjects, obtaining informed consent from older participants, and use of genetic samples for future research. Although the older population is growing in developed countries, they are still underrepresented in health-related research due to several barriers that include poor health, social and cultural hesitations, and impaired decisional capacity to provide informed consent. For successful recruitment and retention of older individuals, studies that maximize benefit–burden ratios, whereby the individual has more to gain than to lose, increases participation. Evidence demonstrates that older subjects have limitations on their capability to provide informed consent based on impaired cognition, hearing, speech, and vision. Their inability to completely understand the implications of the research makes geriatric patients a vulnerable population that needs to have protections and additional safeguards in place. Therefore, strategies should be optimized to provide materials, forms, and procedures that incorporate these aspects into the informed consent process. Older subjects with memory problems may still be able to give consent, so this alone should not be an exclusion from research. Therefore, prior assessment of vision, hearing, and mental status of participants may need to be done, as well as an assessment of reading ability and understanding. In this manner, the informed consent model can be individualized to each geriatric subject to enhance participation. The methodology of capacity assessment is an ongoing subject area in geriatric research. Research on patients declared legally incompetent must show that the outcome has potential benefit to the patient and is subject to consent of the legal guardian. When research is conducted on Alzheimer's disease, consideration must be given to the impact of the research on the patient, as well as on the guardian.

Nursing Home Placement

Sometimes families are unable or unwilling to care for elders, and institutional care poses many ethical problems. There may be a disparity between the view of the geriatric patient and the caregivers charged with the care of the elderly. This contradicts the patient's autonomy and invokes paternalism if the patient was minimally or not at all involved with the decision to enter a facility. A geriatric team of providers can help evaluate the situation. If the assessment points to the desirability of the patient to continue to live in his or her own home, the solution may be provision of increased social services and support for the family. If, however, the decision points to institutional care, this should be discussed in detail with the patient and involve the patient as much as possible in the decision-making. This may include discussions of a choice of facility by allowing the patient to make visits to several institutions and have trial periods in them so that he or she has time to acclimatize to the change in living situation. If the patient is so demented or impaired that he or she is unable to participate in the decision and has been declared legally incompetent, the actual decision rests with the legal guardian who must balance the patient's interests with the implications for the family. A compromise may be a day center that is devoted to care of the elderly demented. The center has the advantage of creating a sense of purpose for the patient by use of social occupational activities, and it shares the burden of caregiving with the family who benefit from the break during the day.

Ethical Considerations in Suicidal Older People

People aged seventy-five and older commit suicide more than any other age bracket worldwide. Depression significantly increases the risk of suicide. This older age group is more likely to have experienced losses that burden them in the period of time before they commit suicide. Seventy percent of older people who commit suicide are thought to have had contact with a caregiver in the month prior to their death, meaning that signals of suicidality in this age group are going unnoticed (20 percent had contact with the caregiver on the day of suicide and 40 percent in the week prior to their death). When people lose the ability to lead an autonomous life, they see themselves as "burdens" and lose self-esteem. This loss of autonomy plays a role in the suicidal ideation of older people. Some are so strongly influenced by the ideal of individual autonomy to that they feel it is their "duty to die." This value of autonomy is closely related to dignity.

Older people associate autonomy and independence with the dignified retention of their mental and physical capacities. The risk of becoming incompetent and being subjected to the arbitrary acts of others is considered a major motivator of suicide before it is too late. Finally, the value of responsibility is another important motive for committing suicide. Many older people fear becoming a financial or emotional burden on their relatives more than they fear death itself. Care of the older patient should promote values of autonomy, dignity, and responsibility. Care that helps geriatric patient maintain themselves as individuals, keeps them connected, engages in activities that gives them responsibility and meaning, and maintains dignity are optimal. Although these issues aren't always the focus in the ED, these values should be remembered not only in the care of a suicidal older patient.

Pain Management in Geriatric Patients

Older patients with dementia are at high risk for underrecognition and undertreatment of pain. Several studies report that fewer than 25 percent of demented patients in pain receive analgesia. Elderly patients traditionally underreport pain, and it is often undertreated because older adults are more susceptible to the side effects of medications that are used to control pain. Undertreatment of pain is associated with poor outcomes including pressure ulcers, functional disability, falls, malnutrition, sleep disturbances, decreased socialization, depression, impaired immune function, agitated behavior, increased health care use and costs, increased morbidity, and increased mortality. Sedation from inappropriate use of pain medication may predispose to further decline. Appropriate pain management that is titrated to patient needs, that is multimodal and includes nonpharmacological treatments, and that is timely can improve outcomes. Self-report of pain using a validated pain scale is the most reliable indicator of pain and need for pain relief, and pain-assessment tools are available for patients who are not able to self-report. Based on practice guidelines from the American Geriatrics Society and American Medical Directors Association, one best-practice approach for assessing pain in the demented patient involves three steps: ASK if they have pain, LOOK for signs of pain, INVESTIGATE for recent behavioral changes that may be due to pain. Including pain assessment as a vital sign has been incorporated in many ED settings. Although challenged by the complexities of managing pain in older patients with chronic conditions and increased vulnerability to medications, alleviation of suffering and the right of elders to adequate assessment and treatment of pain, as promoted by the Joint Commission, is an ethical responsibility. Pain relief promotes beneficence and nonmaleficence; therefore, not treating pain is ethically indefensible.

Palliative and Hospice Care

In geriatric emergencies, the ability to define the terminal phase of life may be challenging. Effective end-of-life care, effective palliative care, and coordination of hospice care are three of the eleven standards of geriatric care that physicians should be skilled at or at least knowledgeable in when assisting patients and their families. This means helping patients choose the most beneficial or least harmful therapies, helping dying patients and their families cope with decisions to limit life-prolonging care, and supporting families in the grief process. If the physician waits until the patient is in extremis, he or she risks being able to support patient autonomy and risks losing the opportunity to involve the patient in decision-making. An important area of patient–physician communication is the discussion of resuscitation preferences. This is best addressed when taking into consideration the patient's values, goals, and beliefs rather than specifics about the technical procedures. When a patient chooses the option to "do everything," the physician can clarify if the goal is to "do everything to keep them feeling well and avoiding discomfort" versus "doing everything to keep them alive for as long as possible." Decisions should be reassessed as patient preferences change, especially in response to changes in their health status. The physician should be skilled in the control of advanced disease symptoms and in the use of palliative care specialists as appropriate. Many illnesses in geriatric medicine produce distressing symptoms such as pain, nausea, shortness of breath, anxiety, and insomnia, and, whenever possible, underlying causes should be diagnosed and treated. But when this is not possible, the symptoms should be managed by medications, nonpharmacologic therapies, and consultations. The goal of effective palliative care is to make sure the patient's wishes are being honored and that the best possible care is being provided. By providing palliative care interventions such as pain and symptom management, quality of life is improved, hospital lengths of stay and ED recidivisim is reduced, patient and family satisfaction is improved, and intensive care is less utilized. Unfortunately, geriatric patients often end up with a terminal illness, and it is important for the physician to refer patients early for hospice care as appropriate. Eventually, all geriatric patients die, and it is well-established that both patients and physicians avoid the topic of dying because it is uncomfortable. This delays important conversations that can deprive patients and families of the opportunity to plan for their care.

APPROACH TO ETHICAL CONFLICT

Ethical controversies at the end of life are common in the elderly. Identifying ways to promote ethical practice includes achieving a level of "ethical competence" and gaining knowledge of the resources that are available to guide ethical conduct. Professional experience, formal coursework, review of relevant professional literature, continuing education in professional ethics, and routine exchange of ideas and experiences among colleagues promotes ethical competence. At a minimum, professional competence for emergency physicians working with older adults requires a working knowledge of the evaluation of changes of normal aging on cognitive and psychological functioning, potential side effects of medications and other treatment options, needs of families and caregivers in the lives of the patient, and an evolving knowledge base of the current scientific, ethical, and legal standards in place. The comprehensive assessment of an older adult's cognitive, psychiatric, and behavioral symptoms is often best addressed through a multidisciplinary process that includes a variety of specialized health care providers. This may include the emergency physician, geriatric specialist, psychiatrist, neurologist, social worker, pharmacist, and other pertinent specialist, depending on the primary acute emergency problem.

Positive ethics challenges an emergency physician to be proactive and pursue the highest ethical potential and promotion of exemplary behavior in all aspects of his or her professional endeavors. Rather than meeting the minimum requirements of an ethics code, the emergency physician is encouraged to integrate his or her personal ideals with his or her professional life because this connection promotes the pursuit of the highest standards of ethical practice.

The guiding principle is determining what is best for the patient. Ideally, the patient should choose what is best for him- or herself. Ideally, the patient has decided ahead of time what he or she would want done in the event he or she is not able to make the decision. Unfortunately, it is often the case that prior discussion has not taken place. The emergency physician must then have an approach, one based on clear ethical guidelines, that can quickly and consistently be used. Foremost, the physician must respect the patient's autonomy and attempt to obtain informed consent, even when the patient is impaired. This often requires great efforts, but identification of the needs and wishes of the geriatric patient and his or her goals can help define resuscitation efforts. As the geriatric population grows, technology advances, and economic pressures mandate justification for costs, emergency physicians are held accountable for the just allocation of resources. Important in geriatric emergency care is appropriate application of technology and resources based on what is best for that individual's needs and a duty to protect from aggressive interventions that may lead to a predicted painful end.

When ethical dilemmas occur, a structured method of information collection and analysis can aid in clarifying the relevant issues and identifying a preferred course of action. Using a decision-making model can assist emergency physicians with documenting pertinent information that demonstrates appreciation of the problem and efforts to identify an appropriate course of action. The common steps in ethical decision-making models include identification of the problem, consideration of the significance of the context and the setting, determination of patient and family/caregiver assets and limitations, identification and use of ethical and legal resources to help clarify what should be done, consideration of personal beliefs and values, development of possible solutions to the problem, evaluation of alternatives and the potential consequences of each solution, implementation of the best course of action, and evaluation of the outcome and implementation of changes as needed to avoid such ethical challenges in the future.

ETHICS TAKEOUT TIPS

- In the ED, ethical challenges in the geriatric patient are common; the emergency physician must become familiar with these common ethical dilemmas.
- Consider medical indications, patient preferences, quality of life, and ethical principles in analyzing each case.
- Age is not a predictor of survival to hospital discharge after CPR.
- Respect patient autonomy, regardless of the age of the patient
- Assess the decisional capacity of all patients.
- Patients with impaired cognitive abilities may still have sufficient decision-making capacity.
- The level of decision-making capacity required may vary depending on the risks and benefits of the decision to be made.
- Effective communication with the patient, the family, and the patient's primary care physician can prevent many ethical dilemmas.

FOR FURTHER READING

Adams, J., & Wolfson, A. (1990). Ethical issues in geriatric emergency medicine. *Emergency Medicine Clinics of North America*, 5(2), 183–192.

Bandman, E. (1994). Tough calls: Making ethical decisions in the care of older patients. *Geriatrics*, 49(12), 1–9.

American College of Emergency Physicians; American Geriatrics Society; Emergency Nurses Association; Society for Academic Emergency Medicine; Geriatric Emergency Department Guidelines Task Force. (2014). Geriatric emergency department guidelines. *Annals of Emergency Medicine*, 63, e1–e25.

De Vries, M., & Leget, C. (2012). Ethical dilemmas in elderly cancer patients: A perspective from the Ethics of Care. *Clinical Geriatric Medicine*, 28, 93–104.

Fromme, E., Zive, D., Schmidt, T., Cook, J. N., & Tolle, S. W. (2014). Association between Physician Orders for Life-Sustaining Treatment for scope of treatment and in-hospital death in Oregon. *Journal of the American Geriatric Society*, 62, 1246–1251.

Gordon, M. (2002). Ethical challenges in end-of-life therapies in the elderly. *Drugs and Aging*, 19(5), 321–329.

Kahn, J., & Magauran, B. (2006). Trends in geriatric emergency medicine. *Emergency Medical Clinics of North American*, 24, 243–260.

Luchi, R., Gammack, J., Narcisse, V., III, & Storey, C., Jr., (2003). Standards of care in geriatric practice. *Annual Review of Medicine*, 54, 185–196.

Martin, T., & Bush, S. (2008). Ethical considerations in geriatric neuropsychology. *NeuroRehabilitation*, 23, 447–454.

Meldon, S., Ma, O., & Woolard, R. (2004). *Geriatric emergency medicine*. New York: McGraw-Hill.

Rosin, A., & Dijk, Y. (2005). Subtle ethical dilemmas in geriatric management and clinical research. *Journal of Medical Ethics*, 31, 355–359.

Seppet, E., Pääsuke, M., & Conte, M., Capri, M., & Franceschi, C. (2011). Ethical aspects of aging research. *Biogerontology*, 12, 491–502.

Snow, L., Rapp, M., & Kunik, M. (2005). Pain management in persons with dementia. *Geriatrics*, 60, 22–25.

Tanner, C., Fromme, E., & Goodlin, S. (2011). Ethics in the treatment of advanced heart failure: Palliative care and end-of-life issues. *Congestive Heart Failure*, 17, 235–240.

Vanlaere, L., Bouckaert, F., & Gastmans, C. (2007). Care for suicidal older people: Current clinical-ethical considerations. *Journal of Medical Ethics*, 33, 376–381.

22

Palliative Medicine

TAMMIE E. QUEST, MD

PALLIATIVE CARE DEFINITIONS AND DOMAINS

Palliative care is the physical, spiritual, psychological, and social support provided to patients and families suffering from a serious, life-threatening illness. The unit of care is the patient, family, and their caregivers. The focus is on optimization of quality of life, relief from the stress of a serious illness, and relief of physical, spiritual, and psychological suffering that can occur when one experiences a serious illness. Palliative care support can and should be provided at any stage of illness and can be provided congruently with any therapy. Palliative care is often confused with hospice care. *Hospice care* is the type of palliative care that is provided when the patient has a terminal illness with a limited life expectancy of six months or less if the disease runs its usual course. Hospice care is the form of palliative care elected under a formal program for patients with terminal illness. *Palliative care includes hospice care*, but palliative care can and is most often provided outside of hospice care. Core elements of palliative care include pain and symptom management, support in complex medical decision-making, assessment of the goals of care, spiritual support, and support in coordination of care. It is common that those who subspecialize medically in the field of hospice and palliative medicine maintain both a palliative care and hospice practice.

Palliative care can be provided by generalists, those who are functioning in the context of their own primary specialty, and by subspecialists, those who have advanced, subspecialty training in the discipline of hospice and palliative medicine. Emergency clinicians most often practice generalist palliative medicine. Core elements and domains of generalist emergency medicine care include assessment of serious illness trajectories, basic formulation of prognosis, difficult communications (breaking bad news/death disclosure), advance care planning, family presence during resuscitation, management of pain and nonpain symptoms, withdrawal/withholding of nonbeneficial treatments, care of the imminently dying, management of hospice patients/palliative care systems referrals, ethical and legal issues, spiritual/cultural competency, and management of the dying child.

Functional status during the serious illness trajectory is one of the most important factors to consider as one considers palliative care interventions. Lunney and Lynn have described four global trajectories of decline that illustrate functional status as a function of time. The four common global trajectories include sudden illness, cancer/terminal illness, solid organ failure, and frailty. Patients present with intercurrent illnesses on these trajectories that can look like heart failure exacerbation, infection, dehydration, trauma (e.g. fracture, intracranial hemorrhage), renal failure, or other clinical syndromes. The emergency clinician can train him- or herself to mentally picture where the patient is on a global illness trajectory based on the patient's best functional status in the days prior to emergency department (ED) presentation. Typically, as patients have functional declines, the burdens and stressors among caregivers rise, the prevalence of symptoms may increase, and the need increases to focus on the core aspects of palliative care assessment and interventions.

PALLIATIVE CARE DELIVERY IN THE ED

Patients with serious illness should have reliable access to quality palliative care. Depending on the resources of the ED, there may or may not be the ability to access subspecialty palliative care if needed, and the focus of palliative care will rest on the ED-based interdisciplinary team to assess and meet palliative care needs. Given the resource and time constraints in the ED, the emergency care team may only be able to focus on the most critical aspects of palliative care. A focused rapid assessment of palliative care for a seriously ill and unstable patient may include the following *ABCD assessment.* Is there an advance plan that we should be aware of? Does the patient has symptoms that can be made better? Does the patient have the capacity to make medical decisions. Is there a surrogate decision-maker? In more stable patients, one can explore other domains of palliative care as appropriate.

An increasing number of initiatives aim to improve palliative care provided to patients in the ED by emergency clinicians as well as by the palliative care consults that interact in the ED. Initiatives in the ED that are focused on palliative care often turn attention to patients who are at end of

TABLE 22.1. *Focused palliative care assessment*

Palliative care for serious ill and unstable patients:

ABCD assessment:
A: is there an **a**dvance plan that we should be aware of?
B: does the patient have symptoms that can be made **b**etter?
C: does the patient have the **c**apacity to make medical decisions?
D: is there a surrogate **d**ecision-maker?

TABLE 22.2. *Useful ED-specific palliative care processes and protocols*

Policies
- Ensuring adequate space for death disclosure policy
- Honoring physician or medical orders for life sustaining therapy (POSLT/MOSLT) or other advance care planning documents

Protocols
- Family presence during resuscitation and invasive procedure,
- Evaluation of patients currently receiving hospice care,
- Referral for hospice care from the ED
- Death of a child
- Care for the imminently dying
- Common palliative care symptom emergencies
  * cancer pain
  * sickle cell pain
  * care of the imminently dying (last hours of living)
  * ventilator withdrawal order set
  * hospice referral order sets

life, due to their high proportion of palliative care needs and the urgent nature of the discussion of deterioration and decline. It has been demonstrated that emergency clinicians can accurately recognize patients with serious life-threatening illness without the additional help of specialists by using trigger assessment tools that rapidly screen and assess activities of daily living, performance, functional staging, symptom burden, and caregiver distress. Early identification of palliative care needs with a plan to address them initially in the ED with follow-up after leaving the ED may lead to a more durable disposition plan.

There is increasing evidence that hospital-based subspecialty palliative care consultation in patients with serious illness leads to improved patient and caregiver reported quality of life, improved symptom control, decreased hospital length of stay, lower costs at end of life, and, in the case that death does occur, improved ratings of end-of-life experience. Hence, algorithms and protocols that can identify patients who might benefit from subspecialty palliative care referral from the ED may lead a better quality patient care experience.

Integrative palliative care models in the ED setting will be needed when the ED delivers primary palliative care to patients and families while looking to the palliative medicine service subspecialty (when available) to enhance the primary palliative care work of the ED. ED personnel should consider using all the ED, hospital-based, and community resources available to them to meet patient needs. In the ED, the use of case management and social work services to meet social and psychological support needs of the patient and the use of on-call or ED-based chaplain services to meet spiritual care needs will complement the primary focus of the ED's evaluating clinician – the patient's physical needs – in the context of globally coordinating care for a quality ED experience with a safe transition-of-care plan. *Consultative models* of palliative medicine in the ED include emergency physicians and nurses who are trained in subspecialty palliative medicine and who focus on consultation in the ED but more commonly rely on the subspecialty hospital-based palliative medicine service to provide subspecialty consultation. Subspecialty palliative medicine services often can provide consultation for patients in the ED, arrange for direct admission to dedicated hospice or palliative medicine bed assignments for focused care, and have the ability to follow patients post-ED discharge through special clinics or home-based palliative or hospice programs. Subspecialty palliative care scope, availability, and ability to respond to the needs of the ED are highly variable across the nation; the use of subspecialty palliative care requires deliberate discussions and planning regarding the integration of hospital-based palliative care consultation services and ED leadership to create a support plan for the ED.

Ensuring Understanding of the Intent of Therapy

An assessment of the understanding of the intent of therapies can provide information to the care team that will become important in decision-making. Fundamental to palliative care and informed consent, patients have the right to know what their condition is, what treatments are available, and the risks, benefits, and burdens of these treatments. Despite being informed, many patients and surrogates may not hear or retain information regarding their diagnosis, prognosis, and the intent of their treatments. Of 1,193 patients who were diagnosed with stage IV lung or colorectal cancer and received chemotherapy, only 31 percent and 19 percent of late-stage lung and colorectal cancer patients, respectively, understood that their chemotherapy was not curative. In patients with advanced dementia, many caregivers are surprised that the illness is irreversible and struggle to understand the associated trajectory of decline. Patients with advanced heart failure may struggle to understand the progressive nature of their disease, with the progressive effectiveness of vasoactive support and intracardiac mechanical devices (e.g. left ventricular assist devices) to relieve symptoms and increase quality of life often by several years.

Because of the complexities of these interventions and the repeated need to educate patients and families regarding their disease process, emergency clinicians should routinely assess patient and family understanding of the intent of any therapies they are receiving. The emergency clinician can sensitively, but effectively, provide information to patients and families regarding the nature of their illness and the general intent of a therapy. Patients often need to hear information from multiple providers and in multiple settings to fully understand its import.

HOSPICE CARE AND THE ED

Hospice care is the most intense form of palliative care provided to patients in the setting of terminal illness. In the United States, hospice care is the system of care designed to care for terminally ill patients who have a limited prognosis of six months or less if the disease runs its usual course; patients may have any diagnosis. It is common for the emergency clinician to encounter patients who either are receiving hospice care or who might benefit from hospice care, and ethical dilemmas typically arise in the care of these patients when clinicians must decide how to best support and care for patients in this system of care.

A comprehensive understanding of hospice as a care system can support the clinician's knowledge base and give him or her a solid foundation from which to work. Patients are eligible for hospice care based on two key principles: (1) limited prognosis and (2) goals of care consistent with comfort care. Currently, 35 percent of patients receive less than seven days of hospice care, and only 8.8 percent of patients receive between 90–179 days in hospice care. Hospice care represents high-intensity palliative care focused at the end of life. Patients without a limited prognosis, as defined by the Medicare Hospice Benefit (MHB), are not eligible for hospice care. Hospice care in the United States is regulated by Centers for Medicare and Medicaid Services (CMS), and, even when financed by commercial payers, the structure and process of hospice care remains the same, although per diem reimbursement may vary between federal and commercial payers.

The Medicare Hospice Benefit

The MHB was introduced in 1983 and its use follows specific federal guidelines. Hospices are paid in a per diem fashion for each day of service that the patient receives care after agreeing to hospice care; the amount received depends on the level of hospice care the patient receives. To elect the hospice benefit under Medicare, the patient (beneficiary) must be eligible for Medicare Part A. Hospice care must be provided by a structured interdisciplinary team (IDT), and the hospice services provided by the IDT must be guided by a specific plan of care (POC). The MHB consists of two ninety-day benefit periods followed by an unlimited number of sixty-day benefit periods. A beneficiary must be recertified that he or she is terminally ill at the start of each benefit period. Prior to the third benefit period, the patient must have a face-to-face visit with a hospice-employed physician or advanced practice nurse. The IDT must include a physician, registered nurse (often termed *hospice care manager*), chaplain, and social worker. Additional team members can include volunteers and therapists.

Hospice Levels of Care

Emergency clinicians should be familiar with the levels of hospice services that can be provided to a beneficiary. Hospices provide four levels of care: *routine care* (typically, patients receiving care at home or in a skilled nursing or assisted-living facility), *general inpatient care* (for a patient in need of acute symptom control or with a condition that cannot be managed at home after interventions have been tried; this care can be delivered for a time-limited episode but is not meant to be residential or custodial in nature); *continuous care* (provided in the home or resident facility for a patient in crisis to maintain the beneficiary in place), and *respite care* (meant to give a break or respite for the patient's primary home caregivers). For continuous care, 50 percent of the total time of care must be provided by a nurse (RN, LPN, or LVN); hence, this is often limited in availability and depends on available hospice staffing. Finally, respite care is available for the beneficiary who lives outside a skilled nursing facility and is provided as a support to the patient's family or caregiver who need temporary relief from caregiving or who will not be able to provide care for the patient for a short period of time (e.g. the caregiver needs to go out of town for several nights). Respite care is covered for no more than five days per benefit period.

FORMAL ELECTION OF HOSPICE CARE BENEFITS: THE INFORMED CONSENT PROCESS

Patients and their surrogates may present for ED care stating that they did not understand that hospice care was care for terminal illness with palliative intent. Although there may have been confusion or lack of understanding in the consent process, by CMS guidelines, for a patient to receive hospice care, he or she must formally elect such care by signing a consent form. CMS guidelines require that a patient or his or her representative consent to the following four core elements: (1) that a specific hospice will care for the patient, (2) acknowledgement that the patient fully understands that treatments are palliative and not curative, (3) a specific start date of services, and (4) signature of the patient or his or her representative. Once hospice care is elected, the hospice agency develops a POC for the beneficiary, and the hospice IDT is then responsible for instituting this POC. The hospice POC must be detailed and specify the frequency and scope of the services provided, and it should be updated as the patient's condition changes. ED visits are either considered within or outside the patient's POC. If the hospice agency is unaware of the ED visit, the ED visit will be outside of the patient's POC. However, if the hospice agency sends the patient to the ED for care, the ED visit may in fact be a part of the patient's POC (e.g. the patient falls, sustains a laceration, and needs sutures; the hospice sends the patient to the ED for sutures). The hospice is financially liable for services that are within the hospice POC, even if they extend to the ED or hospitalized setting.

Life-Extending Therapies and Hospice

Patients (or their designated representative if the patient lacks capacity) may revoke hospice care to seek life-extending therapies. Very often, the intent of revoking hospice services is the desire to seek reassurance that the choice a comfort care plan is in fact the right one. Patients or their surrogates may need to be reassured regarding a patient's condition, reassured that the hospice is properly caring for the patient, and reassured that electing a comfort care course that focuses on symptoms and not the underlying disease does not constitute neglect, torture, starvation, or mistreatment of their loved one.

It is not uncommon that, as a patient receiving hospice care declines as expected on one of the four illness trajectories, the stress of the illness increases. Patients and families often struggle with the question of whether there is more that can be done for the patient's condition. As a patient declines and approaches the end of life, he or she will typically experience decreased appetite, which leads to decreased oral intake, dehydration, and, in its terminality, renal dysfunction and vascular instability manifested by hypotension and tachycardia. Commonly, the patient will experience infection in the course of decline, and, at its culmination, sepsis. It is a common for ED personnel to feel ethical tension when a patient who has consented to hospice care presents to the ED for evaluation. The role of the emergency clinician is to educate, guide, and support a care plan in the best interest of the patient. Sometimes this will lead to a revocation of hospice care for pursuit of life-sustaining therapies, but, most often, the ability to educate the patient and/or their loved ones about the "normal" decline on an end-of-life trajectory is important. The ability to explain that, as the body weakens, normal dying includes the loss of appetite, the inability and lack of desire to take in fluids or nutrition, and often infection can help caregivers understand that the hospice agency is not medically neglecting their loved one but allowing a natural process to occur.

Request for Interventions or Therapies Not Covered by the Hospice

The hospice agency determines the POC, medications, and therapies that will support comfort care, and these are covered within the MHB; those that do not support comfort care are not covered. Many hospice agencies define therapies for comfort as those with which the patient can experience and report tangible relief of a symptom. Common dilemmas include request by patients or providers' for palliative-intent cancer-directed therapy that does not deliver direct symptom relief and may, in fact, induce symptoms.

Common Crossroad: Infection, Dehydration, Altered Mental Status

The decision to treat intercurrent illness – typically infection and dehydration – in a patient who is nearing the end of life should be guided by the assessment of the goals of care. Patients receiving hospice care who have good functional status and are experiencing symptoms that can be helped or relieved by an intervention that would lead to weeks or months of comfort should not be grouped categorically with patients near the end of life in whom the intervention might only provide benefit for hours or days at high cost to the patient's quality of life and deviates from expressed goals. Many interventions may temporize the active dying process but not reverse it. In some cases, those interventions required to temporize are of high burden (e.g. placement of central venous catheter in sepsis) and, although of some benefit, might extend the patient's life for only hours or days and may require a hospital admission. In advanced dementia, it has been shown that antibiotics extend life but do not enhance comfort. The administration of artificial nutrition and hydration in patients very close to the end of life has not been shown to be beneficial. In patients in the last hours or days of life, education regarding the help or harm of these interventions should be discussed (see Chapter 23, End of Life Care).

THE REFERRAL OF A NEW PATIENT TO HOSPICE CARE FROM THE ED

The Challenge of Prognosis Certification for Hospice Care

The emergency clinician may find it difficult to establish patient eligibility for hospice care. To be eligible, two physicians must certify that the patient appears to have a prognosis of six months or less if the disease runs its usual course. The emergency physician can serve as one certifying physician for hospice care, with the patient's attending or the hospice agencies' hospice medical director serving as the other. Patients, particularly those with noncancer diagnoses, can challenge physicians in determining medical eligibility for hospice care. In general, evidence shows that physicians can be both overly optimistic as well as overly pessimistic in their prognostication. Once the prognosis is formulated, it may be contested by patients, families, and surrogates for a variety of reasons, including the desire not to "destroy hope" or the fear that the care team is "giving up." A number of resources are available to estimate prognosis in a patient, and a discussion with the patient's managing clinician can often produce the information needed to make an informed decision.

For hospice patients receiving dialysis for end-stage renal disease (ESRD) under Medicare, the emergency physician should be aware that these patients can elect hospice care and continue to receive dialysis as long as the ESRD is not related to the patient's terminal disease. For example, if a patient has ESRD and is diagnosed with terminal lung cancer with limited prognosis, he or she may elect hospice care for the terminal lung cancer but continue dialysis. If the dialysis would prolong life longer than six months, the beneficiary would not be prognostically eligible unless he or she stopped dialysis.

One the emergency clinician believes that a patient has a prognosis of six months or less, an assessment of goals of care should occur. What are the patient and family goals in the context of terminal illness with limited prognosis? If the goals of care are consistent with a focus on quality of life, symptom control, and care focused typically outside the hospital, then it might be appropriate to initiate a hospice discussion. It is imperative that the emergency clinician contact the clinician or clinical group that has been primarily caring for the patient to gain clinical consensus regarding a hospice recommendation. The patient's primary treating clinician will need to be involved in determining the hospice POC, which often involves decisions regarding modifying the treatment plan to focus on comfort care goals. Often, patients and their caregivers can more readily accept the recommendations of the emergency clinician when they know that their primary clinician also supports the plan of hospice care. Once agreement has been reached regarding the medical consensus and recommended hospice care, the emergency clinician should approach the patient and his or her caregivers with a potential plan to initiate hospice care. Patients or their families may often fear negative experiences with hospice care or equate hospice care with imminent death; some patients with longer prognoses may have trouble picturing hospice care as a good option. Clinicians can reassure patients and surrogates that evidence shows that those who receive earlier hospice care report better symptom control and, in some conditions, improved quality of life.

COMMON DILEMMAS IN PALLIATIVE CARE DELIVERY IN THE ED

Strained Resources and Support

Although showing improvement in the past decades, barriers to palliative care delivery in the ED continue. With changes in health care, patients who visit EDs will do so with more advanced and serious illness. As programs are developed to focus on decreasing ED visits and hospitalizations, those with serious illnesses who do present in the ED are expected to have more complex disorders than in previous decades and require more complex therapies. It is projected that the number of new cancer cases in the United

States will increase by 42 percent by 2025. During that same period, the number of oncologists will increase by only 28 percent, which will lead to a projected shortage of 1,487 oncologists. The emergency clinician will find a changing landscape of younger and older individuals who will survive multiple serious illnesses to eventually succumb. The subspecialty of hospice and palliative medicine is experiencing a workforce shortage that predicts that subspecialty palliative medicine support will not be available to all who need it.

Discomfort with Palliative Care in the ED Team

For the ED interdisciplinary team to function at its most effective level, all members of the team need to have some knowledge, training, and skills in aspects of ED palliative care. (16) Although training in palliative care usually focuses on ED physicians, nurses, and associate providers (nurse practitioners or physician assistants), technicians/assistants, respiratory therapists, administrative clerks, social workers, case managers, chaplains, and volunteers also should receive some aspect of training in hospice and palliative care. All members of the team should be familiar with the core elements of palliative care, how palliative care differs from and is inclusive of hospice care in terminally ill patients with limited prognosis, and what procedures and protocols are in place to care for patients. Clinical care providers responsible for the direct assessment and management of patients need a higher level of focus and training in specific areas. That said, a successful hospice and palliative care initiative in the ED cannot be fully successful without participation on some level by all members of the ED interdisciplinary team. (17)

Institution of ED Procedures, Protocols, and Clinical Orders

With an increasing number of seriously, chronically ill patients in the ED, the ED clinician may become accustomed to evaluating patients with unmet palliative care needs with few resources, processes, or systems in place to support these patients. (18, 19) Similar to other issues that emergency clinician's face with high prevalence in the ED, the processes and protocols that best support meeting unmet needs are important. Common processes and protocols that the ED should consider instituting include (1) ensuring adequate space for death disclosure, (2) a protocol for family presence during resuscitation and invasive procedures, (3) a protocol for evaluating patients currently receiving hospice care, (4) a protocol for patients who need a recommendation of hospice care from the ED, (5) a protocol for handling

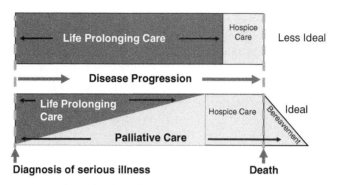

FIGURE 22.1. Interface of Life Prolonging Care and Palliative Care. (Reprinted with permission).

the death of a child, (6) a protocol for care for the imminently dying, and (7) a policy for honoring physician or medical orders for life-sustaining therapy (POSLT/MOSLT) or other advance care planning documents. Common palliative care symptom emergencies and clinical scenarios that would require specific clinical order sets in the ED include cancer pain, sickle cell pain, care of the imminently dying (last hours of life), a ventilator withdrawal order set, and hospice referral order sets. In all these, the ED can consider concomitant observation unit protocols in selected patients.

Integration of Pre-hospital Emergency Care

Emergency clinicians who have oversight of their local pre-hospital care system should ensure that adequate pre-hospital palliative care protocols are in place. In the case of pre-hospital disaster planning, it is important to ensure that special palliative care protocols are in place that support an ethical and empathic response to the needs of the seriously ill or injured who are at significant risk for death.

ETHICS TAKEOUT TIPS

- Palliative care and hospice are often confused and can lead to under-use of either service.
- Palliative care is the physical, spiritual, psychological, and social support given from diagnosis to death or cure of a life-threatening illness; it can be provided at any stage of illness
- Hospice care is a type of palliative care that can be provided under Medicare or other insurers when the patient has a terminal illness with a prognosis of six months or less if the disease runs its usual course.

- Hospice care requires informed consent.
- Early palliative care interventions initiated from the ED can add value to patient care.
- Clinicians can educate patients and families regarding illness trajectory irrespective of the prognosis.

FOR FURTHER READING

Beynon, T., Gomes, B., Murtagh, F. E., Glucksman, E., Parfitt, A., Burman, R., . . . Higginson, I. J. (2011). How common are palliative care needs among older people who die in the emergency department? *BMJ Supportive & Palliative Care*, 1(2), 184–188. PubMed PMID: 24653232.

National Consensus Project for Quality Palliative Care. (2013). *Clinical practice guidelines for quality palliative care* (3rd ed.). Pittsburgh, PA: HPNA.

Finlay, E., & Casarett, D. (2009). Making difficult discussions easier: Using prognosis to facilitate transitions to hospice. *CA: A Cancer Journal for Clinicians*, 59(4), 250–263. PubMed PMID: 19535791.

Glajchen, M., Lawson, R., Homel, P., Desandre, P., & Todd, K. H. (2011). A rapid two-stage screening protocol for palliative care in the emergency department: A quality improvement initiative. *Journal of Pain and Symptom Management*, 42(5), 657–662. PubMed PMID: 22045368.

Goodlin, S. J. (2009). Palliative care in congestive heart failure. *Journal of the American College of Cardiology*, 54(5), 386–396. PubMed PMID: 19628112.

Grudzen, C. R., Richardson, L. D., Hopper, S. S., Ortiz, J. M., Whang, C., & Morrison, R. S. (2012). Does palliative care have a future in the emergency department? Discussions with attending emergency physicians. *Journal of Pain and Symptom Management*, 43(1), 1–9. PubMed PMID: 21802899.

Grudzen, C. R., Richardson, L. D., Major-Monfried, H., Kandarian, B., Ortiz, J. M., & Morrison, R. S. (2013). Hospital administrators' views on barriers and opportunities to delivering palliative care in the emergency department. *Annals of Emergency Medicine*, 61(6), 654–660. PubMed PMID: 22771203.

Lamba, S., DeSandre, P. L., Todd, K. H., Bryant, E. N., Chan, G. K., Grudzen, C. R., . . . Quest, T. E. (2014). Integration of palliative care into emergency medicine: The Improving Palliative Care in Emergency Medicine (IPAL-EM) collaboration. *Journal of Emergency Medicine*, 46(2), 264–270. PubMed PMID: 24286714.

Lamba, S., Nagurka, R., Walther, S., & Murphy, P. (2012). Emergency-department-initiated palliative care consults: A descriptive analysis. *Journal of Palliative Medicine*, 15(6), 633–636. PubMed PMID: 22519573.

Lamba, S., Quest, T. E., & Weissman, D. E. (2011). Initiating a hospice referral from the emergency department #247. *Journal of Palliative Medicine*, 14(12), 1346–1347. PubMed PMID: 22145896.

Lunney, J. R., & Lynn, J. (2010). Trajectories of disability in the last year of life. *New England Journal of Medicine*, 363(3), 294; author reply 5. PubMed PMID: 20647207.

Lupu, D., & American Academy of Hospice and Palliative Medicine Workforce Task Force. (2010). Estimate of current hospice and palliative medicine physician workforce shortage. *Journal of Pain and Symptom Management,* 40(6), 899–911. PubMed PMID: 21145468.

Mahony, S. O., Blank, A., Simpson, J., Persaud, J., Huvane, B., McAllen, S., ... Selwyn, P. (2008). Preliminary report of a palliative care and case management project in an emergency department for chronically ill elderly patients. *Journal of Urban Health,* 85(3), 443–451. PubMed PMID: 18363108. Pubmed Central PMCID: 2329741.

Quest, T. E., Marco, C. A., & Derse, A. R. (2009). Hospice and palliative medicine: New subspecialty, new opportunities. *Annals of Emergency Medicine,* 54(1), 94–102. PubMed PMID: 19185393.

Smith, A. K., Fisher, J., Schonberg, M. A., Pallin, D. J., Block, S. D., Forrow, L., ... McCarthy, E. P. (2009). Am I doing the right thing? Provider perspectives on improving palliative care in the emergency department. *Annals of Emergency Medicine,* 54(1), 86–93, e1. PubMed PMID: 18930337.

Tanner, C. E., Fromme, E. K., & Goodlin, S. J. (2011). Ethics in the treatment of advanced heart failure: Palliative care and end-of-life issues. *Congestive Heart Failure,* 17(5), 235–240. PubMed PMID: 21906248.

van der Steen, J. T., Onwuteaka-Philipsen, B. D., Knol, D. L., Ribbe, M. W., & Deliens, L. (2013). Caregivers' understanding of dementia predicts patients' comfort at death: A prospective observational study. *BMC Medicine,* 11, 105. PubMed PMID: 23577637. Pubmed Central PMCID: 3648449.

Weeks, J. C., Catalano, P. J., Cronin, A., Finkelman, M. D., Mack, J. W., Keating, N. L., & Schrag, D. (2012). Patients' expectations about effects of chemotherapy for advanced cancer. *New England Journal of Medicine,* 367 (17), 1616–1625. PubMed PMID: 23094723. Pubmed Central PMCID: 3613151.

Weissman, D. E., & Meier, D. E. (2011). Identifying patients in need of a palliative care assessment in the hospital setting: A consensus report from the Center to Advance Palliative Care. *Journal of Palliative Medicine,* 14(1), 17–23. PubMed PMID: 21133809.

23

End-of-Life Care

MONICA WILLIAMS-MURPHY, MD

Patients may arrive to the emergency department (ED) dead, dying, or near the end of life. Emergency medicine is a unique profession in which we, the care providers, are essentially strangers to these patients and their families, but yet we very quickly must develop rapport and even intimacy to properly manage one of life's most important events – death. Although emergency physicians are adept at managing complex patients, the skill sets needed for management of end-of-life trajectories are largely interpersonal. Furthermore, these center around communication, respect for autonomy (the patient/surrogate's right to choose or refuse medical therapies offered), and beneficence. Complicated emotions arise for patients and families, as well as for ED staff members, when dealing with the end of life. Great care should be taken to create an atmosphere of open communication, respect, and dignity for all parties. The emergency physician is the team leader for this charge.

THE DEAD PATIENT

When the patient arrives dead to the ED, it is the family who becomes the focus of care, and death disclosure may be the foremost work performed. All emergency physicians should become skillful in death notification. Expert and compassionate death notification is an act of beneficence. What the family and friends hear from the clinician regarding the death of their loved one will become part of the oral history of the patient's life and will be shared throughout their community. As such, emergency physicians should be trained to "tell death" in a way that adds grace and dignity to the extent possible. The GRIEV_ING mnemonic provides a framework for mastery of this conversation.

- Gather: Gather the family; ensure that all members are present.
- Resources: Call for support resources available to assist the family with their grief (i.e. chaplain services, ministers, family, and friends).
- Identify: Identify yourself, identify the deceased or injured patient by name, and identify the state of knowledge of the family relative to the events of the day.
- Educate: Briefly educate the family as to the events that have occurred in the ED, educate them about the current state of their loved one.
- Verify: Verify that their family member has died. Be clear! Use the word "dead" or "died."
- __ Space: Give the family personal space and time for an emotional moment; allow the family time to absorb information.
- Inquire: Ask if there are any questions, and answer them all.
- Nuts and bolts: Inquire about organ donation, funeral services, and personal belongings. Offer the family the opportunity to view the body.
- Give: Give them your card and contact information. Offer to answer any questions that may arise later. Always return their call.

(Hobgood, C., Tamayo-Sarver, J., Hollar, D., & Sawning, S. (2009). GRIEV_ING: Death notification skills and applications for fourth-year medical students. *Teaching and Learning Medicine, 21,* 207–219)

Note that the family's knowledge of the event is elicited and clarified before any details are shared by the clinician. Additionally, as in all forms of communication with the lay population, care should be taken to avoid medical jargon and to use common terminology.

THE PATIENT WHO IS NEAR THE END OF LIFE

When the patient arrives with vital signs but is at high risk for dying or is simply on an end-of-life trajectory, a whole complex of communication goals must be efficiently accomplished to appropriately honor patient autonomy. First, however, the clinician should focus on assessing and addressing the patient's pain or symptom control needs. As a general rule, symptom management should take priority and occur (if the patient is stable enough) before conversations regarding goals of care and decision-making. Other texts are devoted to outlining the treatment of nausea, dyspnea, anxiety, pain, and the like, and specifics will not be detailed here.

After addressing symptomatic care, the emergency physician must next determine the patient's desires for medical treatments in the context of where the patient is located within a trajectory of illness or end-of-life. The

Patient Self-Determination Act of 1991 legally granted patients or surrogates the right to choose or refuse any medical procedure offered to them, including medical interventions that might be viewed as life-saving or time-extending. Thus, ethical and legal autonomy forms the basis for informed consent and advance directives. Given this foundation, it the clinician's duty to establish informed consent and to interpret or create health care directives with the patient or surrogate prior to pursuing a course of medical intervention.

Initially, in supporting patient autonomy in end-of-life decisions, three questions must quickly be answered in the ED setting:

1. Does the patient have decision-making capacity?
2. Is there a health care surrogate available?
3. Is there an advance directive or advance care plan available?

DOES THE PATIENT HAVE DECISION-MAKING CAPACITY?

If the patient arrives conscious to the ED, the clinician must quickly establish whether or not the patient has decision-making capacity. The CURVES mnemonic is a tool for determining capacity in the acute care setting:

- *Choose and Communicate*: Can the patient communicate a choice?
- *Understand*: Does the patient understand the risks, benefits, alternatives, and consequences of the decision?
- *Reason*: Is the patient able to reason and provide logical explanations for the decision?
- *Value*: Is the decision in accordance with the patient's value system?

If the answer to all of these is "yes," then the patient has decisional capacity. If the answer to any of these is "no," then one of the alternative pathways should be selected:

- *Emergency*: Is there a serious and imminent risk to the patient's wellbeing? In the absence of a surrogate decision-maker or directives otherwise, emergency interventions may be performed.
- *Surrogate*: Is there a surrogate decision-maker available? In the absence of directives otherwise, and time permitting, discussion should occur with the surrogate decision-maker before proceeding with medical interventions.

(Chow, C., Czarny, M., Hughest, M., & Carrese, J. (2010) CURVES: A mnemonic for determining medical decision-making capacity and providing emergency treatment in the acute setting. *Chest, 137,* 417–421.)

A patient with decision-making capacity may want to speak with the clinician privately, with family members/caregivers/surrogates present, or may even want the clinician to speak to the family or surrogate only. Many families and cultures prefer shared decision-making or even paternalistic decision-making (by the family "leader") over autonomous patient decision-making. Care should be taken by the clinician to be aware of how to manage differing belief systems in order to optimize relationships and medical care.

If the patient arrives unconscious to the ED, or it is clear that no decisional capacity exists according the CURVES mnemonic, then, as clinicians, it is our duty to seek out a surrogate decision-maker or advance directive to determine next steps. However, if the patient is unstable, and no surrogate or advance directive is available, it is our legal and ethical obligation to attempt all resuscitative measures until such information becomes available. One such common scenario is when a patient arrives in cardiac arrest or is already in the department and arrests unexpectedly with no advance directive or surrogate available: in the absence of direction otherwise, the emergency physician should perform resuscitative or life-prolonging therapies (CPR, intubation, defibrillation, etc.) until further information can be obtained. Recently, arguments have been advanced that aggressive interventions should not be the system default in all scenarios, such as cardiac arrest in the setting of end-stage organ disease. Institutional and organizational policies would need to be in place to support such changes in practice.

IS THERE A HEALTH CARE SURROGATE AVAILABLE?

Officially, a health care surrogate takes on the role of health care decision-maker only when the patient is incapacitated under the conditions stated in an advance directive. (Many state living wills only recognize a health care surrogate under conditions of a terminal or vegetative state leading to the patient's loss of capacity.) Other legal documents (e.g. a grant of guardianship or power of attorney for health care) may expand the surrogate's role to other scenarios as stipulated by the document itself. Furthermore, in theory, health care surrogates should have proper identification correlating with legal paperwork before discussions and decisions proceed. On another note, certain advance directives state whether or not the health care surrogate is granted permission to make decisions beyond the scope of what is documented in the directive itself. Therefore, these clauses should be reviewed and referenced before discussions proceed with the health care proxy.

Often there is no predetermined health care surrogate for a patient who is incapacitated. Health care laws vary by state with regard to who may serve, if at all, in the position of health care proxy and how a grant of guardianship is obtained.

Traditionally, the role of the surrogate decision-maker is to determine interventions and goals of care that the patient would chose if he or she still had decisional capacity. This is known as *substituted judgment* and is grounded in the ethical principle of autonomy. In reality, substituted judgment is very difficult to attain because the surrogate must often wrestle with his or her own emotional reactions or desires for the patient, who is often a loved one.

Clinicians must be willing to guide surrogates, via substituted judgment, in a way that reduces decision-maker regret and increases the likelihood that decisions are consistent with the known values of the patient rather than influenced by the competing desires of other, often well-meaning, family and associates. The operative question is: "What would this patient want us to do or not do next if she was able to make this decision for herself?"

Alternately, a *best interest* standard may be applied where substituted judgment may not be applicable, as in populations who have never had decisional capacity (e.g. pediatrics, adults with severe developmental disabilities). The surrogate, family, and clinician must ask: "What is in the best interest of this patient?" with care taken to evaluate cultural norms for quality of life for persons in similar situations.

As another alternative, the *narrative approach* to surrogate decision-making may be employed, which is grounded in the ethical principal of respect for persons. In the narrative approach, the patient's life story is considered and decisions are made that would be consistent with the pattern of his life.

Table 23.1 provides a sample tool to be administered by the clinician and that may aid the surrogate decision-making process.

IS THERE AN ADVANCE DIRECTIVE OR ADVANCE CARE PLAN AVAILABLE?

Advance care plans may include:

- *Living wills:* Patients may have paper documents available in the ED, accessible as part of an electronic medical record, or online at repository sites. All efforts should be made on the part of ED staff to access

TABLE 23.1. *Fierro's Four R's: A tool for surrogate medical decision-making*

1. Reflect:	Think back and imagine (your loved one) when he or she was still able to make his or her own decisions.
2. Reconstruct preferences:	Answer the following questions: What are his or her favorite things? What is his or her favorite color? What are his or her hobbies? What is his or her favorite meal? What things did he or she dislike?
3. Reconstruct values:	Think about whom he or she was, his or her opinions, his or her beliefs. What were his or her values? How did he or she choose to live his or her life?
4. Review medical options and decide:	Now, imagine that (your loved one) is standing here beside you, looking at himself or herself. He or she hears the diagnosis and the available options the doctor has given. *What does he or she want us to do, or not do next?*

The tool combines substituted judgment with narrative decision-making. Used with Permission.
Williams-Murphy, M., & Murphy, K. (2011). *It's OK to die.* Garden City, AL: MKN LLC.

living wills to assure that autonomous medical decisions, made thoughtfully in advance, are honored.

- *Do Not Resuscitate/Do Not Attempt Resuscitation/Allow Natural Death (DNR/DNAR/AND) order sets:* These must be signed, dated, and witnessed appropriately to be an actionable documents in the pre-hospital and hospital settings. Remember, if you discharge a patient back home or to a facility for end-of-life care and the patient wishes to have DNR/DNAR/AND orders, then they must be discharged with a state or regionally approved document appropriately signed, dated, and witnessed (if applicable) to be valid. Otherwise, should this patient arrest and 911 be called, full resuscitative measures will likely be undertaken by emergency medical service (EMS) providers. This could result in nonbeneficial medical interventions being delivered contrary to the patient's or surrogate's previous wishes – a clear violation of multiple medical ethical principles.

- *Physician Orders for Life-Sustaining Treatment (POLST; paradigm physician order sets)* are advanced-generation patient directives that are quickly becoming the best-practice standard for observing patients' wishes at the end of life. Studies suggest that POLST dramatically increases the likelihood that end-of-life wishes are honored compared to other advance directives. Where available, a valid POLST should accompany the patient across all health care settings to ensure that the patient's wishes are fulfilled (see Figure 23.1).

HIPAA PERMITS DISCLOSURE TO HEALTH CARE PROFESSIONALS & ELECTRONIC REGISTRY AS NECESSARY FOR TREATMENT

Physician Orders for Life-Sustaining Treatment (POLST)

Follow these medical orders until orders change. Any section not completed implies full treatment for that section.

Patient Last Name:	Patient First Name:	Patient Middle Name:	Last 4 SSN:
Address: (street / city / state / zip):		Date of Birth: (mm/dd/yyyy) ___/___/___	Gender: ☐ M ☐ F

A *Check One* — **CARDIOPULMONARY RESUSCITATION (CPR):** ***Unresponsive, pulseless, & not breathing.***

☐ **Attempt Resuscitation/CPR**
☐ **Do Not Attempt Resuscitation/DNR**

If patient is not in cardiopulmonary arrest, follow orders in **B** and **C**.

B *Check One* — **MEDICAL INTERVENTIONS:** ***If patient has pulse and is breathing.***

☐ **Comfort Measures Only** Provide treatments to relieve pain and suffering through the use of any medication by any route, positioning, wound care and other measures. Use oxygen, suction and manual treatment of airway obstruction as needed for comfort. ***Patient prefers no transfer to hospital*** *for life-sustaining treatments. Transfer if comfort needs cannot be met in current location.*
Treatment Plan: Provide treatments for comfort through symptom management.

☐ **Limited Treatment.** In addition to care described in Comfort Measures Only, use medical treatment, antibiotics, IV fluids and cardiac monitor as indicated. No intubation, advanced airway interventions, or mechanical ventilation. May consider less invasive airway support (e.g. CPAP, BiPAP). ***Transfer*** *to hospital if indicated. Generally avoid the intensive care unit.*
Treatment Plan: Provide basic medical treatments.

☐ **Full Treatment.** In addition to care described in Comfort Measures Only and Limited Treatment, use intubation, advanced airway interventions, and mechanical ventilation as indicated. ***Transfer to hospital*** *and/or intensive care unit if indicated.*
Treatment Plan: All treatments including breathing machine.

Additional Orders: ______

C *Check One* — **ARTIFICIALLY ADMINISTERED NUTRITION:** ***Offer food by mouth if feasible.***

☐ Long-term artificial nutrition by tube.
☐ Defined trial period of artificial nutrition by tube.
☐ No artificial nutrition by tube.

Additional Orders (e.g., defining the length of a trial period): ______

D *Must Fill Out* — **DOCUMENTATION OF DISCUSSION: (REQUIRED)** ***See reverse side for add'l info.***

☐ Patient (If patient lacks capacity, must check a box below)
☐ Health Care Representative (legally appointed by advance directive or court)
☐ Surrogate defined by facility policy or Surrogate for patient with developmental disabilities or significant mental health condition (Note: Special requirements for completion- see reverse side)

Representative/Surrogate Name: ______ Relationship: ______

E — **PATIENT OR SURROGATE SIGNATURE AND OREGON POLST REGISTRY OPT OUT**

Signature: *recommended*

This form will be sent to the POLST Registry unless the patient wishes to opt out, if so check opt out box: ☐

F *Must Print Name, Sign & Date* — **ATTESTATION OF MD / DO / NP / PA (REQUIRED)**

By signing below, I attest that these medical orders are, to the best of my knowledge, consistent with the patient's **current** medical condition and preferences.

Print Signing MD / DO / NP / PA Name: *required*	Signer Phone Number:	Signer License Number: *(optional)*
MD / DO / NP / PA Signature: *required*	Date: *required*	Office Use Only

SEND FORM WITH PATIENT WHENEVER TRANSFERRED OR DISCHARGED
SUBMIT COPY OF BOTH SIDES OF FORM TO REGISTRY IF PATIENT DID NOT OPT OUT IN SECTION E

FIGURE 23.1. Sample Oregon Physician Orders for Life-Sustaining Treatment (POLST) form.
Used with permission, Oregon Health and Science University.

Of note, recent TRIAD (The Realistic Interpretation of Advance Directives) studies caution that confusion may exist among health care providers in regard to the interpretation and utilization of advance

HIPAA PERMITS DISCLOSURE TO HEALTH CARE PROFESSIONALS & ELECTRONIC REGISTRY AS NECESSARY FOR TREATMENT

Information for patient named on this form   PATIENT'S NAME: _____

The POLST form is **always voluntary** and is usually for persons with serious illness or frailty. POLST records your wishes for medical treatment in your current state of health (states your treatment wishes if something happened tonight). Once initial medical treatment is begun and the risks and benefits of further therapy are clear, your treatment wishes may change. Your medical care and this form can be changed to reflect your new wishes at any time. No form, however, can address all the medical treatment decisions that may need to be made. An Advance Directive is recommended for all capable adults and allows you to document in detail your future health care instructions and/or name a Health Care Representative to speak for you if you are unable to speak for yourself. Consider reviewing your Advance Directive and giving a copy of it to your health care professional.

Contact Information (Optional)			
Health Care Representative or Surrogate:	Relationship:	Phone Number:	Address:

Health Care Professional Information

Preparer Name:	Preparer Title:	Phone Number:	Date Prepared:
PA's Supervising Physician:		Phone Number:	
Primary Care Professional:			

Directions for Health Care Professionals

Completing POLST
- Completing a POLST is always voluntary and cannot be mandated for a patient.
- An order of CPR in Section A is incompatible with an order for Comfort Measures Only in Section B (will not be accepted in Registry).
- For information on legally appointed health care representatives and their authority, refer to ORS 127.505 - 127.660.
- Should reflect current preferences of persons with serious illness or frailty. Also, encourage completion of an Advance Directive.
- Verbal / phone orders are acceptable with follow-up signature by MD/DO/NP/PA in accordance with facility/community policy.
- Use of original form is encouraged. Photocopies, faxes, and electronic registry forms are also legal and valid.
- A person with developmental disabilities or significant mental health condition requires additional consideration before completing the POLST form; refer to *Guidance for Health Care Professionals* at www.or.polst.org.

Oregon POLST Registry Information

Health Care Professionals:	Registry Contact Information:	Patients:
(1) You are **required** to send a copy of both sides of this POLST form to the Oregon POLST Registry unless the patient opts out.	Phone: 503-418-4083 Fax or eFAX: 503-418-2161 www.orpolstregistry.org polstreg@ohsu.edu	Mailed confirmation packets from Registry may take four weeks for delivery.
(2) The following sections must be completed: • Patient's full name • Date of birth • MD / DO / NP / PA signature • Date signed	Oregon POLST Registry 3181 SW Sam Jackson Park Rd. Mail Code: CDW-EM Portland, Or 97239	**MAY PUT REGISTRY ID STICKER HERE:**

Updating POLST: A POLST Form only needs to be revised if patient treatment preferences have changed.

This POLST should be reviewed periodically, including when:
- The patient is transferred from one care setting or care level to another (including upon admission or at discharge), or
- There is a substantial change in the patient's health status.
If patient wishes haven't changed, the POLST Form does not need to be revised, updated, rewritten or resent to the Registry.

Voiding POLST: A copy of the voided POLST must be sent to the Registry unless patient has opted-out.

- A person with capacity, or the valid surrogate of a person without capacity, can void the form and request alternative treatment.
- Draw line through sections A through E and write "VOID" in large letters if POLST is replaced or becomes invalid.
- Send a copy of the voided form to the POLST Registry (required unless patient has opted out).
- If included in an electronic medical record, follow voiding procedures of facility/community.

For permission to use the copyrighted form contact the OHSU Center for Ethics in Health Care at orpolst@ohsu.edu or (503) 494-3965. Information on the Oregon POLST Program is available online at www.or.polst.org or at **orpolst@ohsu.edu**

SEND FORM WITH PATIENT WHENEVER TRANSFERRED OR DISCHARGED, SUBMIT COPY TO REGISTRY

© CENTER FOR ETHICS IN HEALTH CARE, Oregon Health & Science University   2014

FIGURE 23.1. (cont.)

care plans in critically ill patient scenarios. As such, ABCDE patient safety checklists may be used to clarify previously recorded advance directives (see Figure 23.2 and Mirarchi, F., Doshi, A., Zerkle, S., & Cooney, T., 2015).

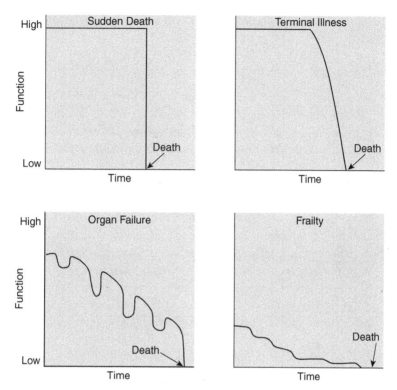

FIGURE 23.2. Theoretical trajectories of dying.
(Lunney, J., Lynn J., & Hogan, C. (2002). Profiles of Older Medicare Decedents, *Journal of the American Geriatrics Society, 50*, 1108–1112.) Used with permission.

DISCUSSING GOALS OF CARE AT THE END OF LIFE: INCREASING PATIENT AUTONOMY

After decision-making capacity has been determined, surrogates identified, and available advanced care plans have been reviewed, if the need for further medical decision-making exists, then the emergency clinician must guide a conversation to elicit goals of care. Informed consent rests on connecting the knowledge of the patient or surrogate with the medical options available in the context of the illness and proximity to the end of life. Furthermore, trajectories of care are often set by the interventions initiated in the ED. As such, it is vitally important to elicit the patient's goals of care before initiating treatment. Most importantly, anyone who is admitted and appears to be near the end of life should have a documented code status at time of admission congruent with intuitional protocols. All of these measures increase patient autonomy.

Some strategies for eliciting goals of care and informed consent followed by clinical respect for patient choices are outlined here:

- After the patient or surrogate has decided who should be present for a goals of care conversation, elicit their understanding of the present illness and "hoped for" prognosis. Encourage support of patient preferences. Avoid medical jargon and speak the truth compassionately.
- Identify the "medical moment." Both the clinician and the patient or surrogate should attempt to honestly answer the question: Where is the patient on the "map of life"? Again, this type of contextual understanding is required for informed consent and accurate medical decision-making by patient and health care surrogate. It is very important to ask the patient or surrogate such questions as: "What have you been told about your health?" "How do you think you are doing?" "How were you hoping we could help?" to understand their perceptions and expectations prior to offering your medical opinion.
- Offer prognosis and risk, benefits, alternatives of treatment options. Make a recommendation, then allow time for decision-making.

  Prognosis: Visual aids such as that shown in Figure 23.2 are often very helpful for enabling laypersons' understanding of end-of-life patterns. Clearly state your expectations of remaining time with or without cure-focused medical intervention, if you are able to do so honestly (in terms of "days-to-weeks," "weeks-to-months," or "months-to-years"). There are two important facts to note regarding life expectancy conversations: (1) as a general rule, clinicians tend to overestimate life expectancy; and (2) patients tend to choose less aggressive intervention when presented with a short life expectancy. Above all, do not offer false hope. It is unethical to do so.

  Risks, Benefits, and Alternatives: Verbal and/or visual descriptions of risk, benefits, and alternatives of emergency interventions should be provided for the patient who is at the expected end of life (intubation, mechanical ventilation, defibrillation, ICU visitation limitations). For example, "CPR involves forceful compressions of your chest which may result in many broken ribs, inhaled vomit, popping one or both lungs, and internal bleeding. CPR may restart your heartbeat, but it is not a cure for your underlying medical condition. You would likely be in worse shape than you are now if CPR is successful in restarting your heartbeat. The alternative to CPR is to allow you to die naturally, and your health care team would focus on creating maximum comfort for you and your family when your time comes." It is important to discuss a range of options, with descriptions of therapeutic alternatives (e.g. from endotracheal intubation to BiPAP to comfort measures). When discussing DNR/DNAR status, it may be preferable to use the term "allow a natural death" (AND) instead. The term "allow a natural death" may be more understandable to the lay person. Avoid presenting limited options in an "all-or-nothing" fashion. Recognize that cultural expectations for the potential success of medical interventions may be much higher than what is supported by scientific data.

Making Recommendations and Allowing Time for Decision-Making.
- Make a recommendation; avoid placing the full burden of decision-making on the surrogate/patient. However, show respect if the decision-maker disagrees with your recommendations.
- Ask many open-ended questions: "What were you hoping for? A miracle? What else?"
- Use verbiage that gives you alliance with the patient: "I wish this were possible for you. I wish that we could cure her. We can't, but we can certainly ensure her comfort."
- Humanize yourself. Share any experiences where you have struggled to help make decisions for someone you love or an experience within your own family. Offer what you would do if the patient was your own loved one.
- Allow time and space for thoughtful deliberation and decision-making.

RESPECTING AUTONOMY OF THE END-OF-LIFE PATIENT

Patients or surrogates may choose full resuscitation, limited medical interventions, or other options for end-of-life care.

- *Full resuscitation.* Even a patient who is clearly near the expected end of life may at times request full-resuscitative measures with a goal of recovering from an acute event despite his or her proximity to the end of life. Physician responses range from full support by the clinician to

conscientious objection with accompanying explanation by the
physician.

- *Limited medical interventions* (e.g. CPAP, BiPaP, but withholding
  CPR or endotracheal intubation) with goal of recovery from the
  acute event despite overall proximity to end of life. A clear record
  should be made regarding the level of intervention requested and an
  order written according to institutional protocols.
- *Comfort care*, with the goal of a natural and peaceful death. A DNR/
  DNAR/AND order should be entered. Discussion of the disposition of
  a patient desiring comfort care is discussed in the next section, "ensuring a good death." Note that a hospital admission for any patient who is
  near the end of life should trigger a palliative care consultation.
- *Organ donation* may be encouraged as a way to directly transform
  death into life. Organ donation may be ethically viewed as an act of
  beneficence on the part of the patient or family and a contribution to
  the stewardship of health care resources on the part of the clinician.
  Refer to your institutional policies regarding recovery of organs and
  tissues for transplantation.

Documentation of the clinician's evaluation of the patient's capacity,
advance directive, surrogate discussions, and resulting medical decisions
should be detailed in the medical record. Finally, an order should be entered
to reflect the patient's wishes according to institutional protocols; for example,
"Mr. Jones appears to have decision-making capacity at the time of my
evaluation. He did not wish for family members to be present during our
goals of care conversation and had not previously created an advance directive
for reference. After discussing the trajectory of his COPD as well as the risks,
benefits, and alternatives to endotracheal intubation, he has chosen to accept
noninvasive respiratory care such as BiPAP but would not want to be
intubated. I have entered a Do Not Intubate order in his chart to reflect his
wishes."

ENSURING A "GOOD DEATH" IS AN ACT OF BENEFICENCE

For all patients who are approaching the end of their lives, it is the duty of
the ED staff to ensure a "good death" to the extent this is possible. This is an
act of beneficence. Indeed, a "good death" should become the ethical
standard of care at the end of life. A "good death" as defined by the
Institute of Medicine is "one that is free from avoidable distress and
suffering, for patients, family, and caregivers; in general accord with the

patients' and families' wishes; and reasonably consistent with clinical, cultural, and ethical standards."

Hospice Care

Early referral to hospice services maximizes quality of time at the end of life and, ultimately, provides a "good death." In addition, studies suggest that hospice care may reduce total health care expenditures, a contribution to the ethical principle of stewardship of health care resources. Hospice provides holistic care for families and patients who are presumed to be in the last six months of life if an illness runs its expected course. Generally, hospice eligibility is suggested by evidence of life-limiting disease progression such as:

- Weight loss: 10 percent or more over the past six months or a serum albumin of less than 2.5 g/L
- Increased pain, nausea, fatigue, dyspnea, dysphagia, or other symptoms
- Increased frequency of medical events including hospital admissions or ED visits. Recurrent infections.
- Increased need for assistance in activities of daily living, decline in functional status, decreased alertness
- Family exhausted from care-giving demands

Note that Medicare does not require hospice patients to have DNR/AND orders. Disease-specific guidelines are available by searching at: http://www.cms.gov.

Many EDs may have access to palliative care consultation services to help in the evaluation of a potential hospice-appropriate patient. However, all EDs should have nursing staff, social workers, or case managers who are qualified to help with hospice referral processing. Also, local hospice agencies may be willing to work closely with EDs. In some areas, hospice agencies may have affiliate privileges and could provide timely consultation while the patient is still in the ED to aid in determining eligibility and disposition for optimal end-of-life care.

If consistent with the goals of care, the hospice patient may be admitted to an inpatient palliative care bed or hospice unit if there is a high symptom burden that cannot feasibly be managed in other settings. Otherwise, the hospice patient may transported back home or to the "home facility" with initiation or continuation of hospice care. When discharging the patient back home or to a "home facility," it is the purview of the provider to organize a seamless transition of care for the patient and family.

Dying in the ED

When a patient is imminently dying, it may be inappropriate to try to arrange transfer from the ED, and instead it becomes our responsibility to create a "good death" for the patient and family. Effective management of a "good death" within the ED setting may augment community trust and satisfaction with care. This may be standardized by creating a departmental protocol for the actively dying patient. Such a protocol should reflect the following action steps and considerations:

- *Physical*: Pain and symptom management are paramount (i.e. oxygen and morphine for dyspnea, ventilator-withdrawal protocols, atropine, oral care etc.). Physical signs of dying should be identified for those present at the bedside. Additionally, family and visitors should be encouraged to have physical contact with the patient. If desired, personal mementos or items of physical comfort or treasured by the patient should be allowed into the room (e.g. blankets, religious icons). Anything promoting comfort and dignity should be considered.
- *Location*: If possible, have a dedicated room that is clean, private, quiet, and absent medical equipment. If medical equipment is present, it should be switched off or set to "comfort care" settings with all monitors silenced. Chairs should be available for family and visitors. A sign on the door may be appropriate to alert others that someone is dying, and this contributes to the privacy of the patient and family.
- *Psychological/Social*: Encourage the presence of family and friends at the bedside, if desired by the patient. Speak to the patient and family compassionately about next steps. This may range from telling the patient that you are about to remove an endotracheal tube to make them more comfortable, to educating the family/visitors about the physical changes to be expected as their loved one dies. Families should be encouraged to speak to the dying person as well. They may be encouraged to offer words of gratitude, love, forgiveness, and release. Finally, a nurse, patient representative, or social worker should check in at frequent intervals to assess needs.
- *Spiritual*: Summon the chaplain or clergy of choice for the patient/family. If there is no religious belief, a social worker or patient representative may offer to provide a special reading or music. These should be offered to those with religious or spiritual preferences as well. Additionally, postmortem care should take into consideration any cultural customs that must be observed.

When these measures are successfully met, surviving family and even ED staff have greater satisfaction with the end-of-life care provided, which may lead to healthier grieving and bereavement processes for all. A "good death" is a death that is well-managed for the patient, the family, and the ED.

ETHICAL DILEMMAS AT THE END OF LIFE

Several ethical dilemmas may present themselves during end-of-life care in the ED:

- *Ethics of withholding, withdrawing, and declining life-saving medical interventions*: When reflecting the clear wishes of the patient, a valid legal surrogate, or a valid advance directive, the withholding and withdrawing of medical interventions, commonly regarded as life-sustaining, constitutes neither suicide nor homicide according to U.S. legal consensus. In the ED setting, this means that intubation, resuscitation, blood transfusions, defibrillation, artificial pacing, antibiotics, medically assisted nutrition or hydration, and the like may be withheld or withdrawn. Comfort-focused care (such as opioids for pain control), however, should never be withheld or withdrawn. To do so would constitute patient abandonment.
- *Hospice patients presenting to the ED*: Hospice patients may present on occasion to the ED for a variety of reasons from poor symptom control to unsafe home conditions to existential distress. Their presentation to the ED should not create the assumption among providers that aggressive or resuscitative intervention is desired. However, every effort must be made to address the needs of these patients and their families and to affirm commitment to creating a peaceful end-of-life pathway for the one who is dying. Communication and collaboration with the primary care provider and hospice agency is paramount to fulfilling this duty.
- *Futile or nonbeneficial care*: Ethicists disagree over many points of so-called futile or nonbeneficial medical interventions; however, there is no argument over physiological futility – meaning that, regardless of intervention, death is the outcome (e.g. traumatic decapitation or a person found with signs of rigor mortis). For cases of such physiological futility, no CPR or intervention is indicated. It may, however, be useful to ask the following questions in other cases involving end-of-life decisions: "How is this intervention beneficial and helpful or not? What are the adverse effects of

this treatment? Does this intervention lead to the life the patient would want to live?" Such questions may allow qualitative exploration of how an intervention may be beneficial or nonbeneficial for the patient who is near the end of life. Relatedly, only appropriate or potentially effective interventions should be offered by the clinician.

- *Physician-assisted suicide (PAS)*: Despite a growing discussion of the merits of PAS in some regions and the actual legalization of PAS in a few states, the American Medical Association regards PAS as unethical, unprofessional, and "fundamentally incompatible with the physician's role as healer." By definition, PAS, in states where it is legal, allows physicians to prescribe, but not administer, a lethal dose of medication to competent, terminally ill patients who have met certain criteria. States draw their authority to legislate support or prohibition of PAS from U.S. Supreme Court rulings that deny constitutional rights to PAS, but leave legislation to the states (*Washington v. Glucksberg* and *Vacco v. Quill*, 1997). Should an emergency physician, practicing in a state where PAS is legal, receive a patient who has legally attempted PAS, palliative care should be provided. However, if the case is medicolegally unclear or there is uncertainty, the clinician should proceed with appropriate care until more information may be obtained.

- *Persistent disagreements over care*: If a thoughtful clinician has considered his or her own biases regarding prognosis or quality of life and there remains a persistent disagreement about the direction of care at the end of life, then it is the clinician's duty to invite the consultation of outside experts and/or an ethics committee to provide a broader atmosphere for discussion and mediation. Institutional policies should be developed to guide end-of-life care disputations and should include two key options: (1) support for physicians to refuse the provision of physiologically futile care, and (2) support for the arrangement of transfer of the patient's care to another physician or institution who is willing to receive the patient.

- *Conscientious objection by physician*: Closely related to persistent disagreements over care is the idea that the physician may object to providing certain medical interventions if (1) the intervention is felt to violate the physician's moral standards, or (2) the physician honestly believes that the risks substantially outweigh the benefits and may harm the patient by causing unnecessary suffering. In such cases, the patient and family should be informed, and there should also be institutional policies in place allowing the physician to withdraw from the case in a way that would not constitute patient abandonment, but that would allow transfer of the patient to another provider or institution.

- *Complexity*: Given that emergency medicine is practiced in a pluralistic, multicultural milieu, ethical end-of-life situations may arise during clinical practice that have no precedent in the mind of the clinician. Such scenarios should prompt legal and/or ethical advisement.
- *Ethics committee*: Many hospitals now have ethics committees available to provide consultation in difficult cases. Furthermore, the majority of those consultations are likely related to end-of-life dilemmas. However, given the imperative of efficiency in emergency medicine, the ED timeline for care is not typically conducive to ethics consultation prior to intervention choices and disposition. This does not preclude the ethics consultation in the ED, yet the focus should be on the expeditious and proper care of a patient with as much ethical certainty as possible. Most often, this may require disposition to admission or observation for full evaluation and recommendations by an ethics consultation service.

ETHICS TAKEOUT TIPS

- Expert and compassionate death notification is an act of beneficence. What the family and friends hear from the clinician regarding the death of their loved one will become part of the oral history of the patient's life and will be shared throughout their community. Memorize the GRIEV_ING mnemonic.
- Patients have ethical and legal rights to autonomy. The Patient Self-Determination Act of 1991 legally granted patients or surrogates the right to choose or refuse any medical procedure offered to them, including medical interventions that might be viewed as life-saving or time-extending.
- The surrogate decision-maker's traditional role is to determine interventions and goals of care that the patient would chose if he or she still had decisional capacity (autonomy).
- Trajectories of care are often set by the interventions initiated in the ED. As such, it is vitally important to elicit the patient's goals of care before initiating treatment to ensure respect for autonomy.
- Ensuring a "good death" is an act of beneficence and should be the ethical standard of care for the dying.

Monica Williams-Murphy

FOR FURTHER READING

American College of Emergency Physicians. (2008). *Ethical issues at the end of life.* American College of Emergency Physicians Policy Statement. www.acep.org/ Clinical-Practice-Management/Ethical-Issues-at-the-End-of-Life/

Anderson, M. (2005). *Attending the dying: A handbook of practical guidelines.* New York: Morehouse Publishing.

Bailey, C., Murphy, R., & Porock, D. (2011). Trajectories of end-of-life care in the emergency department. *Annals of Emergency Medicine,* 57, 362–369.

Chow, C., Czarny, M., Hughest, M., & Carrese, J. (2010). CURVES: A mnemonic for determining medical decision-making capacity and providing emergency treatment in the acute setting. *Chest,* 137, 417–421.

DeSandre, P. L., & Quest, T. E. (2013). *Palliative aspects of emergency care.* Oxford: Oxford University Press.

Forero, R., McDonnell, G., Gallego, B., McCarthy, S., Mohsin, M., Shanley, C., Formby, F., & Hillman, K. (2012). A literature review on care at the end-of-life in the emergency department. *Emergency Medicine International,* 11. http://dx.doi. org/10.1155/2012/486516

Hobgood, C., Tamayo-Sarver, J., Hollar, D., & Sawning, S. (2009). Grieving: Death notification skills and applications for fourth-year medical students. *Teaching and Learning in Medicine,* 21, 207–219.

Institute of Medicine. (1997). *Approaching death: Improving care at the end of life.* Washington, DC: National Academy Press.

Jonsen, A., Siegler, M., & Winslade, W. (2010). Clinical ethics: A practical approach to ethical decisions in clinical medicine *(7th ed.).* New York: McGraw-Hill.

Kehl, K. (2006). Moving toward peace: An analysis of the concept of a good death. *American Journal of Hospice and Palliative Care,* 23, 277–286.

Lo, B. (2013). *Resolving ethical dilemmas: A guide for clinicians.* Philadelphia: Lippincott, Williams and Wilkins.

Marco, C., Savory, E., & Treuhaft, K. (2010). End-of-life terminology: The ED patients' perspective. *AJOB Primary Research,* 1, 22–27. www.bioethics.net/arti cles/end-of-life-terminology-the-ed-patients-perspective/

Mirarchi, F., Doshi, A., Zerkle, S., & Cooney, T. (2015). TRIAD VI: How well do emergency physicians understand physician orders for life-sustaining treatment (POLST) forms? *Journal of Patient Safety,* 11(1), 1–8.

Savory, E., & Marco, C. (2009). End-of-life issues in the acute and critically ill patient. *Scandinavian Journal of Trauma, Resuscitation and Emergency,* 17, 21. www.sjtrem.com/content/17/1/21

Williams-Murphy, M., & Murphy, K. (2011). *It's OK to die.* Garden City, AL: MKN LLC.

Zalenski, R., & Compton, S. (2004). Death trajectories of emergency department patients and palliative care service utilization. *Annals of Emergency Medicine,* 44, S68.

Appendix 1

ACEP Code of Ethics for Emergency Physicians

Revised and approved by the ACEP Board of Directors June 2008.

Reaffirmed by the ACEP Board of Directors October 2001.

Approved by the ACEP Board of Directors June 1997 titled, "Code of Ethics for Emergency Physicians" replacing original statement titled, "Ethics Manual" approved by the ACEP Board of Directors January 1991.

A Compendium of ACEP Policy Statements on Ethical Issues Revised 2002, 2003, 2004, 2005, 2006, 2007, 2008, 2009, 2011, 2012, 2013, 2014.

Contents

I. PRINCIPLES OF ETHICS FOR EMERGENCY PHYSICIANS

The basic professional obligation of beneficent service to humanity is expressed in various physicians' oaths and codes of ethics. In addition to this general obligation, emergency physicians accept specific ethical obligations that arise out of the special features of emergency medical practice. The principles listed below express fundamental moral responsibilities of emergency physicians.

Emergency Physicians shall:

1. Embrace patient welfare as their primary professional responsibility.
2. Respond promptly and expertly, without prejudice or partiality, to the need for emergency medical care.
3. Respect the rights and strive to protect the best interests of their patients, particularly the most vulnerable and those unable to make treatment choices due to diminished decision-making capacity.

4. Communicate truthfully with patients and secure their informed consent for treatment, unless the urgency of the patient's condition demands an immediate response.

5. Respect patient privacy and disclose confidential information only with consent of the patient or when required by an overriding duty such as the duty to protect others or to obey the law.

6. Deal fairly and honestly with colleagues and take appropriate action to protect patients from health care providers who are impaired or incompetent, or who engage in fraud or deception.

7. Work cooperatively with others who care for, and about, emergency patients.

8. Engage in continuing study to maintain the knowledge and skills necessary to provide high quality care for emergency patients.

9. Act as responsible stewards of the health care resources entrusted to them.

10. Support societal efforts to improve public health and safety, reduce the effects of injury and illness, and secure access to emergency and other basic health care for all.

II. ETHICS IN EMERGENCY MEDICINE: AN OVERVIEW

A. Ethical Foundations of Emergency Medicine

Although professional responsibilities have been a concern of physicians since antiquity, recent years have seen dramatic growth of both professional and societal attention to moral issues in health care. This increased interest in medical ethics is a result of multiple factors, including the greater technologic power of contemporary medicine, the medicalization of societal ills, the growing sophistication of patients, efforts to protect the civil rights of disadvantaged groups in our society, and the persistently rising costs of health care. All of these factors contribute to the significance, the complexity, and the urgency of moral questions in contemporary emergency medicine.

1. *Moral pluralism*

In addressing ethical questions, emergency physicians can consult a variety of sources for guidance. Professional oaths and codes of ethics are an important source of guidance, as are general cultural values, social norms embodied in the law, religious and philosophical moral traditions, and professional role models. All of these sources claim moral authority, and together they can inspire physicians to lead rich and committed moral lives. Problems arise, however, when different sources of moral guidance come into conflict in our pluralistic society. Numerous attempts have been made to find an overarching moral theory able to assess and prioritize moral claims from all of their various sources. Lacking agreement on the primacy of any one of these theories, we are left with a pluralism of different sources of moral guidance. The goal of bioethics is to help us understand, interpret, and weigh competing moral values as we see reasoned and defensible solutions to moral problems encountered in health care.

2. Unique duties of emergency physicians

The unique setting and goals of emergency medicine give rise to a number of distinctive ethical concerns. Among the special moral challenges confronted by emergency physicians are the following: First, patients often arrive at the emergency department with acute illnesses or injuries that require immediate care. In these emergent situations, emergency physicians have little time to gather additional data, consult with others, or deliberate about alternative treatments. Instead, there is a presumption for quick action guided by predetermined treatment protocols. Second, patients in the emergency department often are unable to participate in decisions regarding their health care because of acute changes in their mental state. When patients lack decision-making capacity, emergency physicians cannot secure their informed consent to treatment. Third, emergency physicians typically have had no prior relationship with their patients in the emergency department. Patients often arrive in the emergency department unscheduled, in crisis, and sometimes against their own free will. Thus, emergency physicians cannot rely on earned trust or on prior knowledge of the patient's condition, values, or wishes regarding medical treatment. The patient's willingness to seek emergency care and to trust the physician is based on institutional and professional assurances rather than on an established personal relationship. Fourth, emergency physicians practice in an institutional setting, the hospital emergency department, and in close working relationships with other physicians, nurses, emergency medical technicians, and other health care professionals. Thus, emergency physicians must understand and respect institutional regulations and inter-professional norms of conduct. Fifth, in the United States, emergency physicians have been given a unique social role and responsibility to act as health care providers of last resort for many patients who have no other feasible access to care. Sixth, emergency physicians have a societal duty to render emergency aid outside their normal health care setting when such intervention may save life or limb. Finally, by virtue of their broad expertise and training, emergency physicians are expected to be a resource for the community in prehospital care, disaster management, toxicology, cardiopulmonary resuscitation, public health, injury control, and related areas. All of these special circumstances shape the moral dimensions of emergency medical practice.

3.　Virtues in emergency medicine

As noted above, the emergency department is a unique practice environment with distinctive moral challenges. To respond appropriately to these moral challenges, emergency physicians need knowledge of moral concepts and principles, and moral reasoning skills. Just as important for moral action as knowledge and skills, however, are morally valuable attitudes, character traits, and dispositions, identified in ethical theory as virtues. The virtuous person is motivated to act in support of his or her moral beliefs and ideals, and he or she serves as a role model for others. It is, therefore, important to identify and promote the moral virtues needed by emergency physicians. Fostering these virtues can be a kind of moral vaccination against the pitfalls inherent in emergency medical practice. Two timeless virtues of classic Western thought have essential roles in emergency medicine today: courage and justice.

Courage is the ability to carry out one's obligations despite personal risk or danger. The courageous physician advocates for patients against managed care gatekeepers, demanding employers, interrogating police, incompetent trainees, dismissive consultants, self-absorbed families, and inquiring reporters, just to name a few. Emergency physicians exhibit courage when they assume personal risk to provide steadfast care for the violent, psychologically agitated criminal or the infected intravenous drug-user.

Justice or fairness is the disposition to give such person what is due to him or her. Justice helps emergency physicians shepherd resources and employ therapeutic parsimony, refusing marginally beneficial care to some while guaranteeing a basic level of care for all others.

Additional virtues important to the practice of emergency medicine are vigilance, impartiality, trustworthiness, and resilience.

Vigilance is perhaps the virtue most emblematic of emergency medicine. In few other specialties are physicians called upon to assist patients and colleagues, immediately, twenty-four hours a day. Emergency physicians must be alert and prepared to meet unpredictable and uncontrollable demands, despite the circadian disharmony that threatens personal wellness.

The virtuous emergency physician practices impartiality by giving emergency patients an unconditional positive regard and treating them in an unbiased, unprejudiced way. Impartiality is most important in emergency medicine, since many emergency patients are poor or intoxicated and have poor hygiene, little education, and value systems at odds with that of the physician. Emergency physicians must treat perpetrators of violent crime with the same regard as victims and must resist the temptation to use disparaging remarks and gallows humor to ridicule psychotic patients or eccentric colleagues. Emergency physicians must be tolerant of people of different races, creeds, customs, habits, and lifestyle preferences.

Another essential virtue of emergency physicians is trustworthiness. Sick and vulnerable emergency patients are in a dependent relationship, forced to trust that emergency physicians will protect their interests through competence, informed consent, truthfulness, and the maintenance of confidentiality. Emergency physician clinical investigators must also be trustworthy, so that patient-subjects can trust they will not be exploited for power, profit, or prestige.

Finally, emergency physicians require the virtue of resilience in order to remain composed, flexible, and competent in the midst of clinical chaos. A tired, overstressed emergency department staff requires elasticity and optimism in order to stave off cynicism, resignation, disillusionment, numbing and professional burnout. Resilience enables emergency physicians to meet the challenges of difficult situations and enables them to encourage others to do so also. Excellence in emergency medicine requires flexibility, adaptability, and cooperative ability, allowing one to work well with patients and team members of all types. Resilience facilitates one's ability to recover undaunted from change of misfortune. It is also manifest in an ability to not take personally every insult hurled by angry patients, bereft families, or disgruntled coworkers. Resilient persons are hardy, curious, purposeful, and adaptable; they trust in their own power to influence the course of events. Maintaining flexibility and coping with the typical circadian disharmony of emergency work is difficult, but the virtue of resilience, an appropriate sense of humor, and an unsinkable optimism can keep team spirit afloat even in the harshest emergency department environment.

B. The Emergency Physician–Patient Relationship

The physician–patient relationship is the moral center of medicine and the defining element in biomedical ethics. The unique nature of emergency medical practice and the diversity of emergency patients pose special moral challenges, as noted above. Broad moral principles can nevertheless help to categorize the emergency physician's fundamental ethical duties. This section will rely on a prominent principle-based approach to bioethical theory to describe emergency physician duties of beneficence, nonmaleficence, respect for autonomy, and justice.

1. Beneficence

Physicians assume a fundamental duty to serve the best interests of their patients by treating or preventing disease or injury and by informing patients about their conditions. Emergency physicians respond promptly to acute illnesses and injuries in order to prevent or minimize pain and suffering, loss of function, and loss of life. In pursuing these goals, emergency physicians serve the principle of beneficence, that is, they act for the benefit of their patients.

To secure the benefits of health care, patients freely disclose sensitive personal information to their physicians and allow physicians access to their bodies for examination and treatment. Patients retain a strong interest, however, in protecting personal information from unauthorized disclosure and in preventing unnecessary intrusions on their physical privacy. Emergency physicians also respect the principle of beneficence, therefore, by protecting the privacy of their patients and the confidentiality of patient information. Personal information may only be disclosed when such disclosure is necessary to carry out a stronger conflicting duty, such as a duty to protect an identifiable third party from serious harm or to comply with a just law.

2. Nonmaleficence

At least as fundamental as the duty to benefit patients is the corresponding duty to refrain from inflicting harm. This duty, called the duty of non-maleficence, is central to maintaining the emergency physician's integrity and the patient's trust. In contemporary emergency medical care, the potential for significant patient benefit is often inescapably linked with the potential for significant complications, side effects, or other harms. Emergency physicians cannot, therefore, avoid inflicting harms, but they can respect the principle of nonmaleficence by seeking always to maximize the benefits of treatment and to minimize the risk of harm. Physicians who lack appropriate training and experience in emergency medicine should not misrepresent themselves as emergency physicians. Likewise, in order to avoid unnecessary harm to patients, physicians without adequate training and knowledge should not practice without supervision in the emergency department or prehospital setting.

3. Respect for patient autonomy

Adult patients with decision-making capacity have a right to accept or refuse recommended health care, and physicians have a concomitant duty to respect their choices. This right is grounded in the moral principle of respect for patient autonomy and is expressed in the legal doctrine of informed consent. According to this doctrine, physicians must first inform the patient with decision-making capacity about the nature of his or her medical condition, treatment alternatives, and their expected consequences, and then obtain the patient's voluntary consent to treatment. Emergency physicians also should respect decisions about a patient's treatment made by an appropriate surrogate decision maker, if the patient lacks decision-making capacity. Emergency physicians should be expert in the determination of decision-making capacity and the identification of appropriate surrogate decision makers if indicated.

Emergency physicians may treat without securing informed consent when immediate intervention is necessary to prevent death or serious harm to the patient. This is, however, a limited exception to the duty to obtain informed consent. When the initiation of treatment can be delayed without serious harm, informed consent should be obtained. Even if all the information needed for an informed consent cannot be provided, the emergency physician should, to whatever extent time allows, inform the patient (or, if the patient lacks capacity, a surrogate) about the treatment he or she is providing, and should not violate the explicit refusal of treatment, if the patient possesses decision-making capacity. In some cases, for personal and cultural reasons, patients ask that information be given to family or friends and that these third parties be allowed to make treatment choices for the patient. Patients may, if they wish, waive their right to informed consent or delegate decision-making authority for their care to others. Other exceptions to the duty to obtain informed consent apply when treatment is necessary to protect the public health and in a limited number of emergency medicine research protocols where obtaining consent is not feasible, provided that these research protocols are developed in concordance with federal guidelines and are approved by the appropriate review bodies.

To choose and act autonomously, patients must receive accurate information about their medical conditions and treatment options. Emergency physicians should relay sufficient information to patients for them to make an informed choice among various diagnostic and treatment options. Emergency physicians, when speaking to patients and families, must not overstate their experience or abilities, or those of their colleagues or institution. They should not overstate the potential benefits or success rates of the proposed treatment or research.

Significant moral issues may arise in the care of terminally ill patients. Emergency physicians should, for example, be willing to respect a terminally ill patient's wish to forgo life-prolonging treatment, as expressed in a living will or through a health care agent appointed under a durable power of attorney for health care. Emergency physicians should also be willing to honor "Do Not Attempt Resuscitation (DNAR)" orders and other end of life orders, appropriately executed to express the patient's treatment preferences. Emergency physicians should understand established criteria for the determination of death and should be prepared to assist families in decisions regarding the potential donation of a patient's organs for transplantation.

4. Justice

In a broad sense, acting justly can be understood as acting with impartiality or fairness. In this sense, emergency physicians have a duty of justice to provide care to patients regardless of race, color, creed, gender, nationality, or other irrelevant properties. In a more specific sense, justice refers to the equitable distribution of benefits and burdens within a community or society. In the United States, public policy has established a limited right of patients to receive evaluation and stabilizing treatment for emergency medical conditions in hospital emergency departments. This policy indirectly ascribes to emergency physicians a social responsibility to provide necessary emergency care to all patients, regardless of ability to pay. As noted in the Principles of Ethics for Emergency Physicians listed above, emergency physicians also have a duty in justice to act as responsible stewards of the health care resources entrusted to them. In carrying out this duty, emergency physicians must make careful judgments about the appropriate allocation of resources to maximize benefits and minimize burdens.

C. Emergency Physician Relationships with Other Professionals

The practice of emergency medicine requires multidisciplinary cooperation and teamwork. Emergency physicians interact closely with a wide variety of other health care professionals, including emergency nurses, emergency medical technicians, and physicians from other specialties. General ethical rules governing these interactions include honesty, respect, appreciation of other perspectives and needs, and an overriding duty to maximize patient benefit.

1. *Relationships with other physicians*

Emergency physicians, in keeping patient benefit as a primary goal, must participate with other physicians in the provision of health care. Channels of communication between health care providers must remain open to optimize patient outcomes. However, communication may be interrupted when a sick patient requires immediate and definitive intervention before discussion with other physicians can take place. When practical, emergency physicians should cooperate with the patient's primary care physician to provide continuity of care that satisfies the needs of the patient and minimizes burdens to other providers. Concerns regarding the extent of primary care rendered and referral required should be discussed with the primary physician whenever practical. Emergency physicians should support the development and implementation of systems that facilitate communications with primary care providers, consultants, and others involved in patient care.

On-call physicians, like emergency physicians, are morally obligated to provide timely and appropriate medical care. Emergency physicians should strive to treat consultants fairly and to make care as efficient as possible. The choice of consultant by the emergency physician may be guided by the preference of both the primary care physician and the patient or by institutional protocols. If multiple physicians work in the emergency department, each patient should have a clearly identified physician who is responsible for his or her care. Transfer of this responsibility should be clear to the patient, family, and staff involved, and should be clearly documented in the patient's medical record. When a patient is discharged from the emergency department, there must be a clear transfer of responsibility to the admitting or follow-up physician. This transfer must be clearly communicated to the patient when practical.

Contractual relationships between an emergency physician and an emergency physician group should be fair to all parties involved. Emergency medicine business, practices must be transparently ethical, and compensation should take into account both clinical and administrative services rendered by the physician. Disagreements arising from contractual arrangements should be arbitrated appropriately using a due process approach, whenever possible. Physicians with disabilities, injuries, or certain infections, such as HIV, may practice emergency medicine if their conditions do not inhibit proper performance or constitute a threat of harm to patients or others.

2. *Relationships with nurses and paramedical personnel*

Although the emergency physician assumes primary responsibility for patient welfare, emergency medicine is a team effort. For any specific patient, the physician must coordinate the efforts of nurses and support staff. To make the most effective use of the specific skills and expertise of emergency physicians, nurses, and other support staff, all should participate in the design and execution of emergency department care systems and protocols. Neither nurse practitioners nor physician assistants nor doctors in training should be used as emergency physician substitutes without adequate supervision and the consent of patients.

In the prehospital setting, emergency medical technicians of all levels rely on and rightfully expect the cooperation of emergency physicians with whom they work. Base station command physicians and other emergency providers should strive to work harmoniously with prehospital personnel to optimize care for the patient. Patient-centered, nonjudgmental, open communication is an important part of ethical medical command. Hospital and prehospital providers must respect patient confidentiality and the dignity of all personnel involved.

While emergency physicians may have greater expertise in scientific and technical matters, they share equal expertise with other health care workers with regard to moral judgment. Physicians should encourage involvement of other providers and staff when difficult moral issues arise.

3. *Impaired or incompetent physicians*

The principle of nonmaleficence dictates that patients be protected from physicians who are incompetent or impaired. Emergency physicians should strive for technical and moral excellence and should refrain from fraud or deception. When any physician is found deficient in competence or character through appropriate peer review process, it is morally imperative to protect patients and to assist that physician in addressing and, if possible, overcoming such deficiencies. Corrective action may include internal discipline or remedial training. To provide adequate protection for their patients, health care institutions should require appropriate remediation before the impaired physician returns to practice.

Whenever an emergency physician believes that a colleague or consulting physician is incompetent or impaired by drugs, alcohol, or psychiatric or medical conditions, he or she should report the impaired physician to the appropriate institutional and regulatory authorities This should be done with discretion and sensitivity, and with a clear intention to help the impaired physician progress toward treatment and recovery.

Physicians who conscientiously fulfill this responsibility should be protected from adverse political, legal, or financial consequences.

4. Relationships with business and administration

Emergency physicians should be advocates for emergency medical care as a fundamental right. Cost effective and efficient care is important so that resources can be available to provide care when it is needed. Cooperation with persons whose expertise is in the management and administration of health care systems is essential for provision of efficient care. A central role of physicians is to keep patient interests paramount in administrative and business decisions.

Incentives from businesses, including managed care organizations and biomedical drug and equipment manufacturers, should not unduly influence patient-centered clinical judgment. Gatekeeping activities that threaten patient safety are unethical, as are clauses that prevent physicians from informing patients about reasonable treatment alternatives. Physicians should not accept inappropriate gifts, trips, or other items from pharmaceutical or medical equipment companies or their representatives.

5. Relationships with students, trainees, and other learners

Emergency physicians practicing in academic settings have important moral responsibilities to medical students, residents, prehospital care personnel, and learners of all types. Learners depend on their clinical supervisors and professors to teach them both the moral and technical aspects of emergency medical practice. In addition to providing explicit instruction, practicing emergency physicians should serve as role models for ethical behavior in their relationships with patients, students, research subjects, and other health care professionals.

Emergency medicine residents, medical students, and other health care professionals in training must not be mistreated, abused, or coerced for faculty self-interest. Teaching physicians must fulfill their obligation to teach and provide appropriate levels of supervision for students under their tutelage. Performance evaluations and letters of recommendation require a careful assessment of the learners' strengths and weaknesses. Such evaluations must be accurate and clearly identify those individuals who may jeopardize patient care. Patient interests should not be compromised in the education process, and patients should never be required to participate in teaching activities or research without their consent. Emergency medicine residents must strive to master the discipline of emergency medicine, including understanding and accepting their moral duties to patients, profession, and society.

6. Relationships with the legal system as an expert witness

Expert witnesses are called on to assess the appropriateness of care provided by emergency physicians in matters of alleged medical malpractice and peer review. To assure that unbiased expert witness testimony is available to courts and panels that are trying to determine the applicable standard of care, the American College of Emergency Physicians (ACEP) encourages emergency physicians with sufficient expertise to testify in these venues. ACEP believes that these expert witnesses, at a minimum, should be emergency physicians who are certified in emergency medicine by the American Board of Emergency Medicine (ABEM), the American Osteopathic Board of Emergency Medicine (AOBEM), or, in pediatric emergency medicine, by the American Board of Pediatrics (ABP), and who have been actively practicing clinical emergency medicine for at least three years prior to the date of the incident under review.

As an expert witness, the physician has a clear ethical responsibility to be objective, truthful, and impartial, evaluating cases on the basis of generally accepted practice standards. It is unethical to overstate one's opinions or credentials, to misrepresent maloccurence as malpractice, to provide false testimony, or to use the name of the College as prima facie evidence of expertise.

While reasonable compensation for a physician's time is ethically acceptable, physicians should not provide expert testimony solely for financial gain lest this unduly influence their testimony.

7. Relationships with the research community

The emergency physician researcher should abide by basic moral and legal principles contained in federal, institutional, and professional guidelines that govern human and animal research. Basic ethical requirements for research studies include appropriate study goals, scientifically valid design, appropriate informed consent, confidentiality of records, and minimization of risks to subjects. Approval from appropriate institutional review boards is required, but it remains the responsibility of the investigator to protect the rights and welfare of patient-subjects. Federal regulations allow institutional review boards to grant a limited waiver of informed consent in specific emergency medicine research studies, where multiple additional protections for patient-subjects are provided. It is imperative that data be collected carefully, interpreted correctly, and reported accurately; research misconduct and fraud are grounds for disciplinary action and loss of funding. Emergency physician investigators should follow responsible authorship practices; for example, all co-authors should actively participate in all parts of the study, including literature review, study design, data collection, data analysis, and manuscript preparation.

D. The Emergency Physician's Relationship with Society

1. *The emergency physician and society*

The emergency physician owes duties not only to his or her patients, but also to the society in which the physician and patients dwell. Though the emergency physician's duty to the patient is primary, it is not absolute. Emergency physician duties to the general public inform decision-making on a daily basis; for example, the emergency physician has duties to allocate resources justly, oppose violence, and promote the public health that sometimes transcend duties to individual patients. To fulfill demands of equity and justice, society may place limits on the authority of the physician to satisfy an individual patient's interests. Emergency physicians should be active in legislative, regulatory, institutional, and educational pursuits that promote patient safety and quality emergency care.

2. *Resource allocation and health care access: problems of justice*

Both society and individual emergency physicians confront questions of justice in deciding how to distribute the benefits of health care and the burdens of financing that care among the various members of the society. Emergency physicians routinely address these issues when they assign order of priority for treatment and choose appropriate diagnostic and treatment resources. In making these judgments, emergency physicians must attempt to reconcile the goals of equitable access to health care and just allocation of health care with the increasing scarcity of resources and the need for cost containment.

3. *Central tenets of the emergency physician's relationship with society*

A. ACCESS TO EMERGENCY MEDICAL CARE IS A FUNDAMENTAL RIGHT
As noted above, US public policy, as articulated in the federal Emergency Medical Treatment and Active Labor Act (EMTALA), has established access to quality emergency care as an individual right that should be available to all who seek it. Recognizing that emergency care makes a substantial contribution to personal well-being, emergency physicians endorse this right and support the universal access to emergency care. Denial of emergency care or delay in providing emergency services on the

basis of race, religion, sexual orientation, real or perceived gender identity, ethnic background, social status, type of illness or injury, or ability to pay is unethical. Emergency physicians should act as advocates for the health needs of indigent patients, assisting them in finding appropriate care. Insurers, including managed care organizations, must support insured patients' access to emergency medical care for what a prudent layperson would reasonably perceive as an emergency medical condition. Society, through its political process, must adequately fund emergency care for all who need it.

Decisions to limit access to care may be made only when the resources of the emergency department are depleted. If overcrowding limits access to care, that limit must be applied equitably, unless the hospital has a unique community resource such as a trauma center, in which case the selection of a special category of patient may be acceptable.

Prehospital care is an essential societal good that emergency physicians, in conjunction with government, industry, and insurers must continue to make available to all members of society. All patients seeking assistance of prehospital care providers should undergo assessment by emergency medical technicians or paramedics in a timely fashion. Decisions concerning transport to a medical facility should be made on the basis of medical necessity, patient preference, and the capacity of the facility to deal with the medical problem.

B. ADEQUATE INHOSPITAL AND OUTPATIENT RESOURCES MUST BE AVAILABLE TO GUARD EMERGENCY PATIENT INTERESTS

Patients requiring hospitalization for further care should not be denied access to an appropriate medical facility on the basis of financial considerations. Transfer to another appropriate accepting medical facility for financial reasons may be effected if a) the patient provides consent and b) there is no undue risk to the patient. Admission or transfer decisions should be made on the basis of a patient's best interest.

It is unethical for an emergency physician to participate in the transfer of an emergency patient to another medical facility unless the medical benefits reasonably expected from the provision of appropriate medical treatment at another medical facility outweigh the risks of the transfer or unless a competent patient, or a legally responsible person acting on the patient's behalf, gives informed consent for the transfer. Emergency physicians should be knowledgeable about applicable federal and state laws regarding the transfer of patients between health care facilities.

Although the care and disposition of the patient are primarily the responsibility of the emergency physician, on-call consultants should share equitably in the care of indigent patients. This may include an on-site evaluation by the consultant if requested by the emergency physician.

For patients who do not require immediate hospitalization but need medical follow-up, adequate outpatient medical resources should be available both to continue proper treatment of the patient's medical condition and to prevent the development of subsequent foreseeable emergencies resulting from the original medical problem.

C. EMERGENCY PHYSICIANS SHOULD PROMOTE PRUDENT RESOURCE STEWARDSHIP WITHOUT COMPROMISING QUALITY

Emergency physicians have an obligation to ensure that quality care is provided to all patients presenting to the emergency department for treatment. Participation in quality assurance activities and peer review are important for assuring that patterns of inadequate care are detected. Participation in continuing education activities, including the development of scientifically based practice guidelines, assists the emergency physician in providing quality care.

Health care resources, including new technologies, should be used on the basis of individual patient needs and the appropriateness of the therapy as documented by medical literature. Diagnostic and therapeutic decisions should be made on the basis of potential risks and benefits of alternative treatments versus no treatment. The emergency physician has an obligation to diagnose and treat patients in a cost-effective manner and must be knowledgeable about cost-effective strategies; but the physician should not allow cost containment to impede proper medical treatment of the patient.

The limitation of health care expenditures is a societal decision that should ideally be made in the political arena and not at the bedside for individual patients. Lacking a societal consensus, however, emergency physicians must keep the patient's interest as a primary concern while recognizing that the medically non-beneficial testing or treatment is not morally required. Thus, the emergency physician has dual obligations to allocate resources prudently while honoring the primacy of patient's best medical interests.

D. THE DUTY TO RESPOND TO PREHOSPITAL EMERGENCIES AND DISASTERS

Because of their unique expertise, emergency physicians have an ethical duty to respond to emergencies in the community and offer assistance.

This responsibility is buttressed by local Good Samaritan statutes that protect health care professionals from legal liability for good-faith efforts to render first aid. Physicians should not disrupt paramedical personnel who are under base station medical control and direction.

In a situation where the resources of a health care facility are overwhelmed by epidemic illness, mass casualties, or the victims of a natural or manmade disaster, the prudent emergency physician must make important triage decisions to benefit the greatest number of potential survivors. When the numbers of patients and severity of their injuries overpower existing resources, triage decisions should classify patients according to both their need and their likelihood of survival. The overriding principle should be to focus health care resources on those patients most likely to benefit who have a reasonable probability of survival. Those patients with fatal injuries and those with minor injuries should be made as comfortable as possible while they await further medical assistance and treatment.

E. THE DUTY TO OPPOSE VIOLENCE

Serving as a societal resource, emergency physicians have the dual obligation to protect themselves, staff, and patients from violence and to teach EMS personnel under their supervision to do likewise. Hospitals have a duty to provide adequate numbers of trained security personnel to assure a safe environment. Ensuring safety may mean that patients who appear to present a high risk of violence will lose some autonomy as they are restrained physically or chemically. Emergency physicians never should resort to restraints or medication for punitive or vindictive reasons. Restraints are indicated only when there is a reasonable possibility that patients will harm themselves or others. The need for restraint of emergency department patients should frequently be reevaluated.

The emergency physician has an ethical duty to diagnose, treat, and properly refer suspected victims of abuse and neglect, including partners, children and dependent adults, and to report domestic violence to appropriate authorities as permitted or required by law.

F. THE DUTY TO PROMOTE THE PUBLIC HEALTH

Emergency physicians advocate for the public health in many ways, including the provision of basic health care for many uninsured patients. As a safety net both for patients who lack other resources of care and for victims of disaster, emergency departments provide needed care and assistance to many of the most vulnerable members of society. In times of disaster, pandemic, or other public health emergencies, emergency departments serve as a vanguard of preparedness against a constellation of medical and social ills.

Emergency physicians have first-hand knowledge of the grave harms caused by firearms, motor vehicles, alcohol, and other causes of preventable illness and injury. Inspired by this knowledge, emergency physicians should participate in efforts to educate others about the potential of well-designed laws, programs, and policies to improve the overall health and safety of the public.

CONCLUSION

Serving patients effectively requires both scientific and technical competence, knowledge of what can be done, and moral competence, knowledge of what should be done. The technical emphasis of emergency medicine must be accompanied by a corresponding emphasis on character and careful moral reasoning, as emergency physicians increasingly confront difficult moral questions in clinical practice.

In the face of future uncertainties and challenges, ethics will remain central to the clinical practice of quality emergency medicine. Both technical and moral expertise can and should be nurtured through advanced preparation and training. The time and information constraints inherent in emergency practice make reflection on important ethical principles and values challenging. This Code is offered both for thoughtful consideration and as a resource when issues arise in clinical practice. The principles of emergency medical ethics identified herein may serve as a guide for practitioners and students of this developing art. Through the process of moral reflection and deliberation, emergency physicians can make difficult and time-sensitive decisions based on a sound moral framework that benefits both patients and profession.

III. A COMPENDIUM OF ACEP POLICY STATEMENTS ON ETHICAL ISSUES

The policy statements listed in the Compendium section of the Table of Contents of this policy are available on ACEP's website http://acep.org

Appendix 2

The Emergency Medicine Milestone Project

A Joint Initiative of

The Accreditation Council for Graduate Medical Education and The American Board of Emergency Medicine

The Milestones are designed only for use in evaluation of resident physicians in the context of their participation in ACGME accredited residency or fellowship programs. The Milestones provide a framework for the assessment of the development of the resident physician in key dimensions of the elements of physician competency in a specialty or subspecialty. They neither represent the entirety of the dimensions of the six domains of physician competency, nor are they designed to be relevant in any other context.

Emergency Medicine Milestones

Working Group	Advisory Group
Chair: Michael Beeson, MD	Timothy Brigham, MDiv, PhD
Theodore Christopher, MD	Wallace Carter, MD
Jonathan Heidt, MD	Earl Reisdorff, MD
James Jones, MD	
Susan Promes, MD	
Lynne Meyer, PhD, MPH	
Kevin Rodgers, MD	
Philip Shayne, MD	
Susan Swing, PhD	
Mary Jo Wagner, MD	

MILESTONE REPORTING

This document presents milestones designed for programs to use in semi-annual review of resident performance and reporting to the ACGME.

Milestones are knowledge, skills, attitudes, and other attributes for each of the ACGME competencies organized in a developmental framework from less to more advanced. They are descriptors and targets for resident performance as a resident moves from entry into residency through graduation. In the initial years of implementation, the Review Committee will examine milestone performance data for each program's residents as one element in the Next Accreditation System (NAS) to determine whether residents overall are progressing.

For each reporting period, review and reporting will involve selecting the level of milestones that best describes a resident's current performance level in relation to milestones, using evidence from multiple methods, such as direct observation, multi-source feedback, tests, and record reviews. Milestones are arranged into numbered levels. These levels do not correspond with post-graduate year of education.

Selection of a level implies that the resident substantially demonstrates the milestones in that level, as well as those in lower levels (See the diagram on page v). A general interpretation of levels for emergency medicine is below:

Level 1: The resident demonstrates milestones expected of an incoming resident.

Level 2: The resident is advancing and demonstrates additional milestones, but is not yet performing at a mid-residency level.

Level 3: The resident continues to advance and demonstrate additional milestones; the resident demonstrates the majority of milestones targeted for residency in this sub-competency.

Level 4: The resident has advanced so that he or she now substantially demonstrates the milestones targeted for residency. This level is designed as the graduation target.

Level 5: The resident has advanced beyond performance targets set for residency and is demonstrating "aspirational" goals which might describe the performance of someone who has been in practice for several years. It is expected that only a few exceptional residents will reach this level.

Additional Notes

Level 4 is designed as the graduation *target* and <u>does not</u> represent a graduation *requirement*. Making decisions about readiness for graduation is the purview of the residency program director (See the following NAS FAQ for educational milestones on the ACGME's NAS microsite for further discussion of this issue: "Can a resident graduate if he or she does not reach every milestone?"). Study of milestone performance data will be required before the ACGME and its partners will be able to determine whether Level 4 milestones and milestones in lower levels are in the appropriate level within the developmental framework, and whether milestone data are of sufficient quality to be used for high stakes decisions.

Answers to Frequently Asked Questions about the Next Accreditation System (NAS) and milestones are available on the ACGME's NAS microsite: http://www.acgme-nas.org/assets/pdf/NASFAQs.pdf.

The diagram below presents an example set of milestones for one subcompetency in the same format as the milestone report worksheet. For each reporting period, a resident's performance on the milestones for each sub-competency will be indicated by:

- selecting the level of milestones that best describes the resident's performance in relation to the milestones <u>or</u>
- selecting the "Has not Achieved Level 1" response option

EMERGENCY MEDICINE MILESTONES ACGME REPORT
WORKSHEET

1. *Emergency Stabilization (PC1) Prioritizes critical initial stabilization action and mobilizes hospital support services in the resuscitation of a critically ill or injured patient and reassesses after stabilizing intervention.*

Has not Achieved Level 1	Level 1	Level 2	Level 3	Level 4	Level 5
	Recognizes abnormal vital signs	Recognizes when a patient is unstable requiring immediate intervention Performs a primary assessment on a critically ill or injured patient Discerns relevant data to formulate a diagnostic impression and plan	Manages and prioritizes critically ill or injured patients Prioritizes critical initial stabilization actions in the resuscitation of a critically ill or injured patient Reasesses after implementing a stabilizing intervention Evaluates the validity of a DNR order	Recognizes in a timely fashion when further clinical intervention is futile Integrates hospital support services into a management strategy for a problematic stabilization situation	Develops policies and protocols for the management and/or transfer of critically ill or injured patients

Comments:

Suggested Evaluation Methods: SDOT, observed resuscitations, simulation, checklist, videotape review

2. *Performance of Focused History and Physical Exam (PC2) Abstracts current findings in a patient with multiple chronic medical problems and, when appropriate, compares with a prior medical record and identifies significant differences between the current presentation and past presentations.*

Has not Achieved Level 1	Level 1	Level 2	Level 3	Level 4	Level 5
	Performs and communicates a reliable, comprehensive history and physical exam	Performs and communicates a focused history and physical exam which effectively addresses the chief complaint and urgent patient issues	Prioritizes essential components of a history given a limited or dynamic circumstance Prioritizes essential components of a physical examination given a limited or dynamic circumstance	Synthesizes essential data necessary for the correct management of patients using all potential sources of data	Identifies obscure, occult or rare patient conditions based solely on historical and physical exam findings

Comments:

Suggested Evaluation Methods: Global ratings of live performance, checklist assessments of live performance, SDOT, oral boards, simulation

3. *Diagnostic Studies (PC₃) Applies the results of diagnostic testing based on the probability of disease and the likelihood of test results altering management.*

Has not Achieved Level 1	Level 1	Level 2	Level 3	Level 4	Level 5
	Determines the necessity of diagnostic studies	Orders appropriate diagnostic studies Performs appropriate bedside diagnostic studies and procedures	Prioritizes essential testing Interprets results of a diagnostic study, recognizing limitations and risks, seeking interpretive assistance when appropriate Reviews risks, benefits, contraindications, and alternatives to a diagnostic study or procedure	Uses diagnostic testing based on the pre-test probability of disease and the likelihood of test results altering management Practices cost effective ordering of diagnostic studies Understands the implications of false positives and negatives for post-test probability	Discriminates between subtle and/or conflicting diagnostic results in the context of the patient presentation

Comments:

Suggested Evaluation Methods: SDOT, oral boards, standardized exams, chart review, simulation

4. *Diagnosis (PC4) Based on all of the available data, narrows and prioritizes the list of weighted differential diagnoses to determine appropriate management.*

Has not Achieved Level 1	Level 1	Level 2	Level 3	Level 4	Level 5
	Constructs a list of potential diagnoses based on chief complaint and initial assessment	Constructs a list of potential diagnoses, based on the greatest likelihood of occurrence Constructs a list of potential diagnoses with the greatest potential for morbidity or mortality	Uses all available medical information to develop a list of ranked differential diagnoses including those with the greatest potential for morbidity or mortality Correctly identifies "sick versus not sick" patients Revises a differential diagnosis in response to changes in a patient's course over time	Synthesizes all of the available data and narrows and prioritizes the list of weighted differential diagnoses to determine appropriate management	Uses pattern recognition to identify discriminating features between similar patients and avoids premature closure

Comments:

Suggested Evaluation Methods: SDOT as baseline, global ratings, simulation, oral boards, chart review

5. *Pharmacotherapy (PC5) Selects and prescribes, appropriate pharmaceutical agents based upon relevant considerations such as mechanism of action, intended effect, financial considerations, possible adverse effects, patient preferences, allergies, potential drug-food and drug-drug interactions, institutional policies, and clinical guidelines; and effectively combines agents and monitors and intervenes in the advent of adverse effects in the ED.*

Has not Achieved
Level 1

Level 1	Level 2	Level 3	Level 4	Level 5
Knows the different classifications of pharmacologic agents and their mechanism of action.	Applies medical knowledge for selection of appropriate agent for therapeutic intervention	Considers array of drug therapy for treatment. Selects appropriate agent based on mechanism of action, intended effect, and anticipates potential adverse side effects	Selects the appropriate agent based on mechanism of action, intended effect, possible adverse effects, patient preferences, allergies, potential drug-food and drug-drug interactions, financial considerations, institutional policies, and clinical guidelines, including patient's age, weight, and other modifying factors	Participates in developing institutional policies on pharmacy and therapeutics
Consistently asks patients for drug allergies	Considers potential adverse effects of pharmacotherapy	Considers and recognizes potential drug to drug interactions		

Comments:

Suggested Evaluation Methods: SDOT, portfolio, simulation, oral boards, global ratings, medical knowledge examinations

6. *Observation and Reassessment (PC6) Re-evaluates patients undergoing ED observation (and monitoring) and using appropriate data and resources, determines the differential diagnosis and, treatment plan, and disposition.*

Has not Achieved Level 1	Level 1	Level 2	Level 3	Level 4	Level 5
	Recognizes the need for patient re-evaluation	Monitors that necessary therapeutic interventions are performed during a patient's ED stay	Identifies which patients will require observation in the ED	Considers additional diagnoses and therapies for a patient who is under observation and changes treatment plan accordingly	Develops protocols to avoid potential complications of interventions and therapies
			Evaluates effectiveness of therapies and treatments provided during observation	Identifies and complies with federal and other regulatory requirements, including billing, which must be met for a patient who is under observation	
			Monitors a patient's clinical status at timely intervals during their stay in the ED		

Comments:

Suggested Evaluation Methods: SDOT, multi-source feedback, oral boards, simulation

7. *Disposition (PC7) Establishes and implements a comprehensive disposition plan that uses appropriate consultation resources; patient education regarding diagnosis; treatment plan; medications; and time and location specific disposition instructions.*

Has not Achieved Level 1	Level 1	Level 2	Level 3	Level 4	Level 5
	Describes basic resources available for care of the emergency department patient	Formulates a specific follow-up plan for common ED complaints with appropriate resource utilization	Formulates and provides patient education regarding diagnosis, treatment plan, medication review and PCP/consultant appointments for complicated patients Involves appropriate resources (e.g. PCP, consultants, social work, PT/OT, financial aid, care coordinators) in a timely manner Makes correct decision regarding admission or discharge of patients Correctly assigns admitted patients to an appropriate level of care (ICU/Telemetry/Floor/Observation Unit)	Formulates sufficient admission plans or discharge instructions including future diagnostic/therapeutic interventions for ED patients Engages patient or surrogate to effectively implement a discharge plan	Works within the institution to develop hospital systems that enhance safe patient disposition and maximizes resource utilization

Comments:

Suggested Evaluation Methods: SDOT, shift evaluations, simulation cases/Objective Structure Clinical Exam (OSCE), multi-source feedback, chart review

8. *Multi-tasking (Task-switching) (PC8) Employs task switching in an efficient and timely manner in order to manage the ED.*

Has not Achieved Level 1	Level 1	Level 2	Level 3	Level 4	Level 5
	Manages a single patient amidst distractions	Task switches between different patients	Employs task switching in an efficient and timely manner in order to manage multiple patients	Employs task switching in an efficient and timely manner in order to manage the ED	Employs task switching in an efficient and timely manner in order to manage the ED under high volume or surge situations

Comments:

Suggested Evaluation Methods: Simulation, SDOT, mock oral examination, multi-source feedback

9. *General Approach to Procedures (PC9) Performs the indicated procedure on all appropriate patients (including those who are uncooperative, at the extremes of age, hemodynamically unstable and those who have multiple co-morbidities, poorly defined anatomy, high risk for pain or procedural complications, sedation requirement), takes steps to avoid potential complications, and recognizes the outcome and/or complications resulting from the procedure.*

Has not Achieved Level 1	Level 1	Level 2	Level 3	Level 4	Level 5
	Identifies pertinent anatomy and physiology for a specific procedure Uses appropriate Universal Precautions	Performs patient assessment, obtains informed consent and ensures monitoring equipment is in place in accordance with patient safety standards Knows indications, contraindications, anatomic landmarks, equipment, anesthetic and procedural technique, and potential complications for common ED procedures Performs the indicated common procedure on a patient with moderate urgency who has	Determines a backup strategy if initial attempts to perform a procedure are unsuccessful Correctly interprets the results of a diagnostic procedure	Performs indicated procedures on any patients with challenging features (e.g. poorly identifiable landmarks, at extremes of age or with co-morbid conditions) Performs the indicated procedure, takes steps to avoid potential complications, and recognizes the outcome and/or complications resulting from the procedure	Teaches procedural competency and corrects mistakes

identifiable landmarks
and a low-moderate risk
for complications

Performs post-procedural
assessment and
identifies any potential
complications

Comments:

Suggested Evaluation Methods: Procedural competency forms, checklist assessment of procedure and simulation lab performance, global ratings

10. *Airway Management (PC10) Performs airway management on all appropriate patients (including those who are uncooperative, at the extremes of age, hemodynamically unstable and those who have multiple co-morbidities, poorly defined anatomy, high risk for pain or procedural complications, sedation requirement), takes steps to avoid potential complications, and recognize the outcome and/or complications resulting from the procedure.*

Has not Achieved Level 1	Level 1	Level 2	Level 3	Level 4	Level 5
	Describes upper airway anatomy Performs basic airway maneuvers or adjuncts (jaw thrust/chin lift/oral airway/ nasopharyngeal airway) and ventilates/oxygenates patient using BVM	Describes elements of airway assessment and indications impacting the airway management Describes the pharmacology of agents used for rapid sequence intubation including specific indications and contraindications Performs rapid sequence intubation in patients without adjuncts Confirms proper endotracheal tube placement using multiple modalities	Uses airway algorithms in decision making for complicated patients employing airway adjuncts as indicated Performs rapid sequence intubation in patients using airway adjuncts Implements post-intubation management Employs appropriate methods of mechanical ventilation based on specific patient physiology	Performs airway management in any circumstance taking steps to avoid potential complications, and recognizes the outcome and/or complications resulting from the procedure Performs a minimum of 35 intubations Demonstrates the ability to perform a cricothyrotomy Uses advanced airway modalities in complicated patients	Teaches airway management skills to health care providers

Comments:

Suggested Evaluation Methods: Airway Management Competency Assessment Tool (CORD), Airway Management Assessment Cards, SDOT checklist, procedure log, and simulation

11. *Anesthesia and Acute Pain Management (PC11) Provides safe acute pain management, anesthesia, and procedural sedation to patients of all ages regardless of the clinical situation.*

Has not Achieved Level 1	Level 1	Level 2	Level 3	Level 4	Level 5
	Discusses with the patient indications, contraindications and possible complications of local anesthesia	Knows the indications, contraindications, potential complications and appropriate doses of analgesic/sedative medications	Knows the indications, contraindications, potential complications and appropriate doses of medications used for procedural sedation	Performs procedural sedation providing effective sedation with the least risk of complications and minimal recovery time through selective dosing, route and choice of medications	Develops pain management protocols/ care plans
	Performs local anesthesia using appropriate doses of local anesthetic and appropriate technique to provide skin to sub-dermal anesthesia for procedures	Knows the anatomic landmarks, indications, contraindications, potential complications and appropriate doses of local anesthetics used for regional anesthesia	Performs patient assessment and discusses with the patient the most appropriate analgesic/sedative medication and administers in the most appropriate dose and route		
			Performs pre-sedation assessment, obtains informed consent and orders appropriate choice and dose of medications for procedural sedation		
			Obtains informed consent and correctly performs regional anesthesia		
			Ensures appropriate monitoring of patients during procedural sedation		

Comments:

Suggested Evaluation Methods: Procedural competency forms, checklist assessment of procedure and simulation lab performance, global ratings. patient survey, chart review

12. *Other Diagnostic and Therapeutic Procedures: Goal-directed Focused Ultrasound (Diagnostic/Procedural) (PC12) Uses goal-directed focused Ultrasound for the bedside diagnostic evaluation of emergency medical conditions and diagnoses, resuscitation of the acutely ill or injured patient, and procedural guidance.*

Has not Achieved Level 1	Level 1	Level 2	Level 3	Level 4	Level 5
	Describes the indications for emergency ultrasound	Explains how to optimize ultrasound images and Identifies the proper probe for each of the focused ultrasound applications Performs an eFAST	Performs goal-directed focused ultrasound exams Correctly interprets acquired images	Performs a minimum of 150 focused ultrasound examinations	Expands ultrasonography skills to include: advanced echo, TEE, bowel, adnexal and testicular pathology, and transcranial Doppler

Comments:

Suggested Evaluation Methods: OSCE, SDOT, videotape review, written examination, checklist

13. *Other Diagnostic and Therapeutic Procedures: Wound Management (PC13) Assesses and appropriately manages wounds in patients of all ages regardless of the clinical situation.*

Has not Achieved Level 1	Level 1	Level 2	Level 3	Level 4	Level 5
	Prepares a simple wound for suturing (identify appropriate suture material, anesthetize wound and irrigate) Demonstrates sterile technique Places a simple interrupted suture	Uses medical terminology to clearly describe/classify a wound (e.g. stellate, abrasion, avulsion, laceration, deep vs superficial) Classifies burns with respect to depth and body surface area Compares and contrasts modes of wound management (adhesives, steri-	Performs complex wound repairs (deep sutures, layered repair, corner stitch) Manages a severe burn Determines which wounds should not be closed primarily Demonstrates appropriate use of consultants Identifies wounds that may be high risk and require more extensive evaluation	Achieves hemostasis in a bleeding wound using advanced techniques such as: cautery, ligation, deep suture, injection, topical hemostatic agents, and tourniquet Repairs wounds that are high risk for cosmetic complications (such as eyelid margin, nose, ear) Describes the indications for and steps to perform an escharotomy	Performs advanced wound repairs, such as tendon repairs and skin flaps

13. *(continued)*

Has not Achieved Level 1	Level 1	Level 2	Level 3	Level 4	Level 5
		strips, hair apposition, staples) Identifies wounds that require antibiotics or tetanus prophylaxis Educates patients on appropriate outpatient management of their wound	(e.g. x-ray, ultrasound, and/ or exploration)		

Comments:

Suggested Evaluation Methods: Direct observation, procedure checklist, medical knowledge quiz, portfolio, global ratings, procedure log

14. *Other Diagnostic and Therapeutic Procedures: Vascular Access (PC14) Successfully obtains vascular access in patients of all ages regardless of the clinical situation.*

Has not Achieved Level 1	Level 1	Level 2	Level 3	Level 4	Level 5
	Performs a venipuncture Places a peripheral intravenous line Performs an arterial puncture	Describes the indications, contraindications, anticipated undesirable outcomes and complications for the various vascular access modalities Inserts an arterial catheter Assesses the indications in conjunction with the patient anatomy/pathophysiology and select the optimal site for a central venous catheter Inserts a central venous catheter using ultrasound and universal precautions Confirms appropriate placement of central venous catheter Performs intraosseous access	Inserts a central venous catheter without ultrasound when appropriate Places an ultrasound guided deep vein catheter (e.g. basilic, brachial, and cephalic veins)	Successfully performs 20 central venous lines Routinely gains venous access in patients with difficult vascular access	Teaches advanced vascular access techniques

Comments:

Suggested Evaluation Methods: Knowledge assessment using MCQ, checklist driven task analysis, procedure log

15. Medical Knowledge (MK) Demonstrates appropriate medical knowledge in the care of emergency medicine patients.

Has not Achieved Level 1	Level 1	Level 2	Level 3	Level 4	Level 5
	Passes initial national licensing examinations (e.g. USMLE Step 1 and Step 2 or COMLEX Level 1 and Level 2)	Resident develops and completes a self-assessment plan based on the in-training examination results	Demonstrates improvement of the percentage correct on the in-training examination or maintain an acceptable percentile ranking	Obtains a score on the annual in-training examination that indicates a high likelihood of passing the national qualifying examinations	Passes ABEM certifying examinations
		Completes objective residency training program examinations and/or assessments at an acceptable score for specific rotations		Successfully completes all objective residency training program examinations and/or assessments	Meets all the requirements for the ABEM Maintenance of Certification program set forth by national certifying agency
				Passes final national licensing examination (e.g. USMLE Step 3 or COMLEX Level 3)	

Comments:

Suggested Evaluation Methods: National licensing examinations (USMLE, COMLEX), national in-training examination (developed by ABEM & AOA), CORD Question & Answer Bank tests, MedChallenger, local residency examinations

16. *Patient Safety (SBP1) Participates in performance improvement to optimize patient safety.*

Has not Achieved Level 1	Level 1	Level 2	Level 3	Level 4	Level 5
	Adheres to standards for maintenance of a safe working environment Describes medical errors and adverse events	Routinely uses basic patient safety practices, such as time-outs and 'calls for help'	Describes patient safety concepts Employs processes (e.g. checklists, SBAR), personnel, and technologies that optimize patient safety (SBAR=Situation – Background – Assessment – Recommendation) Appropriately uses system resources to improve both patient care and medical knowledge	Participates in an institutional process improvement plan to optimize ED practice and patient safety Leads team reflection such as code debriefings, root cause analysis, or M&M to improve ED performance Identifies situations when the breakdown in teamwork or communication may contribute to medical error	Uses analytical tools to assess health care quality and safety and reassess quality improvement programs for effectiveness for patients and for populations Develops and evaluates measures of professional performance and process improvement and implements them to improve departmental practice

Comments:

Suggested Evaluation Methods: SDOT, simulation, global ratings, multi-source feedback, portfolio work products, including a QI project

17. *Systems-based Management (SBP2) Participates in strategies to improve health care delivery and flow. Demonstrates an awareness of and responsiveness to the larger context and system of health care.*

Has not Achieved Level 1	Level 1	Level 2	Level 3	Level 4	Level 5
	Describes members of ED team (e.g. nurses, technicians, and security)	Mobilizes institutional resources to assist in patient care Participates in patient satisfaction initiatives	Practices cost-effective care Demonstrates the ability to call effectively on other resources in the system to provide optimal health care	Participates in processes and logistics to improve patient flow and decrease turnaround times (e.g. rapid triage, bedside registration, Fast Tracks, bedside testing, rapid treatment units, standard protocols, and observation units) Recommends strategies by which patients' access to care can be improved Coordinates system resources to optimize a patient's care for complicated medical situations	Creates departmental flow metric from benchmarks, best practices, and dash boards Develops internal and external departmental solutions to process and operational problems Addresses the differing customer needs of patients, hospital medical staff, EMS, and the community

Comments:

Suggested Evaluation Methods: Direct observation-SDOT, chart review, global ratings, billing records, simulation, multi-source feedback, and outcome data including throughput numbers and patients per hour

18. *Technology (SBP3) Uses technology to accomplish and document safe health care delivery.*

Has not Achieved Level 1	Level 1	Level 2	Level 3	Level 4	Level 5
	Uses the Electronic Health Record (EHR) to order tests, medications and document notes, and respond to alerts Reviews medications for patients	Ensures that medical records are complete, with attention to preventing confusion and error Effectively and ethically uses technology for patient care, medical communication and learning	Recognizes the risk of computer shortcuts and reliance upon computer information on accurate patient care and documentation	Uses decision support systems in EHR (as applicable in institution)	Recommends systems re-design for improved computerized processes

Comments:

Suggested Evaluation Methods: Direct observation-SDOT, chart review, global ratings, billing records, simulation, multi-source feedback

19. *Practice-based Performance Improvement (PBLI) Participates in performance improvement to optimize ED function, self-learning, and patient care.*

Has not Achieved Level 1	Level 1	Level 2	Level 3	Level 4	Level 5
	Describes basic principles of evidence-based medicine	Performs patient follow-up	Performs self-assessment to identify areas for continued self-improvement and implements learning plans Continually assesses performance by evaluating feedback and assessment Demonstrates the ability to critically appraise scientific literature and apply evidence-based medicine to improve one's individual performance	Applies performance improvement methodologies Demonstrates evidence based clinical practice and information retrieval mastery Participates in a process improvement plan to optimize ED practice	Independently teaches evidence-based medicine and information mastery techniques

Comments:

Suggested Evaluation Methods: SDOT, simulation, global ratings, checklist or ratings of portfolio work products, including a literature review, Vanderbilt matrix evaluation of a clinical issue, critical appraisal

20. *Professional values (PROF1) Demonstrates compassion, integrity, and respect for others as well as adherence to the ethical principles relevant to the practice of medicine.*

Has not Achieved Level 1	Level 1	Level 2	Level 3	Level 4	Level 5
	Demonstrates behavior that conveys caring, honesty, genuine interest and tolerance when interacting with a diverse population of patients and families	Demonstrates an understanding of the importance of compassion, integrity, respect, sensitivity and responsiveness and exhibits these attitudes consistently in common/ uncomplicated situations and with diverse populations	Recognizes how own personal beliefs and values impact medical care; consistently manages own values and beliefs to optimize relationships and medical care. Develops alternate care plans when patients' personal decisions/beliefs preclude the use of commonly accepted practices	Develops and applies a consistent and appropriate approach to evaluating appropriate care, possible barriers and strategies to intervene that consistently prioritizes the patient's best interest in all relationships and situations. Effectively analyzes and manages ethical issues in complicated and challenging clinical situations	Develops institutional and organizational strategies to protect and maintain professional and bioethical principles

Comments:

Suggested Evaluation Methods: Direct observation, SDOT, portfolio, simulation, oral board, multi-source feedback, global ratings

21. *Accountability (PROF2) Demonstrates accountability to patients, society, profession and self.*

Has not Achieved Level 1	Level 1	Level 2	Level 3	Level 4	Level 5
	Demonstrates basic professional responsibilities such as timely reporting for duty, appropriate dress/grooming, rested and ready to work, delivery of patient care as a functional physician	Identifies basic principles of physician wellness, including sleep hygiene	Consistently recognizes limits of knowledge in uncommon and complicated clinical situations; develops and implements plans for the best possible patient care	Can form a plan to address impairment in one's self or a colleague, in a professional and confidential manner	Develops institutional and organizational strategies to improve physician insight into and management of professional responsibilities
	Maintains patient confidentially	Consistently recognizes limits of knowledge in common and frequent clinical situations and asks for assistance	Recognizes and avoids inappropriate influences of marketing and advertising	Manages medical errors according to principles of responsibility and accountability in accordance with institutional policy	Trains physicians and educators regarding responsibility, wellness, fatigue, and physician impairment
	Uses social media ethically and responsibly	Demonstrates knowledge of alertness management and fatigue mitigation principles			
	Adheres to professional responsibilities, such as conference attendance, timely chart completion, duty hour reporting, procedure reporting				

Comments:

Suggested Evaluation Methods: Direct observation, SDOT, portfolio, simulation, oral boards, multi-source feedback, global ratings

22. *Patient Centered Communication (ICS1) Demonstrates interpersonal and communication skills that result in the effective exchange of information and collaboration with patients and their families.*

Has not Achieved

Level 1	Level 1	Level 2	Level 3	Level 4	Level 5
	Establishes rapport with and demonstrate empathy toward patients and their families	Elicits patients' reasons for seeking health care and expectations from the ED visit	Manages the expectations of those who receive care in the ED and uses communication methods that minimize the potential for stress, conflict, and misunderstanding	Uses flexible communication strategies and adjusts them based on the clinical situation to resolve specific ED challenges, such as drug seeking behavior, delivering bad news, unexpected outcomes, medical errors, and high risk refusal-of-care patients	Teaches communication and conflict management skills
	Listens effectively to patients and their families	Negotiates and manages simple patient/family-related conflicts	Effectively communicates with vulnerable populations, including both patients at risk and their families		Participates in review and counsel of colleagues with communication deficiencies

Comments:

Suggested Evaluation Methods: Direct observation, SDOT, simulation, multi-source feedback, OSCE, global ratings, oral boards

23. *Team Management (ICS2) Leads patient-centered care teams, ensuring effective communication and mutual respect among members of the team.*

Has not Achieved Level 1	Level 1	Level 2	Level 3	Level 4	Level 5
	Participates as a member of a patient care team	Communicates pertinent information to emergency physicians and other health care colleagues	Develops working relationships across specialties and with ancillary staff Ensures transitions of care are accurately and efficiently communicated Ensures clear communication and respect among team members	Recommends changes in team performance as necessary for optimal efficiency Uses flexible communication strategies to resolve specific ED challenges such as difficulties with consultants and other health care providers Communicates with out-of-hospital and nonmedical personnel, such as police, media, and hospital administrators	Participates in and leads interdepartmental groups in the patient setting and in collaborative meetings outside of the patient care setting Designs patient care teams and evaluates their performance Seeks leadership opportunities within professional organizations

Comments:

Suggested Evaluation Methods: Direct observation, SDOT, simulation, multi-source feedback, OSCE, global ratings, oral boards

INDEX

Note: Page number in *italics* indicate a table or figure

for wrongful death, 62
manipulative help-rejector, 145
mass casualty incidents (MCIs)
    consent and student participation, 59
    frontline challenges for physicians, 54
    patient privacy and, 67
    triage strategy, 37, 48
    types of, 54, 249
mass triage casualty strategy, 37
medical education. *See* education in emergency
    medicine
medical errors and patient safety
    barriers to disclosure
        liability, 210–211
        patient, 210
        physician, 210
        systemic, 209–210
    case examples, 199–200, 213–214
    competing interests in reporting,
        investigating, prevention, 204–207
        fears of reporting, 206–207
        patient-based interests, 205
        personal interests, 206
        third-party interests, 205–206
    conceptual distinctions, 202–203
    definitions, 201–202, *202*
    disclosure to patients, surrogates
        moral foundations, 20, *34*, 207–209
        'reporting' distinction, 203
        strategies for, 212–213, 215
    electronic communication and, 83
    historical background, 200–201
        AMA ethics opinion, 200, 201
        Institute for Healthcare Improvement
            programs, 200
        Institute of Medicine report, 200, 201
        Joint Commission safety standards, 201
    incidence and distribution, 203–204
    from miscommunication, 93
    patient safety concepts, 202
    reporting, investigation, prevention
        competing interests, 204–207
        moral foundations, 204
    in research, 171
    strategies for disclosure, 212–213
        practice strategies, 213
        public policy strategies, 212
        system strategies, 212–213
    types and categories, 203
medical journals, conflicts of interest of, 187
medical malpractice
    state law variance, 234–235
    U.S. frequency of, 18, 31
Medicare Hospice Benefit (MHB), 320
Medicare Modernization Act (2003), 158
mentally ill patients, and informed consent, 109
mid-level principles, 4–6

Mill, John Stewart, 3, 42. *See also* utilitarianism
    theory; utilitarianism theory (of Mill
    and Bentham)
Minnesota, physician Good Samaritan law, 22
minors (pediatric patients). *See also* pediatric
    end-of-life care
    complications of decision-making for, 125
    confidentiality discussion with patients,
        parents, 130–131, 133
    differences with adolescents, adults, 127–128
    emancipation/state laws (U.S.), 27, 108, 129,
        133
    influence of social media, 128, 133
    informed consent and, 27, 111, 128–130
    and law enforcement in the emergency
        department, 154
    Pediatric Palliative Care Model, 131
    refusal of care and, 125, 129
    and social media, 128
    triage accommodations, 46, 51
MMS (media messaging services), 77
mobile devices. *See* smart phones with built-in
    cameras
Moskop, John C., 45, 213
multiculturalism. *See also* cultural competency;
        racial/ethnic disparities in health care
    avoidance of stereotyping, prejudgments, 98
    barriers to communication, 92
    case history (suspicion of child abuse)
        description of symptoms, 91–92
        facilitation of mutual understanding, 92
        interpretation of physical exam findings,
            92
        outcome of case, 93
        steps to take, 92
    description/implications, 97–98
    interactive, case-based teaching sessions, 97
multisomatoform disorder, 138, 139–140

narcissistic personality disorder, 139
National Association of EMS Physicians, 132
National Commission for the Protection of
        Human Subjects, 5
National Notifiable Infectious Conditions
        (CDC, 2014), 62, 64
National Research Act (1974), 163, 165
natural law system, 4
Navajo belief system, 98
A New Justification of Moral Rules (Gert),
        235–236
next of kin
    and advance directives, 65, 110
    disclosure of medical errors to, 210
    as surrogate decision-makers, 60
nonmaleficence
    conflicts of interest and, 180
    defined, 6, 24, 236, 303